Observations on the Changes of the Air and the
Concomitant Epidemical Diseases in the
Island of Barbadoes, 1752–1758

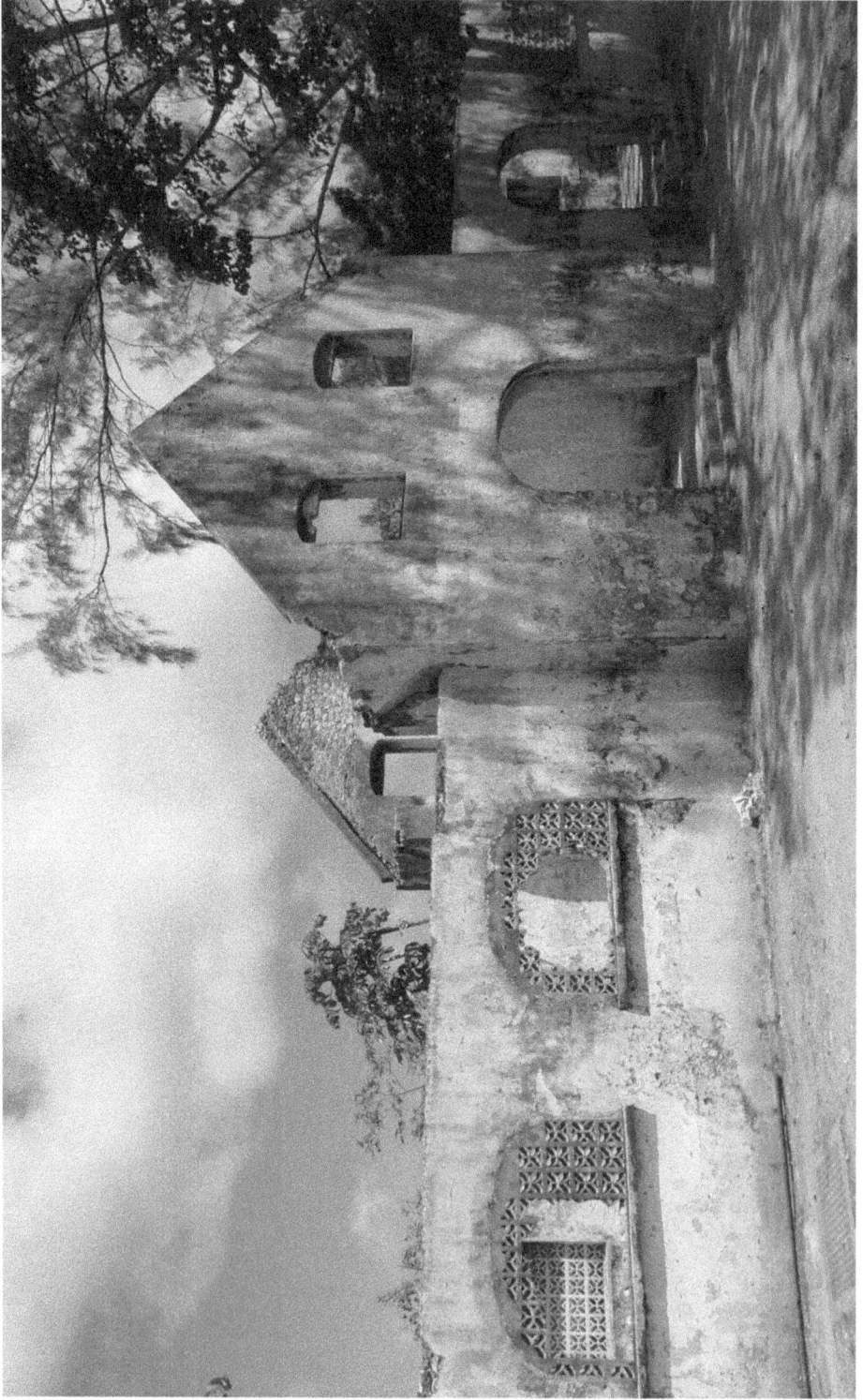

Slave hospital, Grantley Adams School (formerly Blackman's Plantation), St Joseph, Barbados. *Photograph by J. Edward Hutson.*

Observations on the Changes of the Air and the Concomitant Epidemical Diseases in the Island of Barbadoes, 1752–1758

William Hillary, MD

Edited and annotated by

J. Edward Hutson, MB, ChB, DA, MFARCS
and
Henry S. Fraser, GCM, MBBS, PhD, FACP, FRCP

University of the West Indies Press
Jamaica • Barbados • Trinidad and Tobago

University of the West Indies Press
7A Gibraltar Hall Road   Mona
Kingston 7   Jamaica
www.uwipress.com

A catalogue record of this book is available from
the National Library of Jamaica.

ISBN: 978-976-640-263-1

Cover illustration: Henry S. Fraser, watercolour painting of
the slave hospital, Grantley Adams School (formerly Blackman's Plantation),
St Joseph, Barbados.

Book and jacket design by Robert Harris.
Set in Adobe Garamond 11/14 x 24
Printed in the United States of America.

THIS WORK IS DEDICATED TO THE MEMORY OF THOSE
EXCELLENT TEACHERS WHO, DURING OUR DAYS AT THE
LODGE SCHOOL, BARBADOS, INSPIRED US WITH AN ABIDING
INTEREST IN THE ENGLISH LANGUAGE, HISTORY AND THE SCIENCES.

Contents

Foreword

It is a pleasure to write this foreword to the annotated edition of William Hillary's *Observations on the Changes of the Air and Concomitant Epidemical Diseases in the Island of Barbadoes*. However, I confess that I demurred when first asked, as I am certainly no medical historian and indeed wondered why very busy persons such as the two editors should concern themselves with reviewing Dr Hillary's work. But after having read some part of the treatise and the introduction, I must congratulate them and can imagine at least three good reasons why this work should be brought again to the public's attention. I do not include among these reasons to have Barbadians preen themselves on the information given to Hillary before he came there that the people are "more humane and polite than anywhere else".

First, it is good to bring out again and again that the observation of Hippocrates as regards the influence of the external environment is as relevant today as it ever was, and has continued to concern serious physicians throughout the ages. It is fascinating to follow Hillary's attempt to relate the occurrence of disease and particularly the patient's temperature and general condition to the climate. This is more striking when one appreciates that the variation of climate in Barbados is really quite small. But it is not only the climate that concerns him but more particularly the ambient temperature and the prevailing winds. Of course, we must remember that his generation believed that the air itself was a proximate cause of disease.

But a second and perhaps for me more important reason is to have the young physicians and the public at large understand the medical "journey" of the last 250 years. Barbados does not arrive at an infant mortality rate of 14 per 100,000 live births and a life expectancy at birth of 77.5 years through a slow but constant improvement in health. The fevers and epidemical diseases that Hillary described continued for almost two hundred years and it is only in the past fifty or sixty years that we have seen the rapid change in the public's health which we now sometimes take for granted. It is not an empty claim to contend that the University of the West Indies, founded two hundred years after Hillary came to Barbados, has contributed to that change.

The third reason for bringing Hilary's work to the attention of the medical and general public is to give us a sense of humility. We marvel at the conclusions he drew from his observations without the use of the technology which we have at our disposal. We are surprised by the accuracy of the symptomatology he describes. His description of leptospirosis and the variations in its presentation are fascinating. We should bear in mind that future historians may also comment at the apparent inadequacy of our deductions based on what we arrogantly describe now as the best evidence.

In addition, the elegance with which he expresses opinions makes us rue the standard current cold practice of describing clinical data. I suppose it is his Quaker background that makes him so constantly decry the use of "vinous or spirituous liquors", and his admonitions are equally valid today. But the one area in which I find his advice to be most egregious is in his strictures against dancing, which, as he says, "is much too violent an exercise in this hot climate and many do greatly injure their health by it, and I have known it fatal to some". But he goes on to say that "most of the ladies are so excessive fond of it that say what I will, they dance on". Good for them!

I hope this work becomes popular in the sense of being read by others beside medical people, as it is fascinating not only because of the effort Hillary made to relate disease to climatic conditions, but it gives a picture of Barbados health as a frame of reference for what is current today. Dr Hutson and Professor Fraser are to be congratulated for the tremendous effort they have put into this annotated edition and we are very much in their debt.

SIR GEORGE ALLEYNE
Director Emeritus of PAHO/WHO
Professor Emeritus and Chancellor of the University of the West Indies

Acknowledgements

During preparation of this work we received help and direction from several individuals, among whom we would like to particularly acknowledge Peter Homan and Briony Hudson of the Royal Pharmaceutical Society of Great Britain, who provided the translations of Dr Hillary's prescriptions, often rendered in his eclectic Latin; Father Simon Tugwell, OP, of the Istituto storico domenicano, Università S Tommaso, Rome, who translated and disentangled Dr Hillary's Latin renditions of quotations attributed to the first-century Persian physician and author Haly Abbas (Ali ibn Abbas al-Majusi); and Sir Christopher Booth, who first introduced Henry Fraser to the eminent Dr Hillary – his interest in and admiration for Hillary and his published biography inspired this volume.

Editors' Introduction

WILLIAM HILLARY, MD
PHYSICIAN, METEOROLOGIST AND EPIDEMIOLOGIST

> That wise father and Prince of Physicians, HIPPOCRATES, advises all Physicians to examine and duly consider the Situation, Air, and the Water, used by the people of such Cities, or Places, as they are called to, or may practice in.

The presumed relationship between weather phenomena and incidence of disease was a cherished medical tenet, slavishly observed for many centuries after being articulated by Hippocrates. Even today a trace of that relationship persists with recognition of seasonal affective disorder (SAD), a depressive illness associated with diminution of hours of daylight during the dark winter months in temperate climates.[1] In Barbados it persists most strongly in the folklore of older Barbadians, most of whom consider respiratory illnesses, ranging from the common cold to pneumonia, to be related to "damp" weather or being wet by rain.

In his 1750 *Natural History of the Island of Barbados*, Reverend Griffith Hughes[2] reiterates the opinion of Hippocrates that "the Constitution of the

---

1. See T. Dalgleish, K. Rosen and M. Marks, "Rhythm and Blues: The Theory and Treatment of Seasonal Affective Disorder", *British Journal of Clinical Psychology* (1996): 163–82.

2. The enigmatic Reverend Griffith Hughes, FRS, was curate of St Lucy's Parish Church, Barbados. A cleric, naturalist and scholar, after publishing this remarkable book he abruptly disappeared from the island, leaving his horse tethered to a tree. See S. Carrington, H. Fraser, J. Gilmore and A. Forde, *A–Z of Barbados Heritage* (London: Macmillan Caribbean, 2003), 101–2.

Air that preceded pestilential Fevers, was mixed with great Heat, much Rains, and southerly Winds", in addition to that of Lucretius, "*Ubi putrorem humidia nacta est / Intempestivis pulviisq; et solibis icta*" (these diseases either come from the air or rise from the earth). Hughes also observes:

> The South-west Wind . . . , with different Degrees of Circulation gives Birth to various Diseases: Whereas the Trade-Wind, by its Frequency, or rather its Constancy, is not only constitutional to the Inhabitants, but is in itself purer than the other, because it blows upon the Island at East-north-east; and as the nearest Part of the [African] Continent upon that Point, is 3,127 Miles from us, the Air must be far colder by passing over so much more Water than the South-west Wind, and consequently more wholesome.

At the time Reverend Hughes was writing his magnum opus, an eminent Yorkshire physician was also living in Barbados and conducting rigorous research on the relationships between weather and disease: Dr William Hillary.[3]

William, the second son of John Hillary and his wife, Mary, was born on 17 March 1697 at the family farm in Wensleydale, Yorkshire, and named for his paternal grandfather. John and Mary Hillary were fervent Quakers. In December 1715 William, aged eighteen, took his first step towards becoming a physician when he was apprenticed to Benjamin Bartlett, a Bradford apothecary. However, he did not complete his seven-year apprenticeship; in about 1720 he entered the University of Leyden, Holland, where he came under the influence of Herman Boerhaave, "the greatest clinical teacher of the eighteenth-century". Being a Quaker, and therefore considered a religious dissenter, William was excluded from admission to either Oxford or Cambridge; however, no such restriction applied at the University of Leyden. He received his medical degree on 24 July 1722 after defending his thesis, titled "*Dissertatio medica inauguralis practica de febribus intermittenibus*", a dissertation on intermittent fever.

---

3. The summary of Dr Hillary's life is largely extracted from the fascinating biography *A Pupil of Boerhaave*, by Sir Christopher Booth (b. 1924), a British physician and medical historian; past professor of medicine, Royal Postgraduate Medical School; and founding director of the Medical Research Council's research centre at Northwick Park. See also Christopher Booth, *Doctors in Science and Society: Essays of a Clinical Scientist* (London: British Medical Journal Memoir Club, 1987).

Shortly after graduation Dr Hillary established his practice at Ripon, Yorkshire, where he began recording observations of weather phenomena in an attempt to correlate weather and disease patterns. While still in Ripon he published his first book, *A Rational and Mechanical Essay on the Small Pox*; in the introduction he acknowledged his debt "to the sagacious and learned Boerhaave".[4] The second edition of *A Rational and Mechanical Essay* appeared in 1740, and to it Dr Hillary added his observations on the "Principal variations of the Weather and the Concomitant Diseases as they appeared at Ripon and the circumjacent parts of Yorkshire". In addition he explained his reasons for moving to the city of Bath: "About this time d'yd the eminent Dr Bave of Bath, and being weary of the Fatigue of Country Practice, I was advised by some of my friends to remove thither."

Dr Hillary practised at Bath from 1743 to 1746, and while there he published *An Inquiry into the Contents and Medicinal Virtues of the Lincomb Spaw-water, near Bath*. However, as an ardent Quaker, suggests Sir Christopher Booth, he must have found the society and mores of eighteenth-century Bath foreign to his fundamentalist beliefs, because by the summer of 1746 he was making plans to emigrate to Jamaica. In a letter to William's elder brother Alexander, John Fothergill, the famous London physician – and a Quaker and close friend of Dr Hillary – wrote:

> Several persons of note discouraged [Dr Hillary] from going thither, so that all thoughts of that place have been laid aside. Whilst he was here, news arrived of the Death of the only eminent Physician at Barbados . . . I procured him an interview with a person who gave him an exact account of the affairs of that Island, he likewise spoke with several others who jointly recommended the place as much preferable to Jamaica . . . At Barbados there are several [Quaker] meetings, the island pleasant and healthy; the people more humane and polite than anywhere else with a prospect of good employ.

In November 1746 Dr Hillary applied to his regular monthly meeting in Bath for a "Certificate of removal to Barbados", which he duly presented to the meeting in Tudor Street, Bridgetown, Barbados, in early 1747. He established his medical practice in Bridgetown very shortly thereafter. In his practice Dr Hillary would have been consulted by a varied continuum of eighteenth-century Barbadian society, including planters and their families,

---

4. Spontaneous rupture of the oesophagus is known as Boerhaave's syndrome.

military personnel, itinerant mariners whose ships had called at Bridgetown, and undoubtedly plantation slaves.

On 5 November 1751, early in his two-month sojourn in Barbados, nineteen-year-old George Washington recorded in his diary:

> Early this morning came Dr Hillary, an eminent physician recommended by Major Clarke, to pass his opinion on my brother's disorder, which he did in a favourable light, giving great assurance that it was not so fixed but that a cure might be effectually made. In the cool of the evening we rode out, accompanied by Mr Carter, to seek lodgings in the country, as the Doctor advised, and were perfectly enraptured with the beautiful prospects, which every side presented to our view – the fields of cane, corn, fruit trees, all in a delightful green.5

Despite Dr Hillary's favourable prognosis, Lawrence Washington's pulmonary tuberculosis progressed steadily. Following his return to Virginia after spending almost two months in Barbados, he died at Mount Vernon on 24 July 1752.

On 16 November 1751 George Washington developed a skin rash that was diagnosed by Dr John Lanahan, who attended the patient, as smallpox. It is unclear why Dr Lanahan was called in to see George when Dr Hillary was already apparently caring for Lawrence, particularly as Dr Hillary had published a monograph on smallpox while still practising in England; he may simply not have been at home when a messenger was sent to fetch him. However, George's attack of smallpox was comparatively mild and he made a complete recovery. Viewed in retrospect, it can be argued that George's attack of smallpox in Barbados served him well during the American Revolutionary War; it has been estimated that during that war more soldiers died of smallpox than of wounds.

In March 1752, Dr Hillary began recording his observations of Barbados weather patterns and associated patterns of disease, "with Care and Exactness":

> The Degrees of the Heat, or the Coolness, of the Air, were observed by Fahrenheit's Mercurial Thermometer, every Morning at or before the Rising of the Sun, and again between the Hours of Twelve and One o'clock at Noon. And the Height of

---

5. Washington was a habitual diarist, recording his observations until the time of his death but making no diary entries during the Revolutionary War. His "Barbados Diary" was published in 1892, with notes by J.M. Toner. See Carrington et al., *A–Z of Barbados Heritage*, 219.

the Mercury in the Barometer was observed at the same Times, tho' I have only recorded its Station at Noon.

So likewise the Succession, as well as the Variations of the concomitant epidemical Diseases, were as carefully observed in my Practice, at the same time, and recorded at the End of each Month; that I might, if possible, observe how those Diseases were either influenced, caused, or changed, by those Variations of the Weather.

Dr Hillary's *Observations on the Changes of the Air and the Concomitant Epidemical Diseases in the Island of Barbadoes* is divided into two parts. The first is concerned with observations of weather patterns and perceived associated disease patterns, while the second is called "A Treatise on the putrid bilious Fever, commonly called The Yellow Fever; and such other Diseases as are indigenous or endemial, in the West India Islands, or in the Torrid Zone". Dr Hillary's work is of significance for several reasons. First, it is certainly the first comprehensive documentation of an epidemiological nature in English outside Europe and in the Caribbean, justifying the titles "First Caribbean epidemiologist" and perhaps "First Caribbean meteorologist". Since epidemiology is the branch of medicine that investigates the causes and control of diseases, it is clear why Dr Hillary deserves these designations. The medical authors of the era were almost entirely descriptive in their writings, and while there was much conjecture, few attempted, as Dr Hillary did, to carry out extensive investigations looking for correlations of cause and disease, incidence and control. Indeed, he came to Barbados armed with all the weather-related instrumentation at his disposal – thermometer, barometer, hygrometer and rain gauge – and was rigorous in his twice daily measurements and observations. In *Doctors and Slaves*, Richard Sheridan notes that while Dr Hillary's work is chiefly concerned with diseases of Europeans, he also gives attention to diseases of African origin and the "medical ecology" of black slaves in Barbados.[6] And, as a pupil of Boerhaave, he was said to have learned to make the connection between theory and experience in medical practice.

The main authors writing in English in the eighteenth century who described the diseases of the English colonies were Reverend Griffith Hughes of Barbados (1750), Dr James Grainger of St Kitts (1764) and Dr Benjamin

---

6. Richard Sheridan, *Doctors and Slaves: A Medical and Demographic History of Slavery in the British West Indies, 1680–1834* (Cambridge University Press, 1985), 24.

Moseley of Jamaica (1789). The works of these authors have been compiled in an anthology, *On the Treatment and Management of the More Common West-India Diseases (1750–1802)*, edited and annotated by Dr J. Edward Hutson. A comprehensive review of diseases and medical disabilities in the slave era, specifically in enslaved Barbadians, has been written by anthropologist Dr Jerome Handler for the *Journal of Caribbean History*,[7] while Sheridan's *Doctors and Slaves* covers the broader Caribbean but focuses much more on Jamaica.

Dr Grainger's aim was to fill a perceived gap in the recommendations for treatment of African slaves; he referred to differences in their diseases, although he limited himself to noting the greater frequency of leprosy and a few other generalizations. For example, "rheumatism and Sciatica . . . These diseases are even more common in the Torrid Zone than at home", and "Heart-burn. This is a very common disease, and though not deadly, is yet troublesome. It arises from too free use of vegetables, a weak stomach and inert bile." Dr Hillary makes a similar comment as to the causation of dysentery: "[by] their too freely eating the herbs, roots, and fruits of the earth".

Dr Handler's review is comprehensive and provides source material for the many epidemics that occurred in the slave era. But again, many diagnoses are vague, with few causal inferences. For example, he notes Dr Grainger's observation that "more Negroes for some years past have perished by sore throats, than by any other disease". He adds that sore throats were given as a cause of death among Newton Plantation children in the late 1700s and early 1800s, but that from such limited information the diseases included under the rubric "sore throat" cannot be identified. Diphtheria has been the most frequently identified fatal "sore throat" in the pre-antibiotic area, and many older Barbadians, including the editors, have heard family tales of its ravages in the early twentieth century.

Second, and of more general interest, Dr Hillary's work documents the extraordinary sequence of the dramatic rise and fall of the sea flowing into the Bridgetown harbour (the Careenage) after the major earthquake at Lisbon on 1 November 1755, which killed thirty thousand people and triggered a tsunami that reached Barbados, on the other side of the Atlantic. Also of general interest

---

7. J.S. Handler, "Diseases and Medical Disabilities of Enslaved Barbadians, from the Seventeenth Century to around 1838", part 1, *Journal of Caribbean History* 40, no. 1 (2006): 1–38.

are observations on the inappropriateness and discomfort of wearing "a thick rich Coat and Waistcoat" in Barbados, under which he had seen men "melting, preferring the character of a Fop to that of a Man of Sense and Honour".

Third, the book contains a convincing description of tropical sprue, which, according to Hillary's biographer, Sir Christopher Booth, "has earned him an assured place in medical history". Dr Hillary wrote: "within the four last Years past, it is become so frequent that I have seen some Scores of Patients labouring under it". In Sir Christopher's words, "Hillary emphasised the cardinal clinical features of tropical sprue: the chronic nature of the disease, subject to relapse and remissions, the troublesome glossitis, now known to be due to folic acid deficiency, the recurrent diarrhoeas", which, as he states, "gradually wastes the patient, depriving him of his nourishment, leading to anaemia, progressive wasting, and death."

Fourth, Dr Hillary recognized that malaria was not endemic in Barbados and was not seen there except in patients who had come from another island and brought the disease with them. This insightful observation has been reviewed and reported by several later writers, including Sir Rubert Boyce, dean of the London School of Hygiene and Tropical Medicine, in his 1905 report on health conditions of the West Indies.[8] In fact, malaria did become briefly endemic in Barbados between the 1920s and 1940s, after which time it was totally eradicated.[9]

Fifth, Dr Hillary wrote extensively on what he described as "the Putrid Bilious fever, commonly called the Yellow Fever", but noted that it was rarely passed from person to person. He recorded: "its not spreading and infecting others, as the Plague always does; for this Fever very rarely or never is infectious or contagious to others, not even to those who attend the Sick, except a chance Time". Both the eminent twentieth-century Barbadian physician Dr Harry Bayley and Dr Hillary's biographer, Sir Christopher Booth, considered that he was describing leptospirosis, a spirochaetal disease transmitted by rats and dogs which is endemic in the West Indies. The severe form of leptospirosis,

---

8. Sir Rubert Boyce, often incorrectly noted as Sir Robert, was the mosquito expert of the era. Ironically, he considered that "Barbados jaundice" was yellow fever, although it was subsequently shown by Dr Harry Bayley not to be prevalent in mosquito-prone environments but rather in warehouse and sugar-cane workers, and was almost certainly leptospirosis.

9. Frank Ramsey, *Protein Calorie Malnutrition*. Sir Frank was a paediatrician and founder of the National Nutrition Centre, Barbados.

which Dr Bayley described in his 1940 Cambridge University MD thesis, is caused by *Leptospira icterohaemorrhagiae* and is known as Weil's Disease.[10]

The manifestations of a severe case of leptospirosis are indistinguishable from the features described by Dr Hillary, with vomiting leading to dehydration and hypotension, jaundice due to haemolysis, haemorrhages, respiratory problems, kidney failure, cardiac arrhythmias, meningitis and death in a high proportion of inadequately treated cases. Leptospirosis was not recognized until Adolph Weil's seminal description was published in 1898. Identification of the causal spirochaete followed only in 1917, so it is not surprising that Dr Hillary and others should mistake it for yellow fever; by the early twentieth century its unique characteristics and lack of epidemic pattern had earned it the sobriquet "Barbados jaundice". It is noteworthy that Dr Hillary's careful observations led to his conclusion that it was "only infrequently contagious",[11] which was key to its recognition by later Barbadian doctors as lacking the epidemic pattern of yellow fever, the causal virus of which is transmitted by the *Aedes aegypti* mosquito.

Dr Hillary made many other cogent observations – on the endemic "dry bellyache" (lead poisoning), tetanus, elephantiasis (widely known as "Barbados leg" in the eighteenth and nineteenth centuries but in Barbados called "Guyana leg"), leprosy and yaws – and comments on the usefulness of these observations will be found in the notes throughout this work.

It is worth noting that Dr Hillary does not appear to have been attached to any specific plantation, but he may well have been a visiting physician to many. He has little to say about the slave hospital, in spite of the known existence of "Sick-House[s] and a proper Room to confine Negroes" from the inventory of William Belgrove's plantation in Barbados of 1755.[12] A few years later (1769), Dr Grainger described his "model for a complete sick house", while Philip Gibbes, "an absentee planter of Barbados", felt strongly that hospitals were needed "for the preservation of the blacks". He wrote in 1797 that he could not "too much lament the parsimony of the proprietors of plantations, who can behold a regular decrease of their negroes without attention to some of the more obvious means of preserving them".

---

10. Weil's Disease was described in 1898 by H. Adolph Weil (1848–1916), a German physician.

11. Since leptospirosis is transmitted chiefly by rats, cases of the disease may occasionally occur in clusters or in the same household, perhaps explaining Dr Hillary's impression of the disease's contagiousness.

12. Quoted by Sheridan, *Doctors and Slaves*, 270.

Sheridan (*Doctors and Slaves*) opines that Barbados may have had enough medical practitioners to visit the sick slaves daily and states that Governor Parry testified before the Privy Council of 1789 that "the plantations were constantly provided with an apothecary who was paid by the master annually and who generally visited the blacks every day, whether they were sick or well". Moreover, whenever the apothecary "saw a necessity for it, he recommended to the Owners and Overseers to call in the aid of a Physician or Surgeon".

Kipple (*The Caribbean Slave*) states that "most plantations on all [Caribbean] islands did have a [slave] hospital, 'sick house' or 'hothouse' under the daily or at least weekly supervision of a doctor" and that the "doctor generally was contracted for on an annual basis". In addition "each plantation [usually] had one or more slave 'doctors' or 'doctor women' . . . all generally elderly". Kipple estimates that "at the turn of the nineteenth century slaves averaged at least nineteen sick days per year".

Today only one extant Barbadian building has been tentatively identified as a slave hospital. It demonstrates the features recommended by Dr Grainger and Gibbes: a long building with separate, well-ventilated long, narrow rooms on each side of a central two-storey structure. This building – unique for a Barbadian plantation – is at the former Blackman's Plantation site, now Grantley Adams School, in the parish of St Joseph (see frontispiece).

On 16 August 1811 Dr Benjamin Rush, one of the signatories of the American Declaration of Independence,[13] published an annotated version of *Observations on the Changes of the Air and the Concomitant Epidemical Diseases in the Island of Barbadoes*, in which he enthusiastically endorsed most, though not all, of the therapeutic measures and procedures advocated by Dr Hillary. Moreover, he dedicated his work to "The students of Medicine in the University of Pennsylvania", directing their attention to

> another of those fountains of practical knowledge in medicine, which have been opened by the history of epidemic diseases.
>
> The physician [Dr William Hillary], to whose patience and labour we are indebted for performing that useful task by means of the following work, was a pupil of the celebrated Dr Boerhaave, from whom he learned the necessary connection of theory with experience in the practice of physic. It is true, some of

---

13. Rush (1745–1813) was an American physician, author, politician and professor of chemistry at the universities of Philadelphia and Pennsylvania.

the theories he adopted, from his illustrious master, have been discovered to be erroneous, but the facts he has recorded in his history of the weather, . . . will be true, in like circumstances, in all ages and countries . . .

Clearly, theories on the overwhelming influence of weather on diseases of all kinds were still alive and well sixty years after Dr Hillary published his seminal work. What is disappointing is the lack of significant advances in medical knowledge or therapeutic options over those years; the annotations of Dr Rush add little of significance. It was to be at least another sixty years before major discoveries – for example, in anaesthesia, pathology and microbiology – were to have an impact on medical care. But it is instructive to recognize that the rigorous scientific and medical observations made by a lone physician in Barbados were perpetuated, crossed the Atlantic, and were recognized and republished sixty years later with the glowing praise of the United States' most famous physician – a most striking early example of the impact of Barbadian medical research and scholarship upon the metropolis.

It is also instructive for us to review the resolution of one of Dr Hillary's most challenging medical conundrums – the fact that "the putrid bilious fever" did not appear to be contagious – two hundred years later by another Barbadian physician, Dr Harry Bayley. Henry Fraser was introduced to Dr Hillary's work by Sir Christopher Booth, Hillary's biographer and one of Fraser's mentors, early in his medical career at the Royal Postgraduate Medical School in the early 1970s. On obtaining a copy of the second (1766) edition, he realized the accuracy and brilliance of Dr Hillary's observations, not only in relation to his descriptions of tropical sprue but in many other details so lucidly expressed. Sharing this volume and its ideas with his co-editor, Edward Hutson, produced an immediate mutual commitment to bringing Dr Hillary's work to the widest possible medical audience. The recent widespread recognition of the importance of medical history and its inclusion in medical school curricula are most timely and more than validate this effort, not merely as an academic exercise but also as an outstanding example of an early epidemiological approach, rigorous observations and clear deductions that have stood the test of time surprisingly well.

J. EDWARD HUTSON
HENRY S. FRASER

Notes on Editorial Procedures

T HIS VOLUME CONTAINS both footnotes, numbered consecutively within each part of the text, and endnotes, marked throughout by the superscript symbol †. The footnotes, on the relevant pages, are those provided by William Hillary and the endnotes are ours.

We have deliberately kept editing to a minimum, and on the few occasions we have added a word or words for the sake of clarity, we have identified them [thus]. Spelling, grammar and syntax remain as in the original.

Apothecaries' Weights and Measures

The following is extracted from information provided by the Museum of the Royal Pharmaceutical Society of Great Britain and compiled by Peter G. Homan, FRPharmS MCPP, in 2002.

> English weights were evolved by the Romans using a grain of wheat as the standard. Apothecaries' weight, a variation of the Troy weight system, was used in Europe for the measurement of pharmaceutical ingredients from as early as 1270. Henry VIII decreed Troy weights (5,760 grains to the pound) to test coins. Elizabeth I decreed that a pound (weight) of 7,000 grains should be used for selling ordinary goods, and that Troy weights were to be used for precious metals and stones. . . . In 1758 [the British] Parliament legalized only the Troy weight.
>
> The basis of the Apothecary system was the grain. Dispensing and selling [of pharmaceuticals] were permitted using this system. Weights [and symbols] were as follows:
>
> One grain: gr
> One scruple: Э = 20 grains
> One drachm: Ʒ = 60 grains
> One ounce: Ʒ = 480 grains
> One pound: lb = 5,760 grains

OBSERVATIONS
on the
CHANGES of the AIR
and the
Concomitant Epidemical DISEASES
in the
Island of BARBADOES

To which is added
A Treatise on the putrid bilious FEVER,
commonly called
The YELLOW FEVER;
And such other DISEASES as are indigenous
or endemial, in the WEST INDIA ISLANDS,
or in the TORRID ZONE.

By WILLIAM HILLARY, MD
1766
LONDON

Preface

THE FOLLOWING OBSERVATIONS on the Changes of the Air, and Variations of the Weather, were made in the Island of *Barbadoes*, with Care and Exactness, and are truly related.

The Degrees of the Heat, or the Coolness, of the Air, were observed by *Fahrenheit's* Mercurial Thermometer,[†] made at *Amsterdam*, every Morning at or before the Rising of the Sun, and again between the Hours of Twelve and One o'clock at Noon. And the height of the Mercury in the Barometer[†] was observed at the same Times, tho' I have only recorded its Station[†] at Noon; and I should have begun these Observations some Years sooner, if an Accident had not deprived me of my Barometer; but if I had known that the Variations in it had been so very little, within the Torrid Zone,[†] as I found them afterwards, I should have made them without it; as the greatest Variation in it, in six Years time, was never more than four Tenths of an Inch, *viz.* from twenty-nine, six Tenths of an Inch high, to thirty Inches. I also made use of a Hygrometer[†] to observe the Degrees of Moisture and Dryness of the Air, but found its Variations to be so immaterial, except when the Rains fell, and were visible to our Senses, as not to be worth recording; especially as the Quantity of Rain which fell in each Month is recorded: But as it is observed that much more Rain usually falls in mountainous Places, than in flat, low, level Countries, and *Bridgetown* being on a level Plain, they often had Rain on the Hills when we had little or none; and my worthy and ingenious Friend[†] *Andrew Drury*,[†] whose Seat[†] is on the rising Hills near the Medium[†] between them, having carefully measured the Quantities of the Rain which fell in each Month, for some Years, and reduced it into cubic Inches and the decimal Parts of an Inch in its Depth; his Observations and Measurements, where he is situated, may be taken as a Medium† for the whole Island; and he readily obliged me with a Table of the Quantities of Rain which fell in six Years, for which I now return him my grateful Acknowledgements. And I think that the Changes of the Air and Weather, as well as the Quantity of Rain falling, may be depended on, as being very exact.

So likewise the Succession, as well as the Variations of the concomitant epidemical Diseases, were as carefully observed in my Practice,† at the same time, and recorded at the End of each Month; that I might, if possible, observe, how those Diseases were either influenced, caused, or changed, by those Variations of the Weather; which, when they were evident, material, or important, I have occasionally observed and remarked; as also such Variations, either in the Method of curing those Diseases, or such Alterations in the Medicines given, as I found were necessary, and the Success they had; all which I have endeavoured carefully to relate. I do not here mean such Alterations, either in the Methods of Cure, or in the Medicines, or their Doses, as are necessary to be made, in different Patients, or different Ages and Constitutions;† [such] as the Difference between a Patient who has strong, rigid, and elastic Solids, and a dense Blood; and one who has a delicate, slender, or a relaxed weak State of his Solids, and a lax, loose, unconnected State of the Globules of his Blood; nor the Difference between one who has a viscid, sizzy, or buff-like Blood,† from one who has a lax, putrescent, dissolved State of Blood; for all these different Constitutions may possibly have the same epidemical Disease, at the same time, but with different Symptoms, and may require different Methods of Cure, both as to the Quantity of Bleeding† and other Evacuations,† as well as different Medicines, tho' it be the same Disease, and arises from the same epidemical Cause; as every judicious Physician knows. But I mean such Changes in Diseases, as arise from the Variations in the Weather, and either produce different Symptoms in the same Disease, or such as may determine† the morbid Matter to a different Part of the Body; or lastly to be carried off by a different critical Discharge, than it was before; all which should be carefully observed by the attending Physician, and Nature should always be assisted by him, to effect such Ways and Methods as she indicates and endeavours to do, if it can be done; these I have endeavoured to observe: As also when those Changes in the Weather have either put an end to the then reigning epidemical Diseases, or have produced some other Diseases which did not appear before; and when these Changes were any way considerable, or of any Importance, I have taken care to mention them, as well as such Changes in the Methods of Cure, or in the Medicines, as I found necessary to be made, especially those which I found to be the most successful.

Though I have given but few or no *Formulæ* or *Prescriptions*, because the same Form† or Prescription can but suit a few Patients, or Constitutions, without some Alterations in them *pro re nata*;† and therefore could not be of much service to such Practitioners as are qualified either to prescribe, or administer any Medicines; and a Prescription to the Judicious is unnecessary, because, as the great *Hippocrates*† says, "He, who knows the Disease, knows what is proper to cure it." And as for those who will neither read, nor yet know how to reason on the Causes, or the manner of their Production of Diseases, and yet will boldly practise by rote, and prescribe by guess at a Venture, though the Life of the Patient depends on the right or wrong Method of prescribing; I must, with the learned and judicious Dr *Huxam*,† seriously advise them, at least to peruse the sixth Commandment.†

Introduction

T HAT WISE FATHER and Prince of Physicians, *HIPPOCRATES*, advises all Physicians to examine and duly consider the Situation,† Air, and the Water, used by the people of such Cities, or Places, as they are called to, or may practice in. It is therefore necessary that I should say something concerning the Situation, Air, Water, *&c.*, of this Island, before I give an Account of the Observations made on the epidemical† and endemial† Diseases in it, at least for the Satisfaction of such of my Readers as are Strangers to it.

BARBADOES is a small Island, near [twenty-six] Miles long, and near [fourteen] broad,† situated in the West-Indies, in Lat. 13°N and Long. 59°W from London, and is one of the Caribbee Islands. It is, most of it, pretty high rocky dry Land; the Soil is usually about two Feet deep, in some Places less, in others more, and mostly consists of a blackish Mould, in some Places red. It has but few Springs of Water, and only one Rivulet which deserves that Name: No marshy or wet Lands of any Importance, the whole Island being in general rocky and dry; yet the Inhabitants have Plenty of good Spring-water, by digging into the Rock, all over the Island, though it is most commonly a little hard: The Rock is in general composed of a soft porous white Freestone,† in some Places a little Lime-stone;† in others it consists of Brain-stones,† Astroites,† and stalactite† Concretions.† In the North-east part of the Island there are Mun-jack† Pits, from which the Petroleum, called *Barbadoes Tar*, is gotten, and near them Iron-ore is found. The Air is generally pure, serene, and dry, except in the rainy Seasons, but always very warm.

The Inhabitants who live temperately, and are prudent in the Use of the six Non-naturals,† if they have tolerable good natural Constitutions, live to as great an Age as the Europeans. Some have died here lately, who were above an hundred Years old; but those who live irregularly, and are too free in the Use of vinous† and other spirituous Liquors, generally hasten their End more expeditiously, than they who live in the same manner in Europe. But I must observe, in Justice to, and Honour of, the Fair-sex, that they all in general are exceeding temperate, and very few or any of them drink any thing but Water, and generally live to a good old Age.

The Europeans and North-Americans, from the colder Parts of it, and especially the Britons, when they first come to this or the other West-India Islands, are, by the great increased Heat of the Climate, usually not long after their Arrival there, seized either with a Fever, or with a Sort of Efflorescences,† which most commonly first appear on the Legs, in pretty large Lumps of reddish Colour, which are sometimes as large or larger than a Shilling, but of an irregular Figure,† and itch violently, especially towards Night, if they are either rubbed or scratched; and from doing which it is difficult to refrain, though doing either much increases both the Itching and the Swelling, and often either rubs the cuticle† off, or causes little Blisters to rise, and a saltish yellow Serum to ouse† out, which makes them smart;† after which a Scurff† or Scab ensues, which after a few Days falls off: These Lumps commonly rise on the Hands, Arms, Legs, Thighs, Neck, and Face, and usually continue three, four, or five Days, then turn to a yellowish Colour, and soon after disappear; but are soon succeeded by others in or near the same Places, and so continue successively for several Weeks, or Months, in most Strangers which come into this hot Climate.

These exanthematous† Eruptions, are vulgarly,† but erroneously, ascribed to the stinging or biting of Mosquitoes. It is certain that these Insects do bite, and that little Lumps or Swellings will rise where they bite, but these are neither so large, nor do they usually continue so many Hours, as the other Lumps do Days: These being only the Bite of a small Insect, which is not more offensive than the Bite of the Midge† in England; whereas the others are Efflorescences cast out by Nature, or the Vis Vitæ,† and proceed from the great increased Heat of the Climate, which continuing rarifies and expands the circulating Fluids, and so exalts,† semi-volatilizes, and alkalizes† their natural soft, mild, semi-ammoniacal† neutral animal Salts, as to render them very acrid,† and unfit to pass through the small subcuticular Vessels and secretory Pores, without obstructing them, and producing those troublesome itching Tumours.

Whilst these Efflorescences continue, there are also other but smaller eruptive Pustulæ, or little red Pimples, which arise from the same Cause, often come out all over the rest of the Body, called *Essera* by the Arabians, *Sudamina* by the Romans, and the Prickly-heat† by the English, which cause great Itching and Prickling, as if with small Needles: This usually continues several Weeks, and in some Persons for some Months, in the hotter Months, and then declines, and cause the Cuticle to fall gradually off in small white Scales. The Prickly-heat seizes most of the Inhabitants, both Natives and Strangers, either in a greater or lesser Degree, every Year during the hot Summer-months. It seldom causes any Sickness or Disorder, except the troublesome Itching and Prickling, but every one goes about his Business with it, as if he was well; unless it be imprudently repelled† and struck suddenly in, either by rubbing it with Lime-juice, Vinegar, camphorated Spirits,† or by washing the Body with cold Water, which some are so imprudent as to use, to take that troublesome itching and prickling Heat off, whereby they have repelled those acrid saline Humours into the Blood again, when kind Nature had thus cast them out, and so have produced a Fever, which has sometimes been attended with bad Consequences. For going into a cold Bath, or the Sea, is not so bad or dangerous in this Case, as washing the Body with cold Water is; for though the Humour may be repelled, whilst they are in the Cold bath, yet the glowing Heat which usually follows it, strikes it more effectually out again after, which washing with cold Water does not. The best Method is to live temperately, use moderate Exercise, and encourage the Eruption by taking small warm Liquids and Nourishments, [such] as Gruel,† Tea, Coffee, Wine-whey,† Broth and plain Meats; and to avoid suddenly exposing themselves when warm to a Current of cool Air, Night-dews, and damp wet Places,† and the too freely drinking [of] spirituous Liquors, as they increase this as well as inflammatory Diseases.

For I have observed, that not only the yellow Serum which those little Tumours or blisters ouse out, but the common Sweat, even of Persons who are well, when tasted in this hot Climate, is so very salt and acrid, that it tastes like the Salt or Spirit of Hartshorn† mixed with Water in a considerable Proportion, which being retained in, or repelled into, the Blood, must attenuate and dissolve it, and stimulate the Solids also, and produce not only this depuratory† Fever, but if continued, the yellow putrid Fever,† or other putrid Fevers† also.

Moderate Bleeding, and a free Use of gentle acid Antiphlogisticks,† and sometimes other Evacuations, and encouraging a free Diaphoresis,[†] generally takes this Fever off; but a great Languor,[†] and want[†] of Spirits and Strength, often continue for some time after it. And it is remarkable, that in this hot Climate the Sick seldom recover from any Fever, or other Sickness, so soon as they usually do in England, or other colder Countries.

Notwithstanding that the Air is generally clear and serene, (except in the rainy Seasons) yet the Heat is generally so great, as never to cause the Mercury in *Fahrenheit's* Thermometer to fall lower than 70°F, in the coolest Mornings, or higher than 86°F in the Day time; yet as the greater Degree of Heat usually continues eight or nine Months in the Year, it must greatly relax the animal Fibres, especially when it is accompanied with Moisture, as in the rainy Seasons, and give a putrescent[†] Diathesis[†] to the Fluids, both which must greatly tend to attenuate and dissolve the circulating Fluids: And it is observed, that the Blood in general is much more lax, loose, and attenuated, even in Health here, than it is in England: Hence the Disposition to putrid Fevers, and other Diseases from thence arising, may be seen. But this lax State of the Fibres has its Advantages in this Climate, as well as its Disadvantages: For if the Fibres were not thus relaxed, but were to continue in that elastic active State, which they are usually in, in colder Countries, every extraordinary Motion and Exercise, accompanied with that great Heat, would bring on a Fever of the inflammatory Kind, with greater or less Violence, as these procatarctic Causes[†] were greater or less. But let us not imagine, that a general Relaxation of the Solids attends every one, in the same Degree, because the same Degree of Heat equally affects all; for some are much more relaxed than others from the same Cause, and different Constitutions differ as much here as they do in England, or elsewhere, though none may have their Solids so elastic here, as the same Person would have them there.

Having said thus much on the Climate, and the Effects of the Variations of the Weather on the human Body, I must make some Remarks on the Customs of the Country, particularly on those which do, or may, affect the Health of the Inhabitants.

I am well informed, that it was the Custom of the first Comers hither, to wrap and swaddle up their new-born Infants in Linen and Flannel in this hot Climate, as they did in England, by which it is probable that several of them must have lost their Lives innocently and ignorantly; and those who were strong enough to survive it, must have been so relaxed and weakened by it, as to render them weak and sickly a great part of, and some of them all, their

Life-time after. But this Practice is, in a good measure, left off, though not near so much as it should be; for the Midwives and Nurses still continue to use a great deal more Clothing and Wrapping than is proper, and do not use Washing and Bathing their Infants in cold Water, near so much as they should, whereby many are rendered sickly, weak, tender, and pale, all, or a great Part of their Life-time after. Whereas, if they used cold Bathing in a proper manner, not only to Infants, but all others, except the very ancient People, it would greatly contribute not only to brace-up and strengthen their relaxed Solids, but to prevent all those Diseases which arise from thence: And we find that all the Eastern warm Nations use cold Bathing frequently, if not daily, and no doubt have found the Benefit of it for many Ages past; and if the Inhabitants of the West-India Islands would follow the same Practice, they would find the same Advantage from it also.

Fashion and Custom are two prevailing Things, which enslave the greatest Part of Mankind, though often both contrary to Reason and Conveniency, and particularly in our Dress: For no doubt but the loose cool easy Dress of the Eastern Nations, a thin, loose, Gown or Banjan,† is much easier, and better fitted for us in the hot Climate, than the English Dress; and all who have tried both find it so: But such is the Influence of Fashion and Custom, that I have seen many Men loaded, and almost half melting, under a thick Coat and Waistcoat, daubed and loaded with Gold, on a hot Day, scarce able to bear them, little considering how much they injured their Constitutions thereby, as well as their being troublesome.

A Banjan is the dress of the *Mandareens*,† at the Courts of China, Japan, Indostan,† and Persia, and some other Courts; and why it may not be so at Barbadoes, and the other hot Islands, I see nothing but Custom to hinder it: And if any one cannot part with his Finery, and thinks the Character of a Fop† preferable to that of a Man of Sense and Honour, he may daub his Banjan with as much Gold as he pleases. But after all, I think it is the most convenient Dress in all hot Countries, and the best suited to preserve their Ease and Health.

I must also say something of Exercise, as that when prudently used contributes much to the Preservation, and in some Cases to the Restoration, of Health. But as no rural Diversions, such as are used in England, can be followed here, because we have little or no Game,† and if we had the Country is too hot to pursue them; wherefore Riding, Walking, and Dancing, are the only Exercises here used: The two first, when taken in moderation, at suitable

Hours, *viz.* Mornings and Evenings, when the Air is a little cooler, do, no doubt, contribute much both to the Preservation and Restoration of Health in some Cases, as also does Navigation[†] in some others; but Dancing is much too violent an Exercise in this hot Climate, and many do greatly injure their Health by it, and I have known it fatal to some; neither is it used in the Eastern hot Countries: But most of the Ladies are so excessive fond of it, that say what I will they will dance on.[†]

As to the Diseases of this and the other West-India Islands, there are several both acute and chronical, which are indigenous or endemial in them, and probably to such other Countries as are situated within the Torrid Zone, which are scarce ever seen, and are but little known, in England, or the other European Nations. I have endeavoured carefully to observe those Diseases, and strictly enquired into them, and shall delineate them in such a manner, that they may be known when seen by those who have not seen them before. I have also recommended such Methods of Cure as I have found to be the most successful, as also the manner of giving those Medicines which I have found to be the most efficacious in their Cure; and I have added some *Formulæ* or *Prescriptions* in the Second Part, for the Benefit of such young Practitioners as may not be acquainted with the usual Method or Manner of giving them. But I must observe, that neither these, nor any other *Formulæ* or *Prescriptions* that can be given, can no more suit all Constitutions or Cases in the same Disease, than one Coat can be made to fit all Men; for these must be varied according to the different Causes, Circumstances, and Natures of the Symptoms of the Disease, as well as to the different Ages, Strengths, and Constitutions of the Patient, by the judicious Physician, as he may see necessary.[†]

In the first Part I have given an Account of the Weather, and all its material Changes, as I observed them by *Fahrenheit's* Mercurial Thermometer, and a common portable Barometer, and also have given an Account of the Quantities of Rain which fell in each Month and Year, and the other visible Changes in it; and an Account of all the concomitant endemial and epidemical Diseases, and such Variations as happened in them, as were any way remarkable or material, together with their Indications[†] and Intentions[†] of Cure, generally taken *ex ipsa re et ratione*,[†] and such Methods and Medicines as I found to be the most successful in their Cure. And I have remarked wherein those Diseases differed from the same Diseases in England, when any such happened to appear, that were any thing material or remarkable, arising from the Heat, or other Variations of the Climate; as also such Variations as I found it necessary to make, either in the Method of treating those Diseases, or in the Medicines, when it was different from the Method of treating them in England; and I have mentioned such as I found to be the most successful, in as plain, clear, and full a manner as I could, without being too tedious, in order to adapt it to the Capacity of the Unlearned, as too many of the Apothecaries[†] in this Part of the World are too much so, that it may be more generally useful to Mankind, and in particular to the Inhabitants of the Island of Barbadoes, for whose Benefit and Service I have chiefly taken all this Labour; and I sincerely wish that this Performance[†] may be as useful and beneficial to them, and all the other West-India Islands, as either they or I can desire.

Part I

A.D. 1752†

THE MONTHS of MARCH, APRIL, and MAY, were more than usually warm and dry, little Rain falling in all that time, insomuch that the whole Quantity which fell in those three Months, was only equal to 1.22 cubical Inches deep.

And the lowest that *Fahrenheit's* Thermometer was, at Sun-rise, was in the MONTH of MARCH at 74°F; and the highest in the Morning at 78°F; and the lowest at Noon was at 80°F; and the highest at Noon was 82°F. In APRIL the lowest in the Morning was 76°F; and the highest in the Morning at 79°F; and the lowest at Noon was 81°F; and the highest at Noon was at 82°F. In MAY the lowest in the Morning was 77°F; and the highest in the Morning at 81°F. And the [lowest the] Barometer in these three Months was 29.8 [inches of mercury]; the highest 29.9 [inches of mercury].

During this warm dry Season, inflammatory Diseases were very frequent, chiefly Ophthalmies,† Quincies,† Peripneumonies,† and Pleurisies;† in all which the Pulse was mostly full, quick, and hard, and their Blood generally inflamed; and in most it was covered with a Starch† or Buff-like inflammatory Pellicle:† But I must observe, that their Blood in these inflammatory Diseases, is seldom so much sizzy or buff-like in this warm Climate, as it usually is in

England, when the Pain and Height of the Inflammation, and the other Symptoms are nearly the same.[1]

These generally required larger Bleeding than in most other Years, unless equally hot and dry; but by bleeding pretty freely, and by a liberal Use of antiphlogistic[†] Medicines, with Sal. Nitre[†] and crude Sal. Ammoniac,[†] as hereafter mentioned, and diluting[†] plentifully, they were generally relieved; and I found emollient Fomentations, with crude Sal. Ammoniac,[†] were of great Service.

The Small Pox[†] also were epidemical at this Time, but were in general of the distinct Kind; and those few who had the confluent Sort, were generally of a good Kind, notwithstanding that the above inflammatory Diseases were then epidemical.

The Beginning of JUNE was also very dry and warm; but from the Middle of it to the End of it, and during the MONTHS of JULY and AUGUST, we had frequent and much Rain.

The Quantity of Rain which fell in JUNE was [equal] to 10.03 cubic Inches deep. The lowest that the Thermometer was in the Mornings was at 77°F; and the highest it was at or before Sun-rise in the Morning was 80°F. The lowest it was at Noon was at 82°F; and the highest at Noon was 84°F.

The Quantity of Rain which fell in [the MONTH of] JULY was [equal] to 8.48 cubic Inches deep; and the lowest that the Thermometer was at in the Mornings was at 78°F; and the highest that it was at in the Mornings was at 80°F. The lowest it was at Noon was at 82°F; and the highest at Noon was 86°F.

The Quantity of Rain which fell in the MONTH of AUGUST was [equal] to 8.72 [cubic] Inches deep. The lowest the Thermometer was in the Mornings was at 79°F; and the highest that ever it was in the Mornings was at 82°F. The lowest it was at Noon was 83°F; and the highest at Noon was 86°F; and the lowest that the Mercury fell in the Barometer in these three Months was to 29.8 [inches of mercury]; and the highest that it ever did arise to was 29.9 [inches of mercury].

Upon this Change of the Weather from very dry to very wet, Dysenteries

---

1. *Query.* Does not this Difference most probably arise from their Solids here being more relaxed by the Heat of the Climate, than they are in England? Whence their Fluids are more lax, and more readily attenuated, or dissolved, by the alkaline Acrimony of the semivolatilized animal Salts.

became very frequent and epidemical; as they do usually every Year upon much Rain falling at this Time of the Year, and seized many both white and black People, but especially the latter, who are often but little clothed, and more exposed to the Inclemency of the Weather, and some of them but poorly fed. We had still some few Pleurisies and Peripneumonies, but these became less frequent, and the Quincies and Opthalmies ceased to appear upon the falling of the Rain.

A Cholera Morbus† also seized several, but I think its Symptoms are less violent here, than they usually are in England: And some were seized with Apoplexies† and Palsies,† and some of the First died before any proper Assistance could be called in.

Many Children were seized with an Aphthous Fever,² in which the Aphthæ† were most commonly of the white or yellowish Kind, and rarely black, or of a bad Kind, unless they were wrongly treated; it usually came on with a moderate Fever, a quick† but not very high† Pulse, and was attended with Diarrhœa, but not much Pain in the Bowels; and as Dysenteries were then frequent, some ignorant Practitioners treated it as such, and gave them strong Restringents† (tho' not good Practice in that case†) which increased the Fever and Inflammation of the Bowels, and brought on a Mortification† which proved fatal. But when this Fever was treated with small Doses of Rhubarb† with gentle Anodynes,† to carry off the acrid Humours, and abate the Irritation and Pain, and gentle Antiphlogisticks with Anodynes, to take off the Fever, and restrain or prevent the too violent Purging; and then giving soft, smooth, healing Balsamicks,† [such] as *Sperm. Cet. Cremor. Lactis,*† or the *Wax Emulsion,* with a little *Syr. Meconio,*† to heal the *Primæ Viæ,*† they generally recovered. As the morbid Humours, being rendered acrid by the preceding

---

2. *Query.* Was not both the Dysentery and this Aphthous Fever, caused by the falling of so much Rain, and rendering the Air cooler, by which the great Perspiration and Sweating, caused and continued by the long continued Dryness and Heat before, being suddenly abated and stopped; were they not now turned upon the Bowels, and the Humours being rendered acrid by that Heat, so produced these Diseases? And,

Query 2. Were not the Apoplexies and Palsies also produced by the same Causes, *viz.* a Diminution or Stoppage of Perspiration and Sweat, by which a Plethora or Fullness, and the Quantity of the circulating Fluids was too much increased, and the Vessels of the Brain making the least Resistance, the Fluid too violently distended or broke them; as no other Evacuations were sufficiently increased to carry off that Plethora; either from a want of more Acrimony in the Fluids, or too great a Relaxation and Inability of the Solids, to produce such Evacuations.

Dryness and Heat, and now being turned upon the Bowels, by the cooler Rain stopping or diminishing the free Perspiration and Sweating; it was necessary to assist Nature to discharge those acrid Humours, by such ways as she indicated, and not to hinder her; tho' it might be necessary to prevent the Evacuation from being too violent, or too sudden and great.

The MONTH of SEPTEMBER continued to be very wet, and more cool than the preceding Months, tho' we had some calm hot Days in which we had much Thunder and Lightning, and much Rain.[†]

The Quantity of Rain which fell in this Month, tho' it had but 19 Days in it, by reason of the Change of Style made this Year, and begun in it,[†] was [equal] to 7.89 cubic Inches deep; and the lowest the Thermometer was in this Month in the Morning was 79°F; and the highest it was in any Morning was at 84°F; the lowest it ever was at Noon was 82°F; and the highest was 86°F. The Barometer was never lower than 29.75 [inches of mercury]; nor higher than 29.9 [inches of mercury].

A Catarrhous Fever[†] seized several People in this Month; they at first complained of a Pain in their Heads, and all over in their Limbs, accompanied with a violent Cough, by which a thin acrid Phlegm[†] was expectorated, tho' but little in Quantity, and brought up with much Difficulty; some had a brisk Fever with it, others had only a small Fever, their Pulse small, quick, and in some a little languid,[†] and their extreme Parts[†] rather cold than warm, sometimes with flushing Heats, and then cold again, and sometimes shooting, darting Pains, which were soon over, and often returned again.

Bleeding those who were more plethoric[†] and the Fever higher, with Pectorals[†] and Antiphlogisticks and a few Volatiles,[†] generally took it off; but more attenuating[†] and warmer Pectorals, with a more liberal Use of Volatiles, as also Vesicatories,[†] were necessary to those who were more low and languid, and where the Pulse and Fever were lower, were of great Service and generally successful; and the Dysentery still continued to be epidemical, and we had some few inflammatory Diseases still, tho' but few of these now.

The MONTH of OCTOBER continued to be very wet, and much cooler than usual at this Time of the Year. The Quantity of Rain which fell in this Month, was [equal] to 12.14 cubical Inches deep; and the lowest that the Thermometer was in any Morning in it, was 78°F; and the highest that it rose in any Morning was to 82°F. The lowest it was at Noon was 81°F; and the highest at Noon was 85°F: And the lowest the Barometer was at 29.8 [inches of mercury]; and the highest was at 29.9 [inches of mercury].

The Weather continuing to be wet and cool, several were seized with an irregular, ingeminated,[†] intermitting,[†] quotidian[†] Fever; which at the first generally put on the Appearance of a continued remitting[†] Fever; but in two or three Day's time usually changed to in ingeminated Quotidian, with all the Symptoms of that Fever, as usual in England.[3]

When this Fever was treated by bleeding once, and an Emetic[†] after it, at a proper Distance; and then with saline, saponaceous[†] Draughts[†] after that; [such] as *Sal. Absinth. Succus Limon.*[†] *&c.*, or rather with *Sal. Absinth.* brought to a neutral State with *Elixir. Vitrioli Acid.*[†] *q.s.*[†] in a little *Aq. Menthæ,*[†] *&c.*, which I found to be better in this Case, the Fever was generally carried quite off by a critical Sweat on the Seventh or Ninth Day: or in some few it came to intermit regularly after that time, and then was soon cured by the *Cortex Peruv.*[†] given with the above saline Draughts, and rarely effectual without them. Though these irregular ingeminated Fevers often remitted, and sometimes seemed to intermit, yet if the *Cortex Peruv.* was given too soon in the Disease, before it intermitted regularly (as I have more than once seen where it had been injudiciously given) it generally caused the Fever to become continual, and *mali Moris;*[†] which sometimes produced obstructions in some of the Glands of the Viscera, or elsewhere, which were irremovable, and either ended in a Suppuration, or a Mortification of the Part, as I have several times seen and predicted, that it would be so; as the learned Dr *Boerhaave*[†] very judiciously observes.

The Symptoms of this Fever here, were much the same as they usually are in the continued remitting Fever in England; except only, that the Urine in this hot Climate, never deposits any latericious[†] Sediment in this Fever, nor very rarely in any intermitting, or any other Fever, except sometimes when a Crisis[†] happens that way, as it is commonly observed to do in England; where a latericious Sediment in this Fever generally denotes the Fever either to intermit, or so far to remit, that the *Cortex Peruv.* may be safely given with Success; but no so here.

I must observe, that intermitting Fevers, especially Tertians[†] and Quartans,[†] are very rarely or never seen in this Island now,[†] unless they are brought hither

---

3. *Query* 3. Were not these irregular remitting or intermitting Fevers, as well as the preceding Catarrhous Fever, produced by the Continuance of the moist, wet Season relaxing the solids, and rendering them less active, and a Diminution of the Perspiration and Sweat at the same Time?

from some of the Leeward Islands, or some other Places which are less cultivated, and not yet cleared of the Woods; where intermitting Fevers are said to be much more frequent, and are often attended with Obstructions of the Glands of the Viscera; and when injudiciously treated, and the *Cortex* [*Peruv.*] too hastily given before the Obstructions are removed, they are frequently thereby rendered irremovable, and are changed into chronical Diseases, which are at the best extremely difficult to be cured, or too often become fatal.

Some were seized with Ophthalmies, and several with Tumors about the Jaws, Neck and Head; others seized with a moderate Fever at the first, attended with a dull heavy Pain in the Head; the Pulse was quick, but low and oppressed, tho' no great degree of Heat attended it, yet in a little time they became delirious, and insensible of their Condition; their Strength soon sunk, uncommonly, and a Stupor came on which gradually increased, and took them off in four or five Day's time; as if all the vital Springs were stopped at once by the Afflux† of the Humours upon the Brain.[4] Neither did Bleeding, or other Evacuations downwards,† seem to make that Revulsion,† or give that Relief, which they usually do in similar Cases; nor was the use of Volatiles, *&c.*, or Vesicatories of that Service as they generally are in such Cases.

The Rain still continuing, the before mentioned inflammatory Diseases totally disappeared; but the Dysenteries still continued to be very frequent and epidemical, seizing many of the Negroes and several of the white People also: In some it came on gradually, with little or no Fever at the first, nor any violent Symptoms, but the stools became more and more frequent, and the Fever gradually increased, though some had not much external Heat, yet inwardly they were feverish and hot: In others the Fever came on sooner, and with more acute Symptoms, and the Griping and Pains were great, the Pulse very quick, and in some full: They generally had a Sickness and a Load,† or Loathing† at their Stomachs, Pain in their Heads, and often all over the Body; not much Griping at the Beginning, but it gradually increased, and became severe and painful; especially before going to stool; great Quantities of Blood were generally discharged that Way, and a bloody Mucus after it: And as the

---

4. *Query 4.* Were not those Humours which produced those Tumors and Swellings in the others, turned or cast upon the Brain or its Meninges, in these, and produced these Effects? As the Humours seemed to have an unusual Tendency and Afflux towards the Head at this Time.

Disease advanced, most of the Symptoms increased, and sometimes a Singultus,† with a Coldness of the extreme Parts came on, which are always in this Disease very bad, and sometimes fatal Symptoms, and if not timely relieved too often prove mortal. Also as the Disease increases, a terrible Tenesmus† comes on, and increases so as to be very painful, and often will continue several Days, even after the Frequency of the Stools is abated.

This Distemper† may be truly said to be Endemial in the hot Climate, and this Island, as we have it more or less every Year, when the rainy Seasons come on: As the heavy Rains which usually fall at those Times, and the Coolness and Moistness in the Air which they produce, too suddenly check and stop the Discharge by Perspiration and Sweat, which in this warm Climate are usually very great, the Humours are thereby too suddenly turned upon the Bowels; to which may be added as a concomitant Cause, their too freely eating the Herbs, Roots, and Fruits of the Earth, which are too hastily and luxuriantly produced in this warm Climate, upon the falling of such Rain, and are then crude and waterish, which the Negro Slaves too voraciously devour; and who are at the same time too much exposed to the Inclemencies of the Weather, and hard Labour in the Fields, and some of them ill-cloathed; all which jointly contribute to produce this Disease: And I have observed that the Negro Slaves are generally the first seized with such Diseases as are epidemical or endemial in this Island.

As this Disease is always attended with a Fever in a higher or lower Degree, and is caused by too sudden a Stoppage or Diminution of Perspiration or Sweat, which are turned upon the Intestines, with sometimes the Addition of infectious Effluvia† from others labouring under it, where the Humours become more acrid and irritating by the Heat of the Body; they produce *Inflammation* of the *Tunica Villosa Intestinorum*,† in a greater or less Degree, which being increased by the Continuance of the Disease, extends itself to the other Coats of the Intestines, and too often ends in a Mortification of them, if not timely relieved; as is but too evident from the Symptoms which attend them to the last, who die of this Disease, as well as from the Inspection of their dead Bodies. From whence it is evident that unless a Revulsion be made, and the Inflammation taken off, all the boasted Specifics,† or famed Restringents, how much so ever extolled, are in vain, and too often do but hasten the Death of the Patient. But Bleeding accordingly, as the Strength of the Patient, the Quickness, Fullness, and Hardness of his Pulse, and the Height of the Fever, and the other Symptoms indicate, and that repeated as the Strength of the Patient and the above Symptoms require, at proper Intervals; and after giving a Dose of *Ipecacuanha*† to cleanse the Stomach, and probably to revulse the Humours from the Bowels, and a dose of torrified† Rhubarb with an Anodyne; giving *Antiphlogisticks* with gentle Subastringents, and moderate Anodynes at proper Distances, and diluting moderately with subastringent cooling Liquids, given warm to encourage a free Perspiration, I have always found to be the most successful Method. In some Cases, where the Stools continue to be bad, and a free Diaphoresis is not obtained, a Dose or two of *Stibium Ceratum*† after sufficient Bleeding, *&c.*, may be given, but I have often found that giving a few small doses of *Ipecacuanha,* and an Anodyne after them, is much preferable, and has often succeeded when that much celebrated Medicine would not. *See the Treatise on* Dysentery.

The MONTH of NOVEMBER continued to be very wet, and much Rain fell, and it was also much cooler than usual in other Years. The Quantity of Rain which fell in this Month was [equal] to 12.96 cubic Inches deep. The lowest the Thermometer ever was in any Morning this Month, was at 74°F; and the highest it ever was in the Morning, was at 80°F. The lowest it ever was at Noon was 78°F; and the highest at Noon was at 83°F. The lowest the Barometer ever was this month was at 29.7 [inches of mercury]; the highest at 29.9 [inches of mercury].

We still continued to have some Dysenteries, though much fewer than we had in the preceding Months: And a few were seized with a continued slow Fever of the *Synochus*† kind; it first came on with a moderate Rigor,† which was succeeded by a great Heat, a very quick Pulse, Pain all over the Body, but most severe in the Head, and in some few was attended with a Catarrh and a Cough, then came on large profuse Sweats, which did not relieve, but brought on a Languor† and sunk them much; their Blood was florid† and a little lax, but not dissolved. Bleeding these moderately once, or those who had more elastic strong Fibres and a more full hard Pulse, twice, and giving Antiphlogisticks in cooling Pectorals, kept the Fever moderate, and generally brought it to a Crisis on the [twenty-first] Day, when it was usually carried off by a large warm, critical Sweat, and in some few by three or four loose Stools, or in some by both. But this Fever soon disappeared; and in general this Month was more healthful than the preceding Months.

DECEMBER was much more dry than the preceding Months were, though we had a few small showers of Rain, more than usual in this Month in other Years, but in general the Days were Dry. The Quantity of Rain which fell in this Month was but [equal] to 2.25 cubic Inches deep. The lowest the Thermometer ever was in the Morning in this Month was at 74°F; and the highest it ever was in the Morning was at 78°F. The lowest it ever was at Noon was 80°F; and the highest was at 82°F. The lowest the Barometer was at 29.7 [inches of mercury]; and the highest was at 29.9 [inches of mercury].

Upon the coming of this dry Weather, the Dysenteries which were frequent and epidemical all over the Island in the three last Months, now totally ceased and disappeared; and the inflammatory Diseases also, were very few: But towards the latter End of the Month, we had some few inflammatory Quinsies; and many were seized with Catarrhs† and Coryzas,† so that few escaped them; they all had a Cough, Hoarseness, and a great Defluction† of Rheum† on the Nose, Bronchia and Lungs, coughed much, and expectorated a great Quantity of tough viscid Phlegm, and some had a Fever with it; and young Children were in great danger of being suffocated with it.

Bleeding those who were Plethoric and Feverish, and pectoral attenuating Medicines, which promoted a free Expectoration, and diluting with pectoral Liquids warm, soon relieved them: But to those Children who were in danger of being suffocated, it was necessary to give a little *Oxymel Scilliticum*† once or twice a Day, and a little *Syr. Scillitic.*† often in a pectoral Tea, which brought up the tough Phlegm, and gave them immediate Relief; I saw none that died of it, tho' I was told that some died of it; and we had but few other Diseases this month.

This Year from January 1st, 1752, to January 1753, was a more than common wet Year; and the whole Quantity of Rain which fell in this Year was equal to 67.35 cubical Inches deep; which is a very great Quantity of Rain.

A.D. *1753*

THE MONTH of JANUARY was very dry, but moderately cool; the Quantity of Rain which fell in it, was only equal to 0.37 parts of a cubic Inch deep.

The lowest that the Thermometer ever was in the Morning, was at 73°F; and the highest it ever was in the Morning this Month, was at 77°F. The lowest it was at Noon was 78°F; and the highest was at 80°F. The lowest the Barometer was at 29.75 [inches of mercury]; and the highest 29.8 [inches of mercury].

The catarrhal Fever mentioned in the last Month, continued and increased, both in its being more frequent and more inflammatory in this [month], and spread all over the Island; so that few either white or black People escaped having it, either in a greater or less Degree, and as the Time advanced, it became more inflammatory. In some the Inflammation fell upon the Glands of the Throat, and produced an *Angina Inflammatoria*,† attended with a strong Fever, a quick, full, strong, hard Pulse, great Pain in the Head, and Throat, great Thirst, and great Heat and Inflammation in those Parts: Their Blood generally was highly inflamed, and when it stood till cold, was covered with a sizzy Starch or Buff-like Pellicle, and the Serum of a yellowish Colour, all which indicated plentiful Bleeding. And accordingly I found that Bleeding plentifully at the Beginning of the Disease, some cooling Catharticks,† and a liberal Use of Antiphlogisticks internally, and Fomentations of the same Nature externally, with emollient repelling Cataplasms,† with Vinegar and *Crude Sal. Ammoniac*, and sometimes letting them receive the Fumes of Vinegar through a Funnel into their Mouths and Throats, and Gargarisms† of the same Nature, the Fever and all its Symptoms were generally carried off, and they recovered in a few Days. But when Bleeding freely, and the liberal Use of Antiphlogisticks were neglected at the Beginning, they generally suppurated (but not without Danger of suffocating the Patient) in six or seven Day's time, and when they broke, most commonly left a hard Tumour in the external Integuments† of the Throat, which continued a considerable Time (though they generally could breath and swallow pretty well) and were difficult to be discussed† and removed afterwards. In some the Inflammation fell first upon the Throat, where it continued a Day or two, and then was translated† from thence and fell upon the Lungs and produced a violent Peripneumony, and in some it fell upon the Lungs at the first; in both it was attended with a quick, hard, and sometimes a pretty strong Pulse, great Difficulty of Breathing, a Cough, with which they expectorated a tough viscid Phlegm with much Difficulty, their Thirst great, and the Fever high. In some others this Inflammation fell upon the Pleura, and produced a Pleurisy with all the Symptoms of that Disease.

It was remarkable that the Inflammations ran much higher in all these Diseases, and their Blood was generally more inflamed and sizzy in this Year, than ever I observed it to be in this warm Climate before, where the animal Solids are generally more relaxed; and the Sick in general required more large and oftener repeated Bleedings, before the Fever and Inflammation could be taken off, and the Disease conquered, than ever I observed in this warm Climate before.[5]

I must also here observe, that I found the *Crude Sal. Ammoniac* to be a much more powerful *Attenuant,*[†] and a greater *Refrigerant*[†] or *Antiphlogistic* when mixed with *Nitre*, than any that we have; and I found that it was more effectual in dissolving this inflammatory sizzy Lentor[†] of the Blood, than any other Medicine that we have in the whole *Materia Medica*;[†] and though I had given it as a cooling Attenuant for many Years, yet I never had such remarkable Opportunities of observing its extraordinary Effects in these inflammatory Cases, as I had this year. It cools greatly, and I think is more attenuating than the *Spir. C.C.*[†] *vel*[†] *Spir. Salis Ammon. Vol.*[†] or their *Volatile Salts*, which stimulate and heat much at the same Time. I usually give it when it is indicated to be given, from gr.v. to gr.xv.[†] mixed with *Sal. Nitre*, from ʒi to ʒji *vel* ʒi[†] *in Decoct. Pectoral*[†] with *Spr. Nitri. Dul.*[†] *et Sprir. Mindereri*[†] and *Syr. e Meconio*[†] to lessen the Stimulus and Irritation of the Heat and Fever.

This Method I found to be the most successful in the Pleurisy, when assisted with antiphlogistic Fomentations to relax the pained Parts; and with the Addition of *Syr. Scillitic. vel Oxymel Scillit.* to assist Expectoration in the Peripneumonic Fever.[†] And the same antiphlogistic Method was no less successful, with the Addition of cooling Catharticks and Clysters,[†] with the before mentioned Medicines and Cataplasms in the Quincey.

Some few had an inflammatory Fever, attended with a full, quick, hard Pulse, and Pain all over them, without fixing in any one Part or Place. These were generally relieved by large, plentiful Bleeding, and the abovementioned antiphlogistick Medicines. As to the Quantity of Blood to be taken away, either in these, or in any other Cases, it cannot be said how much is necessary, because a Person formed with delicate, weak, or relaxed Fibres, cannot often bear the Loss of nine or ten Ounces[†] of Blood, so well as a plethoric Person with strong elastic Solids, can bear the Loss of sixty or eighty Ounces[†] of Blood.

---

5. *Query 5.* Did not this arise from the continued moist, wet Season, in the latter Part of the last Year, which had much relaxed the Solids, and diminished the Perspiration in this warm Climate; and the sudden Change from that, to the great Dryness and Coolness of the two last Months, which braced up the Solids again and rendered them more rigid and elastic than they were before, without sufficiently restoring a free Perspiration?

The MONTH of FEBRUARY also continued to be very dry, though we had sometimes some small showers of Rain, though of little Importance; for the whole Quantity of Rain which fell in this Month, was but equal to 1.03 Inches deep.

The lowest the Thermometer ever was in the Morning in this Month, was at 74°F; and the highest it ever was in the Morning this Month, was at 76°F; the lowest it was at Noon was 78°F; and the highest at Noon was at 80°F. The lowest that the Barometer was, was at 29.8 [inches of mercury]; and the highest at 29.9 [inches of mercury].

Few Catarrhs appeared after the Middle of the last Month, and now they totally ceased: But the Numbers in the above inflammatory Diseases increased during this Month, and required very large Evacuations by Bleeding, &c., before the Inflammation and Fever could be taken off; which reduced some Patients pretty low. To these as well as to those who were naturally weak, I found it necessary to give some Cardiacs;† but I soon found that the usual Cordial Waters,† and Cardiac Medicines of the Shops, heated and inflamed the Blood too much, and increased the Fever in this warm Climate; wherefore I used the rich sweet Wines made from mature Grapes, [such] as Canary and Frontigniac,† and found them to be much better Cordials in this Case, than the hot fiery Spirits of the Shops are, and that they heated and inflamed much less; to which I sometimes added *Sp. C.C.* or *Spir. Mindereri*, thus,

℞ *Decoct. Pectoral.* lb. i *Vini. Canar. (vel Frontig.)* ʒv. *Elix. Paragoric* ʒss. *Spir. Mindereri* ʒij. *Syr. Scillitic.* ʒiss. *Micse. Capiat æger Sal. Nitri* ʒss. *cum Sal. Ammon. Crud. Pur. gr.* x. *commixt. in Cochl. tria vel quatuor hujus Decoct. tertia quaq; hora.*†

This revived them and encouraged the Expectoration, abated the Fever and Inflammation, and answered the desired success.

And to some I ordered Vesicatories to be applied, which were of Service now at the latter end of the Disease, tho' they would have been hurtful and prejudicial towards the Beginning of it, by increasing the Fever.

About the Middle of February a *slow continued nervous Fever*† seized some few Patients; it usually came on with a slight Chilliness, or a gentle Rigor, and uncertain flushing Heats, a Loss of Appetite, Nausea, and sometimes a Reaching† to vomit, a Lassitude and Listlessness, with Dejection and Anxiety, a Giddiness with Pain in the Head and Back; an Exacerbation of all these Symptoms,† with a low quick Pulse generally towards the Evening: This usually continued for five or six Days without the Patient's being quite cast down, or his being willing to be confined to his Bed, or Chamber, in this warm Climate, in hopes of getting the better of it; but the Rigor returning, and the Fever and its Symptoms increasing, at last obliged them to it. The Pain in the Head and Giddiness increased, with a Torpor† or Sense of Weight and Coldness in the Occiput,† and along the Coronary Suture,† accompanied with a great Lassitude and Watching,† or if they did sleep, they were neither refreshed by it, nor sensible that they did sleep; their Urine was pale and always without a Sediment, as usual in most Fevers in this Climate; the Pulse was usually low but quick, and often unequal or irregular; the Giddiness and Pain in the Head increased much, and they were often delirious for a few Hours and then sensible again, and it returned again in the same Manner; and sometimes a Tinnitus Aurium† came on, after which a Deafness and a Delirium followed; the Tongue was sometimes dry, tho' often moist, but white and a little brown in the Middle, but rarely any Complaint of Thirst; a great Faintness, and sometimes a Deliquium Animi† came on, especially if they sat up too long, though in the Bed; cold partial Sweats came on, especially on the Face, Neck, and the Backs of the Hands, and sometimes about the Præcordia:† Some had a few loose Stools, but they were so far from having Relief from them, that the Dejection and Weakness was increased by them: The Deleriums were not great but often returned, and sometimes were rather a Confusion of Action and Incoherency of Words, with a dosing† and muttering to themselves; and they sometimes deposited their Urine and Excrements† without being sensible of it. When the Delirium increased, the Extremities generally grew cold, and their Nails livid, and the Pulse became very quick, small, weak, and irregular, and then they swallowed their Food with a difficult Gulping, and these were soon followed with great Tremors, Twitchings and Catchings,† a Subsultus Tendinum,† and the Delirium either soon turned to a profound Coma, or Convulsions came on, which soon snapped the Thread of Life.

But on the contrary, if the Sweats were brought to be equal over all the Body, and warm, and copious, or if a plentiful Spitting came on, and the Pulse became fuller, softer and freer, and vibrated with more Liberty, and all the Symptoms changed for the better, the Fever generally ended by a large, copious, warm Sweat on the nineteenth Day.

A Vomit† given at the Beginning of this Fever, when the Sickness, Nausea or Vomiting indicated it, was of singular Service; after which, saline attenuating Medicines, with the Volatiles and gentle Cardiacs were the most efficacious and successful, with Variations *pro re nata*; Vesicatories were also of great Service to some: But Bleeding was in general very prejudicial, unless where the Patient was of a plethoric, robust Constitution, and then only in the Beginning of the Disease, where some inflammatory Symptoms indicated it, which sometimes, though very rarely, happened, and then the Blood was to be taken in a very moderate Quantity, but not without great Caution and Judgment.

I have found that the following Method was both the most rational and the most successful also, *viz.* giving the *Spir. Mindereri* plentifully, and *Spir. C.C. vol.* and sometimes a little *Tinct. Cantharid.*† in warm Wine-whey, made a little stronger than usual in other Fevers; and sometimes the volatile Salts, and Camphor, Saffron, &c., or a Draught of this Nature, which I used the most frequently;

℞ *Sal. C.C. vol.* ℈ss. *Succi. Limon* ℨiij. *Aq. Menthæ Simp.* ℥iss. *Spir. Mindereri* ℨij. *Vini. Crocei* ℨj. *Syr. Crocei* ℨij. *Micse, fiat Haust. Tertia vel quarta, quintave quaq; Hora fumendus.*†

To this Draught I sometimes, in particular Cases, added *Tinct. Cantharid. gut.* xx.† and I found these of the greatest Service, especially if the Patient diluted plentifully with warm Wine-whey, made a little stronger than usual.

Some few had the putrid bilious, or yellow Fever in this Month, though the Season was so cool; and the now reigning epidemical, inflammatory Fevers were attended with such a great inflammatory Lentor, or Viscidity of their Blood; but it is probable that this Fever may arise from Exercise and Intemperance of those who had it now, as they were not many.

The MONTH of MARCH was in general moderately dry, though we had at times some considerable Showers of Rain, so that it was not so dry as the preceding Months were. The Quantity of Rain which fell in this Month was equal to 2.21 cubical Inches deep. The lowest the Thermometer ever was in the Morning in this Month, was at 72°F; and the highest it ever was in the Morning was at 78°F; and the lowest it was at Noon was 78°F; and the highest at Noon was 82°F. The lowest the Barometer was in this Month was at 29.8 [inches of mercury]; the highest at 29.9 [inches of mercury].

We had a few of the inflammatory Fevers, and but a few, for they were now greatly abated; and the slow nervous Fever seemed to cease for this, and the four or five Months following; neither had we many chronical Diseases, so that this Month was more than usually healthful.

APRIL was very dry and warm, and we had very little Rain, the whole

Quantity which fell in this Month, was only equal to 0.24 Tenths of a cubical Inch deep.

The lowest the Thermometer was in any Morning was at 76°F; and the highest it ever was in the Morning was at 78°F; and the lowest it ever was at Noon was 80°F; and the highest at 83°F. The lowest the Barometer was at, was 29.8 [inches of mercury]; the highest was 29.9 [inches of mercury].

This Month, though very dry and warm, was not very sickly; we had only some few inflammatory Diseases, [such] as a few Pleurisies and Peripneumonies, and some inflammatory Fevers; and also some Rheumatisms of the inflammatory Kind, though the last are not near so frequent here as they are in England; neither are they usually in other years attended with so great a degree of Inflammation as they were in this Year, or as they usually are in England: But this Year they appeared with the same Symptoms as they usually do in England, and their Blood was most commonly as much inflamed, and covered with a buff-like Pellicle as it is there, and required the Same Method of Treatment, *viz.* Bleeding, cooling Cathartics, and an Anodyne after them (as Dr *Sydenham*† advises) and Antiphlogistics in the intermediate Days; and I found the Crude *Sal. Ammoniac* and *Nitre* were of great Service; and by this Method they generally soon recovered.

The MONTH of MAY was also very dry and warm, though we had some Rain towards the latter end of it. The whole Quantity which fell in this Month was only [equal to] 1.31 cubic Inch deep. The lowest the Thermometer ever was in the Morning, was at 77°F; and the highest it was at in the Morning, was at 81°F; the lowest it was at Noon, was 80°F; and the highest at 86°F. The lowest the Barometer was 29.85 [inches of mercury]; the highest was at 29.95 [inches of mercury].

The Diseases we had this Month were of the inflammatory Kind, as in the last; a few Pleurisies and Peripneumonies, and some had Tumors about the Fauces,† Neck, or in other glandulous Parts, which suppurated slowly and with difficulty, and some of them left hard Tumors in those Parts for a considerable time after; as observed before: And the Humours seemed now again to have a greater Tendency towards the Head and Breast, as they had then; and we had some few Apoplexies and Palsies.

JUNE was very warm and mostly dry, tho' we had some considerable great Showers of Rain in some Days, but the intermediate Days were very warm and dry. The Quantity of Rain which fell in this Month, was equal to 2.44 cubical Inches deep. The lowest the Thermometer was any Morning was at

77°F; and the highest it ever was in the Morning was at 80°F; the lowest at Noon was at 82°F; and the highest at 86°F. The lowest the Barometer was at 29.85 [inches of mercury]; the highest was at 29.9 [inches of mercury].

Though this Month was very warm, yet it was in general pretty healthful, for we had few sick, except a few who had some of the above-mentioned inflammatory Fevers; and these were much less violent, and more easily relieved by moderate Bleeding and the above-mentioned antiphlogistic Method, than in the preceding Months.

But towards the latter End of the Month, some few had *Diarrhœa Febrilis*,† and a few had a Dysentery, but neither of them were very bad, nor were they difficult to cure. Some had the dry Belly-ach,† which now was attended with some degree of Inflammation, and some inflammatory Symptoms, which are not usual in that Disease, nor did I ever meet with it before or since: This rendered its Cure a little more difficult, and less expeditious than the Cure of that Disease now usually is; for some in this required Bleeding and the use of Antiphlogistics, to be given with those Medicines which are known to relieve, and take off that painful Disease at other times, and their Blood was more or less sizzy in this, though I rarely or never found it so in the true *Cholica Pictonum*† before now.

Several, both Strangers and Natives, were seized with the *putrid bilious Fever*,† in which I found the Method of treating it (hereafter mentioned) very successful. See: Part II.

Some were seized with a Rigor which did not continue long, but was succeeded by a brisk hot Fever which usually continued three or four Days, when a Tumor began to rise usually either in the Parotid, Submaxillary, or Inguinal Glands, or in some other Parts of the Body; upon the Appearance of which the Fever began to abate, and gradually went off as the Suppuration of the Gland advanced, without any malignant or other bad Symptoms, and they soon recovered.

In JULY we had a good deal of Rain, often with Thunder and Lightning, though the intermediate Days were hot and dry. The Quantity of Rain which fell was equal to 6.67 cubic Inches deep. The lowest the Thermometer was in the Morning was 78°F; and the highest 80°F; the lowest it was at Noon was at 80°F; the highest was at 86°F. The lowest the Barometer was at 29.9 [inches of mercury]; the highest was at 29.9½ [inches of mercury].

After the falling of this Rain, the Number of the Sick was considerably increased; Pleurisies, Peripneumonies, and inflammatory Fevers were more frequent, especially the last. Dysenteries also now became frequent, as usual after the falling of the Rain. And the slow continued fever now returned again, with much the same Symptoms as it had in February, and was cured by the same Method and Medicines as then, only Blistering more freely or frequently, as the Sick were generally more sunk and their Pulse usually lower, was necessary, and was of very great Service: But as the Fever then usually went off by a manifest Crisis, by Sweating or Stools on the nineteenth Day, it now gradually declined after the twentieth Day, and went off without any manifest Crisis.

Several were seized with Apoplexies and Palsies this Month, more than I have ever seen here in any one Year before.

The Pertussis or hooping Cough also seized many Children in this Town and Island. This is a Disease, which from all the Observations that I have been able to make, seems to be equally infectious to Children, as either Small-pox or Measles are; tho' I think it has not been mentioned as such, by any one yet that I have seen: For whenever it comes into a Family or Town, I have observed that it generally infects and seizes all the Children in the Town who have not had it before, as the Small-pox and Measles usually do: Neither have I ever observed, or heard from others, that they have known any Person to have it twice; therefore does it not arise from some infectious Miasmata[†] as they do? and is so far analogous to them; as also in this that it chiefly affects Children, rarely Adults as they do; though I have known several ancient People both here and in England to have it, but they all said that they never had it before. And as this Disease has not been known to be in this Island for many Years past, neither could I find by the strictest Enquiry that I could make, that any Child or elder Person did bring it hither; now, must we not conclude that it is a Disease which proceeds from some peculiar Disposition in the Air to generate its Infection or Miasma, or that they can be carried in the Air from some other Place to this great Distance, which being taken with the Saliva or otherwise into the circulating Fluids, as other infectious Diseases are; it there generates a peculiar Viscidity in the serous, lymphatic, or yet finer Fluids, and particularly those of the Bronchia and Lungs, which at the same time do greatly irritate those sensible nervous Parts, so as to cause that convulsive Cough, and convulsive Spasms which usually attend it, which again are increased by the Viscidity of the finer Fluids.

This being the Cause, and these the Effects of it, the Intentions of Cure must be to lessen the Quantity and attenuate the Viscidity of the Fluids, and abate the Stimulus. Wherefore bleeding such Children as are of a sanguine plethoric Constitution, and keeping the Body moderately open,[†] are necessary, and to attenuate the viscid Fluids as much as we can; for which Purpose I have found something of the following Nature, with Variations *pro re nata*, the most effectual.

℞ *Milleped. viv. bene lot. ℥ss. contund. in Mort. vitreo. et superaffund. Infusionis Rad. Glycyrrhiz ℥viii. Probe conterent. deinde cola, Colaturæ adde Aq. Sem. Fœniculi ℥ij. Aq. Nuc. Moscat Spir. Nitri Dul. ana ℥ss. Tinct, Cantharid ʒij Syr. e Mecon. ℥ss. vel ℥i. Misce, exhibe Colch. unum subinde urgente Tusse. Auget. dos. pro ratione ætatis ægei.*[†]

And if the Symptoms increase and the Patient's Pulse will permit, more Blood may be taken away; but if the Pulse be small and low, a Vesicatory may be applied and kept open, or the Quantity of the Tinct. Cantharid. increased, if the Symptoms of a Stranguary[†] do not forbid it: And if Convulsion-Fits come on, I usually give *Musk*[†] with a little *Syr. e Mecon.* or *Elix. Paragoric*;[†] but the first seldom fails to render the Disease more moderate, and in time takes it off.

The MONTH of AUGUST was more dry and warm than the last Month, though we had some wet Days towards the latter End of it. The Quantity of Rain which fell in this Month was equal to 3.47 cubic Inches deep. The lowest the Thermometer was in the Morning was 79°F; and the highest was at 83°F; the lowest it was at Noon was at 83°F; and the highest was at 86°F. The lowest the Barometer was at 29.9 [inches of mercury]; the highest at 29.9 [inches of mercury].

The inflammatory Diseases which reigned in the preceding Months continued, and rather increased in this; especially Pleurisies, Peripneumonies, Pleuro-peripneumonies, and the inflammatory Fevers, and Dysenteries became more frequent; and their Blood in all these was generally full as sizzy, or rather more so, than in the last Year. The hooping Cough also continued to affect Children, and we had a few Apoplexies and Palsies: And some had the slow continued Fever, as in the last Months; in which I found the *Acetum Camphoratum,*[†] *Spiritus Mindereri, vel Haustus è Volatilibus Fullerii,*[†] or the learned Dr *Huxham's*[†] Draught of *Sal. C. C. et Succus Limon.*[†] as before, and *Vesicatories*, were the most efficacious Medicines, and were of the greatest Service.

A Cholera Morbus also seized several, especially Children; in which I found that giving *Rad. Ipocacuanh. gr.* i. *vel gr.* ij. *vel Vini Ipocacuanh. gut.* xx. *vel* xxx.[†] in a little Green Tea, or Chicken Water, to encourage the Vomiting;

and *Tinct. Thebaic. a gut.* v. *ad* x.† and more to Adults, after it; and a small Dose of *Rad. Rhei*† with an Anodyne a few Hours after that; and then a saline Julep with an Anodyne generally took it quite off: But if the Vomiting still continued, a *Fotus ex. Fol. Menthæ, Theriac. Androm. cum paul. Vini Rubri*† applied to the Region of the Stomach, with the use of the saline Julep,† constantly took it off, and they soon recovered.

We had much Rain in SEPTEMBER, though we had some intermediate Days which were dry and very warm, as this is usually the hottest Month in the Year. The Quantity of Rain which fell in this Month was equal to 8.77 cubic Inches deep. The lowest the Thermometer was in the Morning was at 77°F; and the highest was at 82°F; the lowest it was at Noon was at 80°F; and the highest was at 86°F. The lowest the Barometer, was at 29.8 [inches of mercury]; and the highest was at 29.9 [inches of mercury].

The epidemical Diseases of this Month were the same as in the last Months; and notwithstanding that we had so much Rain in this Month, yet the Dysentery was not altogether so frequent as it was in the last Month: But the Peripneumonies, and Pleuro-peripneumonies, were usually attended with more Pain in the Head, the Fever higher, and the Pulse usually more tense and hard, and their Blood was much inflamed and covered with a thick Starch or Buff-like Pellicle.

The slow continued Fever was also more frequent, but their Blood never was inflamed, nor ever had the least Appearance of a Sizziness in it.

OCTOBER also continued to be wet, more than usual in that Month, though we had several interposed Days that were dry and very warm. The Quantity of Rain which fell in this Month was equal to 8.17 cubic Inches deep. The lowest the Thermometer was at in the Mornings was 76°F, and the highest was at 80°F; the lowest it was at Noon was at 80°F; and the highest at Noon was at 86°F. The lowest the Barometer ever was, was at 29.6 [inches of mercury]; and the highest this Month was at 29.8 [inches of mercury]. I never saw the Barometer thus low as it was on the 1st day of this Month, at 29.6 [inches of mercury], and on that Day we had a Storm, or very high Wind, and great Showers of Rain.

The inflammatory Diseases, which reigned in the preceding Months, were much less frequent in this; but the Dysentery was both more frequent and more violent in its Symptoms, and more difficult to be cured. The Hooping-cough was also more frequent among Children; and a few were seized with the slow continued Fever, as in the last Month.

Likewise some had the putrid, bilious, or yellow Fever, but it was either more mild and in its Symptoms less violent than it usually is, or it was rendered so by the Method of treating it; which see, Part II. For tho' its Symptoms at the first were as usual, yet they soon became more moderate by being thus treated; and all I did see, recovered.

NOVEMBER was very dry, and warmer than usual in other Years. The Quantity of Rain which fell this Month was only equal to 1.33 cubic Inch deep.[†] The lowest the Thermometer was in the Mornings, was at 75°F; and the highest was at 78°F; the lowest it was at Noon was 80°F; and the highest at Noon was 86°F. The lowest the Barometer was, at 29.8 [inches of mercury]; and the highest 29.8 [inches of mercury]. It did not alter in this Month but was always the same.

The Dysentery which was very frequent in the last two Months, upon the Season being more warm and dry, became much less so, and towards the latter end of the Month it totally ceased: But the inflammatory Diseases, especially Pleurisies, Peripneumonies, Opthalmies, and some Quinseys, still continued, and now were attended with more Pain in the Head than usual; for the Humours now again had a greater Disposition or Tendency towards the Head, than usual at other Times. The Hooping-cough also still continued among the Children; and some few had the putrid, bilious, or yellow Fever.

DECEMBER also continued to be very dry, and considerably warmer than usual in this Month; though we had a few small Showers in some Days. The Quantity of Rain which fell this Month was equal to 2.11 cubic Inches deep. The lowest that the Thermometer was in the Mornings was at 73°F; the highest at 78°F; the lowest it was at Noon was at 80°F; and the highest at Noon was 82°F. The lowest the Barometer was at 29.8 [inches of mercury]; and the highest was at 29.8½ [inches of mercury].

The Hooping-cough, and the above-mentioned inflammatory Diseases, almost totally ceased and disappeared in this Month also.

Some few were seized with Pain in their Heads, and swellings about the Fauces, and the Humours still continued to have a more than usual Tendency towards the Head and the superior Parts of the Breast, in this as well as in the last Months; but in general both this and the last Month were more than usually healthful: For the only Disease which could properly be called Epidemical, was an Inflammation of the Mediastinum,[†] which most commonly seized the superior Part of it above the Pericardium,[†] and only seized the Negroes, and few if any white People: It first came on with a cold

Rigor and Tremor, which continued one, and sometimes two Hours, and was then succeeded by a hot Fever, with great Heat and acute Pain in the upper Part of the Breast, with darting Pains from the superior Part of the Sternum, through the upper Part of the Mediastinum to the Spine; great Pain in the Head, with a quick, hard, full Pulse, a laborious, difficult, quick Breathing: Some had a Cough and a great Anxiety at their Breast, others had not; those who had, generally had a very quick, small, hard, Pulse, which usually after Bleeding became more full, a dry Tongue and great Thirst, and as the Disease advanced they generally grew delirious. The Heat about the Præcordium and upper Part of the Chest, as also in the Head, was very great; they expectorated little; their Urine was high coloured without a Sediment; their Blood was florid and red on the first Day, but sizzy on the second and after. Bleeding plentifully at the first Beginning of the Disease, and repeating it if the Symptoms indicated it, and a liberal Use of the antiphlogistick Medicines, with a cooling diluting Regimen, and the use of cooling emollient antiphlogistick Fomentations to the Breast, most commonly relieved them, and carried it off in four or five Day's time. But if Bleeding copiously at the first, and the above antiphlogistic Method was not timely used, they usually became delirious on the third Day, and their Pulse became exceeding quick, small and irregular, and their extreme Parts cold, and they died.

In some it did not fall upon the Breast, but upon the Head and Brain, and first one Eye swelled as if from a Stroke or Contusion,[†] and then the other Eye in the same manner, the Fever great, and they soon became delirious, which increased and was a certain Sign that the Brain or its Meninges[†] were inflamed as well as the Eyes; soon after this the Pulse became quick, small and irregular, and their extreme Parts cold; and most of these who were seized thus died.

The whole Quantity of Rain which fell in this Year 1753 was equal to 38.12 cubical Inches deep.

A.D. *1754*

THE MONTH of JANUARY was cool and pleasant, but very dry till the 21st Day, on which and the three following Days we had much Rain, and then it was dry to the End of the Month. The Quantity of Rain which fell in this Month was equal to 5.36 cubic Inches deep. The lowest the Thermometer was any morning was 72°F; and the highest was 76°F; the lowest it was at

Noon was at 76°F; and the highest at 80°F. The lowest the Barometer was at 29.7½ [inches of mercury]; and the highest at 29.9 [inches of mercury].

The slow, continued nervous Fever still continued in some Parts of the Island; and some Negroes had the inflammatory Fever described in the last Month; and we had a few Quinseys of the inflammatory Kind, but upon the falling of the Rain in the latter End of the Month, both these last soon after ceased and disappeared. But the Hooping-cough still continued in the remote Parts of the Island, and also Small-pox, but they generally were of a benign, distinct Kind.

FEBRUARY was very dry and moderately cool, and we had no Rain except on the 10th Day; the whole Quantity of Rain which fell in this Month was only equal to 0.89 Parts of a cubical Inch deep. The lowest the Thermometer was any Morning, was at 72°F; the highest was at 76°F; the lowest it was at Noon was at 78°F; and the highest was at 82°F. The lowest the Barometer, was at 29.7½ [inches of mercury]; and the highest was at 29.9 [inches of mercury].

The slow nervous Fever still continued in Some Parts of the Island, and the Hooping-cough also in some remote Parts of it; but the Small-pox now totally ceased. We had some few inflammatory Fevers, and but few, and they totally disappeared about the Middle of this Month, and it was pretty healthful.

MARCH was also dry till near the latter End of the Month, when we had a considerable Quantity of Rain; it was also moderately cool. The Quantity of Rain which fell was only equal to 3.53 cubic Inches deep. The lowest the Thermometer was in the Morning, was at 73°F; the highest was 77°F; the lowest it was at Noon was 78°F; and the highest at Noon was 82°F. The lowest the Barometer was at 29.8 [inches of mercury]; and the highest at 22.9 [*sic*] [inches of mercury].

I cannot say that we had any Diseases that were epidemical in this Month, but the slow nervous Fever,[†] which now was much more frequent than it was in any of the preceding Months: Its Symptoms were much the same as before described, except that the loose Stools, or slight Diarrhœa, which usually came on towards the Beginning of the Disease, were now less frequent; and the Delirium, Tremors, Startings,[†] Catchings, and the Subsultus Tendinium, were both greater and more frequent than they were before.[6] And the Fever now put on and appeared in this warm Climate, with all the same Symptoms as it usually does in England; and as they are accurately described by that learned and able Physician Dr *Huxham* in the cooler Climate of Plymouth,[†] which therefore I need not here repeat. I shall observe, that this Fever now came constantly and regularly to a Crisis on the nineteenth Day, unless it was injuriously wrongly treated; neither would a small matter divert it from coming to its Crisis on that Day: For I saw a worthy and ingenious Gentleman, who on the sixteenth Day of the Fever lost above two Quarts[†] of Blood in half an Hour's time, by the bursting of one of the internal Hæmorrhoid Veins, which sunk him as low and as near Death as possible; but the Hæmorrhage being instantly stopped by Stypticks,[†] and some cardiac and volatile Medicines[†] given immediately after, and suitable cordial Nourishment;[†] his Pulse, which was scarce perceptible for some considerable time after it, did so rise on that and the next Day, that on the eighteenth Day it was more full than ever before, tho' he was of a slender, thin, dry Constitution; and on the nineteenth Day his Fever came to a regular and compleat Crisis, and he perfectly recovered. I also saw another Patient who lost as much Blood, or more, in the same manner; but his Hæmorrhage caused the coming on of the Crisis to be deferred to the twenty-sixth Day, and yet he recovered; but the Crisis in all the others constantly came regularly on, on the nineteenth Day.

I found that giving an Emetic at the Beginning of the Disease, and a Dose of Rhubarb after it, or in some Cases only the latter; and then giving *Spir. Mindereri* ʒss in any fit simple Water with a little *Vini Crocei*[†] or *Acetum Camphoratum* to some Patients, or saline Draughts with Volatiles, or Dr *Huxham's* saline Draught to others, every three, four, or six Hours, as the Fever was higher or lower, or sunk too low, and diluting plentifully with warm Wine-whey, sometimes made pretty strong of the Wine, especially when they were weak and low, were of the greatest Service; as also were Vesicatories: So likewise were *Musk, Camphor,* and *Tinct. of Cantharides,* when the convulsive Spasms were great; as these attenuated the Viscidity of the Lymph and finer Fluids, without too much inflaming the Blood; whereas the *Rad. Serpentar.*

---

6. *Query 6.* Were not some of the infectious Miasmata, or of the morbid Matter, discharged and carried off by those loose Stools, which rendered the above Symptoms more moderate and milder after? And when Nature did not so carry the morbid Matter off, were not these Symptoms more violent? And did not Nature thus shew us the Way we ought to follow and assist her? At least I thought so; and found that such as I saw in time to give a Dose of Ipocacuanha and a little Rhubarb after, I generally found that the Symptoms were more moderate after.

Virg. Confect. Cardiac.† and such hot Medicines, heated and inflamed more, without attenuating the Fluids so much, as I observed; which confirms the Opinion of the learned Dr. *Huxham*, that the Cause and Seat of this Disease is chiefly in the Lymph and finer Fluids, in which it produces a Viscidity and Inaptitude to Motion.

This slow nervous Fever was certainly infectious, for I observed that many of those who visited, and most of them that attended the Sick in this Fever, were infected by it and got the Disease, and especially those who constantly attended them, and performed the necessary Offices for the Sick.

The MONTH of APRIL was also dry in general, though we had some Showers of Rain sometimes; but from the Middle of it to its latter End, it was more warm than usual in other Years. The Quantity of Rain which fell in this Month was equal to 4.22 cubic Inches deep. The lowest the Thermometer was in the Mornings, was 76°F; the highest 80°F; the lowest it was at Noon was at 80°F; and the highest at Noon was 85°F. The lowest the Barometer, was at 29.8 [inches of mercury]; and continued the same all the Month.

The slow nervous Fever still continued in some remote Parts of the Island, though they were but few that had it. We also had a few Pleuro-peripmeumonies, but the Inflammation that attended it was not very great, neither was it commonly very dangerous.

Some were seized with a violent Pain and Inflammation at the Scrobiculum Cordis,† which extended to the Stomach, attended with Sickness and Vomiting; a quick Pulse, though in some it was small and oppressed, though commonly hard, and accompanied with cold clammy Sweats, and some had a few loose Stools with it at the Beginning; it differed from a Cholera Morbus in most of its Symptoms, though it had some of them, and was really an Inflammation on those Parts, which Nature attempted to relieve by the Vomiting and Stools, but could not: The Pulse being low, though quick, and the Extremities cold, it deterred many from bleeding them; yet they could not be relieved, nor the Pain removed, without it: But upon Bleeding, the Pain abated, and the Pulse became more full, and softer, and the Coldness on the Extremities went off, so that it might be repeated where it was necessary; and by the use of Fomentations to the pained Parts, and giving Antiphlogisticks liberally, and some Volatiles, they were generally pretty soon restored to Health. This Disease came in with the hot Weather, and did not continue long.7 The Hooping-cough still continued in some remote Parts of the Island.

The Beginning of MAY was very warm and dry, but from the 8th Day to the End of the Month we had a great deal of Rain, more than the most ancient People could remember to have seen at this time of the Year. The Quantity of Rain which did fall was equal to 14.65 cubic Inches deep. The lowest the Thermometer was in the Mornings, was at 77°F; the highest at 80°F; the lowest it ever was at Noon, was at 78°F; the highest at Noon was at 86°F. The lowest the Barometer, was at 29.7½ [inches of mercury]; the highest was at 29.9 [inches of mercury].

So much Rain falling rendered the Air more cool and temperate, and the Season more healthful; and we had no Diseases which could be properly called Epidemical, except a few Pleurisies of the Nothus Kind,† and an uncommon kind of Jaundice which seized several Children.[8] The first was most commonly carried off by bleeding once or twice, a cooling Purge or two, and Antiphlogisticks with Volatiles after.

The Jaundice which seized Children, chiefly from three or seven to eight Years of Age, usually came on with an Indisposition to play, and an Indolence to Motion, a Loss of Appetite, with costive Stools, a small dull Pain at the Region of the Liver; some were a little feverish, but none had any Symptoms of an Inflammation of the Liver, or of the biliary Ducts; others had no feverish Heat, but they all had a considerable degree of Yellowness in their Skin and their Eyes.

This uncommon Jaundice was generally carried off by gentle opening Catharticks, and a few saponaceous Medicines, with a few gentle, easy Stomachics to restore the Appetite after.

After these Rains the nervous Fever ceased in the Town† and near it.

The MONTH of JUNE was uncommonly wet, and more Rain fell than any Person living here could remember to have ever seen at this Time of the Year; for we had several great Floods which did considerable damage to several

---

7. *Query 7.* As the nervous Fever was then Epidemical, were not some of its infectious Miasmata received by the Sick at the same time as they were seized with the Inflammation, and produced that small low Pulse, and cold clammy Sweats, which are Symptoms which do not usually attend an Inflammation, at least the Beginning of it? As this certainly was an Inflammation both from its Symptoms, and from some that I saw who had been treated with hot Medicines, and died of it with all the Marks of a Mortification on those Parts.

8. *Query 8.* As this Jaundice seized several Children in the same Town, and sometimes in the same House, at or near the same Time, and some time after ceased or disappeared; may we not conclude that it was Epidemical?

Houses. The Quantity of Rain which fell in this Month was equal to 19.78 cubic Inches deep. The lowest the Thermometer was in the Morning, was at 76°F; the highest at 80°F; the lowest it ever was at Noon, was at 78°F; and the highest at Noon was 85°F. The lowest the Barometer was, was at 29.8 [inches of mercury]; and the highest was at 29.9 [inches of mercury].

We had much Thunder and Lightning with these great Rains.

So much Rain falling rendered the Air cooler and moister than usual, and it was pretty healthful; for we had no Diseases which could be said to be Epidemical, except a few Pleurisies, some of them of the Nothus Kind, and some Pleuro-peripneumonies, and some few who had an Inflammation of the Stomach, and of the Intestines; but these were seldom inflamed in any great Degree, nor the Fever violent in any of them, therefore they were generally pretty soon relieved by Bleeding, and the Use of Antiphlogisticks internally and externally, and recovered pretty soon. The Hooping-cough still continued among Children in the North-west Part of the Island, and some Adults had it there also, who had not had it before.

In JULY we had frequent showers of Rain, though not near so much as we had in the last Month, nor so much Thunder and Lightning, though we had some about the Middle of the Month. The Quantity of Rain which fell in this Month, was equal to 7.52 cubical Inches deep. The lowest the Thermometer was in the Morning, was 76°F; the highest was at 80°F; the lowest it was at Noon was at 81°F; and the highest at Noon was 86°F. The lowest the Barometer, was at 29.8 [inches of mercury]; the highest was at 29.9 [inches of mercury].

This Month was also much cooler than usual in other Years, and also more healthful; though we had a few Pleurisies and Peripneumonies, and some Diarrhœas and Dysenteries: But these were but few, and were rarely attended with either so great a degree of Inflammation or Malignity, as they usually are in a more warm wet Season, coming upon a long hot dry Season. Several were seized with a hard dry Cough, they expectorated little, and that was clear, tough, viscid and unconcocted,[†] and was brought up with violent Coughing and Difficulty.[9] Neither emollient Pectorals, oily Mixtures, nor yet Opiates

---

9. *Query 9.* Did not this uncommon Cough arise from that unusual degree of Moistness and Coolness of the Air, at this time of the Year, introducing such a degree of Viscidity into the circulating Fluids, and falling upon the Bronchia and Lungs? Or was that Viscidity produced by the same Cause which produced it in the Hooping-cough, which was then Epidemical?

were of much Service: But Volatiles, as *Sal. C.C. vol. Flor. Benzoin,*[†] *&c.* mixed with a little *Theriac. Adrom.*[†] given two or three times a Day, soon relieved them, and repeating it two or three Days, took it quite off.

Some few had the slow nervous Fever in the remote Parts of the Island, and the Hooping-cough still continued among the Children in those Parts.

We had frequent Showers of Rain in AUGUST, and sometimes Thunder and Lightning with great Showers, intermixed with calm hot Days, so that it might be called a moist hot Season. The Quantity of Rain which fell in this Month, was only equal to 4.69 cubic Inches deep. The lowest the Thermometer was in the Morning, was 77°F; the highest was at 80°F; the lowest it was at Noon was at 81°F; and the highest at Noon was at 85°F. The lowest the Barometer, was at 29.8 [inches of mercury]; and the highest was at 29.9 [inches of mercury].

This moist warm Season continuing, Diarrhœas and Dysenteries were more frequent, especially among the Negroes; though some white People had it also, but it was more malignant than in most other Years.

We had also some few Pleurisies and Peripneumonies; and several were seized with an Inflammation of the Pelvis and Peritoneum about the lower Region of the Belly, which often extended to the Neck of the Bladder, attended with acute Pain in those Parts, and a Difficulty of making Water, and sometimes great Pain in going to Stool: Their Pulse was quick and hard, though generally small, and sometimes attended with a Coldness and cold Sweats on the extreme Parts,[10] which often deterred the Apothecaries from bleeding them: Though it was a true Inflammation on those Parts, and upon bleeding them the Pain abated, and the Pulse became more full, and the Heat was equally diffused all over the Body. By Bleeding, Fomentations to the pained Parts, cooling emollient Clysters,[†] and a free Use of Antiphlogisticks, they generally soon recovered. Here the Acuteness of the Pain was the principal indication for Bleeding, and its causing the Pulse to rise, the cold Sweats to go off, and its Success, confirmed its being an Inflammation of those Parts, and this Practice to be right.

---

10. *Query 10.* Did not this continued moist warm State of the Air, so relax the Solids as to bring on this small Pulse and cold Sweats, *&c.* in this Inflammation, as also in that of the Scrobiculum Cordis, or Stomach and Diaphragm before mentioned, with the same Symptoms? As they are Symptoms which usually do not attend an Inflammation at its Beginning, as in these, which were both Inflammations.

Some few Patients were seized with a continued remitting Fever, which here usually came to a Crisis on the fourteenth Day, but in some it did not come to its Crisis till the seventeenth or nineteenth Day, and then went off: But it never came to intermit regularly here in any, as it frequently used to do in England.

The slow nervous Fever still continued in the North-east Parts of the Island, with the same Symptoms, and came to its Crisis on the nineteenth Day, when in or near the Town in the Winter or cooler Months; but it has not appeared in, or near the Town, since the Month of May.

We had frequent Showers of Rain, and sometimes Thunder and Lightning, and much Rain in the MONTH of SEPTEMBER; tho' the intervening Days were generally very warm, and either calm, or we had small variable Winds, mostly from some of the Southern Points, which are usually hot. The Quantity of Rain which fell this Month, was equal to 6.10 cubic Inches deep. The lowest the Thermometer was in the Morning, was 77°F; the highest was 80°F; the lowest it was at Noon was 81°F; and the highest at Noon was 85°F. The lowest the Barometer, was at 29.7 [inches of mercury]; and the highest at 29.9 [inches of mercury].

The Weather continuing to be moist and warm, Dysenteries were more frequent, especially among the white People; and were now attended with a greater degree of Inflammation than they were in the last Months. But bleeding once or twice, an Emetic, and toasted Rhubarb with an Opiate after, and Antiphlogisticks with gentle Restringents and Opiates, to abate the Pain and refrain the Violence of the Flux, till the Inflammation was taken off, were generally successful. The Inflammation of the Pelvis and Peritoneum, also continued to seize several in this Month, as well as in the last; and I observed that the Humours had an unusual Tendency and Afflux towards the lower Parts of the Belly, in these two Months, as they had towards the Head and Breast, or the upper Parts of the Body, in the preceding hot and dry Months.[11]

---

11. *Query 11.* Does not the continued Dryness of the Season brace up the Solids, and dispose them to Inflammations; and the continued Heat of the Sun affect the Head and upper Parts of the Body, so as to cause a greater Afflux of the Humours to those Parts, in long continued dry, hot Seasons? And do not the continued moist, warm Seasons, relax the Solids, especially those of the Abdomen, which are naturally more moist, and so cause a greater Afflux of the Humours to them in such Seasons, to which a Diminution of Perspiration in such Seasons, may contribute?

Arthriticks also suffered much in this Month, by the Gout appearing with anomalous† Symptoms, and often attacking the Bowels, or falling upon the Pelvis and the Neck of the Bladder: But they were generally relieved by bathing their Feet in a Decoction of Piemento leaves,† or other warm stimulating Aromaticks,† and applying stimulating Fœnigmi† to the Soles of the Feet, or Vesicatories to the remote Parts which it used to attack when regular; and giving some Aromaticks with light Chalybeats† and Volatiles, by which Methods it was generally brought to be regular, and was carried off as usual.

We had a few Pleurisies, Quinseys, and Ophthalmies, and but few; and these were generally of a mild, benign Kind, and pretty easily cured.

The slow nervous Fever which had continued eighteen Months in this Island, in one Part or other of it, now totally disappeared, and left the Island, and I think has not been seen in it since; tho' some have been pleased to call some other Fevers by that Name.

OCTOBER this Year was much hotter than usual in other Years, and also very dry, except that on the 18th, 19th, and 31st Days, we had much Thunder and Lightning, and a considerable deal of Rain: So that the Quantity of Rain which fell in this Month, though mostly dry, was equal to 4.07 cubic Inches deep. The lowest the Thermometer was in the Morning, was at 76°F; the highest was at 82°F; the lowest it was at Noon was at 82°F; and the highest at 86°F, and mostly at 85°F or 86°F. The lowest the Barometer, was at 29.7 [inches of mercury]; and the highest was at 29.9 [inches of mercury].

This Month being very dry and warm, Dysenteries became much less frequent, and more mild and moderate; and the inflammatory Fevers fewer and much less violent also;[12] and it was in general more healthful.

A Febris Ephemera† seized some few, with a cold Rigor, which usually continued about an Hour, and was then succeeded by a brisk hot Fever, a quick full Pulse, seldom hard, the Heat great, which usually continued about fourteen or sixteen Hours, when a general copious Sweat came on, and carried the Fever quite off in the Space of twenty-four Hours time, as a true simple Ephemera does.

---

12. *Query 12.* Did not this proceed from the long Continuance of the moist warm Season in the preceding Months, by which the Animal Solids were relaxed, and rendered less fit, or less liable to produce inflammatory Diseases? And, did not the coming of the warm dry Weather after that, produce a free Perspiration, without inflaming the Body, turn the Humours from the Bowels that way, and abate the Dysenteries, &c.

In the MONTH of NOVEMBER we had frequent Showers of Rain, and it was much cooler in general than the Months last past. The Quantity of Rain which fell in this Month was equal to 4.66 cubic Inches deep. The lowest the Thermometer was in the Morning, was at 76°F; and the highest was at 80°F; the lowest it was at Noon, was at 79°F; and the highest at Noon was at 84°F. The lowest the Barometer, was at 29.7 [inches of mercury]; and the highest was at 29.8 [inches of mercury].

This Month also continued to be pretty healthful; but towards the latter End of it we had a few Diarrhœas, and some Dysenteries, mostly among the Negroes, and a few inflammatory Fevers; and we had no Diseases but these, which could be said to be Epidemical.

The MONTH of DECEMBER is usually, in other Years, a dry Month, but this was very wet, for we had Rain almost every Day more or less, and some Days much Rain, which rendered it more cool than usual. The Quantity of Rain which fell in this Month was equal to 11.27 cubic Inches deep. The lowest the Thermometer was in the Morning, was at 75°F; the highest was at 78°F; the lowest it was at Noon, was at 77°F; the highest at Noon was at 82°F. The lowest the Barometer, was at 29.6½ [inches of mercury]; the highest was at 29.8 [inches of mercury].

The whole Quantity of Rain which did fall in this Year 1754, was equal to 87.01 cubical Inches deep; which is equal to 7 Feet, 3.01 Inches deep, which is a very great Quantity, as it was an uncommon wet Year.† Upon so much Rain falling, Dysenteries were more frequent, and were attended with some Symptoms which were of a malignant Nature, tho' not more inflammatory; wherein moderate Bleeding once, *Ipocacuanha*, *Rhubarb* and *Opiates*, with gentle Restringents and Sudoricks not too much heating, were the most successful: And when the Disease proved more obstinate, the *Ipocacuanha* in small doses, several times repeated (as mentioned in the following Treatise) generally procured a free Diaphoresis, and carried the Disorder off. To some a Dose or two of the *Stibium Ceratum*, when the Fever and Inflammation were taken off, was of great Service; as this Medicine seldom succeeds till that is abated or taken off: An Observation which has not been taken Sufficient Notice of in giving the *Stibium*.

The Febricula† also seized some few, and when properly treated was not dangerous; and those who were not bled, or but very sparingly, recovered much sooner: But where the Launcet was too hastily and too freely used, it was of bad Consequence; as I saw in some Cases where they had been too hasty with the Launcet before I came: Though I saw none that died, yet some were in great Danger from it, and I heard of some who died by it.

Many were afflicted with Boils, and some with larger Imposthumations;† and we had no other Diseases but these, which could be called Epidemical.

A.D. *1755*

THE MONTH of JANUARY was generally dry, though we had a few small Showers at times, and it was also more cool than usual; and the most pleasant Weather that I ever saw in the West Indies. The Quantity of Rain which fell in this Month, was only equal to 1.20 cubical Inch deep. The lowest the Thermometer ever was in the Morning, was at 72°F; the highest at 77°F; the lowest it ever was at Noon, was at 77°F; the highest at Noon was at 81°F. The lowest the Barometer, was at 29.8 [inches of mercury]; the highest was at 29.9 [inches of mercury].

And as this Month was cool and pleasant, it was also the most healthful; so that I cannot say that we had any Diseases that were epidemical.

FEBRUARY was rather more cool, and full as pleasant as the last Month; and I found *Fahrenheit's* Thermometer in the Mornings as low as 70°F, which I never saw it [at] before, or since, in eleven Years time.

The Quantity of Rain that fell in this Month, was only 1.41 cubic Inch deep. The lowest the Thermometer was in the Morning, was at 70°F, the highest at 75°F; the lowest it ever was at Noon, was at 77°F; and the highest at Noon was at 81°F. The lowest the Barometer, was at 29.8 [inches of mercury]; and the highest was at 29.9 [inches of mercury].

February was as dry, pleasant, and cool, as the last Month, and no less healthful, for we had no epidemical Disease till near the latter End of it, when a catarrhal Fever seized several; first with a cold Rigor, which in some continued four or five Hours, in others no longer than one or two, then was succeeded by a hot Fever, with great Pain in the Head: Some had Pain in their Backs and all over them, but most of them had Pain only in the Head, which continued in some but one Day, in others two or three Days, and in some longer, and then in some went off by a critical warm Sweat; but in most an Inflammation came on in one Leg (something like the Fever which produces the Elephantiasis,† but without any Swelling in the inguinal Glands, or the Red Stroke† from it to the Leg, neither was it that Fever) and it became much inflamed, and looked very red, like the Skin of one in the scarlet Fever;† and in some, little small Blisters rose in the Leg like an Erysipelas,† upon which the Fever abated and went gradually off by this imperfect Crisis, and the Cuticula† peeled off after as in an Erysipelas, or the scarlet Fever, and they soon recovered: In others, when the morbid Matter was not thus cast upon the Leg, or some other Part, the Fever continued a little longer, and was carried off by once moderate bleeding, and encouraging a free Diaphoresis with cooling Sudorificks [such] as *Sal. Nitre, Camphor. Spir. Mindereri, Acetum Camphorat.* and diluting plentifully with warm Wine-whey, most commonly in four or five Day's time. Their Blood was generally very florid, and a little inflamed, but rarely sizzy.

Asthmatical and phthysical† People suffered much from this Catarrh; others had it and a Cough more like a common Cold, and so escaped having either more or less of it; so that it might be said to be truly Epidemical, and most probably did arise from this unusual Coolness and Dryness of the Air, rarely felt in this warm Climate.

The MONTH of MARCH was rather more dry than the two preceding Months; and more cool than usual in such dry Weather. The Quantity of Rain which fell in it, was only equal to 0.66 Parts of a cubic Inch deep. The lowest the Thermometer was in the Morning was at 72°F; the highest was at 77°F; the lowest it was at Noon, was at 78°F; and the highest at Noon was at 82°F. The lowest the Barometer, was at 29.8 [inches of mercury]; and the highest was at 29.9 [inches of mercury].

Catarrhs, Coughs, Pleurisies, and Peripneumonies, now became more frequent, especially the last: Their Blood was now generally more or less sizzy and less inflamed, and both it and the and the Pleurisies required pretty large repeated Bleedings, with antiphlogistick Pectorals, and expectorating Medicines; for in general they expectorated little without the Assistance of the last.

Several Children had that exanthematous Eruption, called the Chicken-pox, and some few on the East Side of the Island, still had the Hooping-cough: And we had no other Diseases that were epidemical.

APRIL was dry, except for a few Showers which fell on three or four Days, but it was warmer than the three preceding Months; though some Days were suddenly cool, then warm again. The Quantity of Rain which fell in this Month, was equal to 2.17 cubical Inches deep. The lowest the Thermometer was in the Morning, was 75°F; the highest was 79°F; the lowest it was at Noon was at 79°F; and the highest at Noon was 84°F. The lowest the Barometer, was at 29.8½ [inches of mercury]; and the highest at 29.9½ [inches of mercury].

These sudden changes in the Air, produced Catarrhs, Coughs, and some Peripneumonies, and Quinseys, but not of a bad Kind, nor the Inflammation attending them very great; and if taken in time were not difficult to be cured, by Bleeding and the above-mentioned antiphlogistick Method. The Chicken-pox continued among Children: Some had the Pictonic Cholic, or dry Belly-ache, which was generally removed in four or five Day's time, by the Method hereafter mentioned.[13]

In the MONTH of MAY we had frequent Showers of Rain, which with the Clouds intercepting the hot rays of the Sun, always cool the Air considerably; so that this Month was more cool than usual in other Years. The Quantity of Rain which fell in this Month, was equal to 6.62 cubic Inches deep. The lowest the Thermometer was in the Mornings, was 76°F; and the highest was 80°F; the lowest it was at Noon, was at 80°F; and the highest was at 85°F. The lowest the Barometer, was at 29.8 [inches of mercury]; and the highest at 29.9 [inches of mercury].

This Month was also cool; it was likewise in general healthful. We had only a few Catarrhs, Coughs, and Pleurisies; and some Dysenteries among the Negroes: But this, as well as the four preceding Months, [was] more than usually cool and healthful.

We also had frequent Showers of Rain during the MONTH of JULY, but it was more warm than the last Month. The Quantity of Rain which fell in this Month was equal to 5.70 cubic Inches deep. The lowest the Thermometer was in the Morning, was 78°F; the highest was 80°F; the lowest it was at Noon, was at 82°F; and the highest at Noon was 86°F. The lowest the Barometer, was at 29.8 [inches of mercury]; and the highest was at 29.9½ [inches of mercury].

The Diseases we had this Month, principally affected the Abdomen; for now the Humours had an uncommon Tendency towards the Viscera of the lower Belly, as in the last Year at this Time: And some were seized with an Inflammation of the Bowels; others with a Cholera Morbus; and several with Diarrhœa with much griping Pain; in some with a Fever: In both they usually had a Sickness at their Stomachs, and their Stools were mixed with a good

---

13. See the following Treatise.

deal of viscid pituitous† Mucus. This Diarrhœa seized Children more frequently than Adults; tho' several of the latter had it. Those who had not a Vomit given at the Beginning of the Disease, generally had it in a more severe degree, and were more difficult to cure; especially when they were reduced low by it. Some had Dysenteries with very bloody Stools, &c. and several had the putrid bilious Fever, especially Strangers.†

Arthriticks also suffered much from this Disposition of the Humours towards the Viscera, which usually carried the gouty Humour to them, from whence it was sometimes difficult to remove it to its proper Place, the extreme Parts.

The MONTH of AUGUST was warmer than the last Month, tho' we had more Rain in this, than in the last. The Quantity of Rain which fell in this Month was equal to 6.28 cubical Inches deep. The lowest the Thermometer was in the Morning, was at 78°F; and the highest at 81°F; the lowest it was at Noon, was at 83°F; the highest at 86°F. The lowest the Barometer, was at 29.8 [inches of mercury]; the highest at 29.9 [inches of mercury].

This frequent Rain, as usual here, produced many Dysenteries, especially among the Negroes; though several white People were seized by it also, but it was neither so frequent, nor so malignant, as it was in the last and some other Years. We also had some Quinseys, Ophthalmies, and inflammatory Fevers, but they were neither attended with so high a degree of Inflammation, nor so difficult to be cured, as in some other Years; for they were generally removed and taken off by Bleeding and Antiphlogisticks, without much danger.

The Essera, or Prickly-heat, and Boils, were frequent, especially among Children, as usual on the coming in of the hot Season; though it was not so sickly as it usually is in most other Years at this Time.

SEPTEMBER was very hot, though we often had Showers of Rain, most commonly in the Nights, which cooled the Air a little. The Quantity of Rain which fell in this Month, was equal to 4.56 cubic Inches deep. The lowest the Thermometer was in the Morning was at 78°F; the highest at 80°F; the lowest it was at Noon, was at 80°F; and the highest at Noon was 85°F. The lowest the Barometer, was at 29.8 [inches of mercury]; and the highest was at 29.9 [inches of mercury].

Diarrhœas and Dysenteries were frequent, as usual at this Time of the Year; though they were not so violent or malignant, nor so difficult to cure as in some other Years. Inflammatory Fevers, Quinseys, Ophthalmies, Pleurisies, and Peripneumonies, though not so very frequent, yet were so frequent that they might justly be deemed Epidemical: Their Blood in general was a little sizzy, and when it stood till cold, was covered with a thin Starch-like Pellicle; yet not so thick, or so much inflamed, as it is in these Diseases in some other Years.

Arthriticks suffered much in this Month also, from the Gouty Humour being turned upon the Bowels, and the Diarrhœa caused thereby, was not easily stayed, or the Gout turned into its proper Course and Place. A small dose of *Ipocacuan.* viz. *gr. iij. in Theriac. Androm.* Ɔ*i. Vel.* Ʒ*ss.*† given and repeated two or three times, at proper Distances; then warm Aromaticks with Volatiles, and a gentle Opiate, commonly answered, with the Assistance of the Pedeluvium† and Fœnigmi to the Soles of the Feet, as before mentioned, to carry the gouty Humour to the remote Parts of the Body; but in some Cases they would not so effectively answer, without the Assistance of some Preparations of Steel, as the learned Dr *Musgrove* so judiciously observes.[14]

The Middle of OCTOBER was dry, but in the Beginning, and towards the latter End of it, we had a great deal of Rain. The Quantity of Rain which fell in this Month, was equal to 9.54 cubic Inches deep. The lowest the Thermometer was in the Morning, was at 78°F, the highest was 80°F; the lowest it was at Noon, was at 82°F, the highest at Noon was at 85°F. The lowest the Barometer, was at 29.8 [inches of mercury], the highest was at 28.8½ [*sic*].

As the falling of so much Rain rendered the Air cooler than it was in the last Month, a catarrhal Fever seized many, especially Children, for of these few or none, either White or Black, escaped it; and all had it in either a greater or less degree: Some had it so slightly, that they eat, drink, and play as if well, then coughed pretty much, and after it returned to their Play again as if well: Some had it in a greater degree; and others were seized with a Chilliness or gentle Rigor, though not observed by some, which was succeeded by a hot Fever, accompanied with Pain in the Head and Back, a Sickness at their Stomachs, and Vomiting; but in some the Vomiting did not come on till the third, fourth or fifth Day, and then it usually was more frequent and more violent, and was attended with some Symptoms of an Inflammation of the Stomach; the Fever and Heat continued great, the Pulse full, quick, tense, and hard; they breathed quick and some with Difficulty; their Blood was florid and much inflamed, and in some very sizzy: The Cough increased as the

---

14. *De Arthritide Onomola.*

Disease advanced, and they brought up a tough viscid Phlegm, some a concocted† thicker Matter, which they usually swallowed down into the Stomach, and after a little time vomited up as Children who are not of Age and Sense to spit it out, usually do: Some had it so slightly as to require no Medicines; others had it so violently as to be in great Danger, and some died of it. Bleeding those once or twice, and some thrice, with a liberal Use of Antiphlogisticks and Pectorals, most commonly relieved them, and carried it off, if taken in time. This Fever did not go off by any regular Crisis; but the Inflammation being abated, and taken off by the above Methods, the remaining Part of the morbid Matter was discharged gradually from the Lungs and Bronchia, by coughing and expectorating, and they recovered; though it reduced some of them very low before they recovered. Some few Adults had it, but most commonly in a more moderate degree; yet some had it more violently.

We had some Peripneumonies, and a few Quinseys; but except these and the above catarrhal Fever in Children, it was a tolerable healthful Season.

NOVEMBER was much drier, and some Days were much warmer than any in the last Month,[15] though we had some Rain about the Middle and at the latter end of the Month. The Quantity of Rain which fell in it being only

---

15. On the 1st of November 1755, which was three Days before the new Moon, a very extraordinary Phænomenon happened at *Bridgetown* in *Barbadoes*. At 20 Minutes after 2 o'Clock after Noon, above an Hour after it was High-water there, the Sea suddenly flowed and rose more than two Feet higher than it does in the highest Spring Tides, and in three Minutes Time it ebbed so as to be as much lower than the usual lowest Ebb; and then it flowed again as high as it did before: And thus it continued to ebb and flow to this uncommon Height, and to fall to that uncommon Lowness, every five Minutes, so as to leave the Sides of the Channel dry to a considerable Distance; but the Times between its Ebbing and Flowing decreased, so as to be a little longer, and the Water to rise a little less each Time, almost in an arithmetical Progression, after the first four or five Times, till near seven o'Clock in the Evening, when I returned out of the Country, and had this Account of it from several Gentlemen who carefully observed it: And it then continued ebbing and flowing, though it did not then rise above one Foot higher, and fall one Foot lower, than its usual Ebbing and Flowing in the common Tides, and it was then about twenty Minutes between each time of Flowing; and so it continued gradually to abate in each Oscillation, till after nine o'Clock in the Evening, when the return of the usual Tide put an end to this extraordinary Motion of the Sea.

This Day was remarkably serene, warm and dry; we had little Wind, and that from the East; the Face of the Sea was calm and smooth before it came, and the Ships in the Bay were not moved by it; but the small Craft in the Channel over the Bar, were driven to and fro with great Violence, and some of them up against the Bridge: And the Water flowed in and out of the Harbour with such a Force, that it tore up the black Mud in the Bottom of the Channel, so

equal to 4.40 cubic Inches deep. The lowest the Thermometer was in the Morning, was at 74°F; the highest at 81°F; the lowest it was at Noon, was 80°F; the highest at Noon was 85°F. The lowest the Barometer, was 29.7 [inches of mercury]; the highest was at 29.8 [inches of mercury].

The catarrhal Fever[†] continued most of this Month also, and spread itself all over this small Island, so that few or no Children escaped it; tho' some had it so mildly as not to be confined in the House by it, when others were in the greatest Danger in it, or died of it. And in this Month several who had it, had an inflammatory Quinsey accompanying it, the Inflammation falling upon the Throat at the same time.

I found the *Crude Sal. Ammoniac.* joined with *Nitre,* to be the most powerful Attenuant of that viscid Lentor, in the Blood of those who have these inflammatory Diseases, and the greatest Antiphlogistick at the same time.

This Fever did not go off by any regular Crisis, but went off gradually in this Month, as it did in the last. I also observed, that it did not in all Patients fall upon the Sneiderian Membrane, and on the Bronchia and Lungs; but in some particular Constitutions, it fell upon such other Parts of the Body, as were either naturally weaker, or had been rendered so by some preceding

---

15. (*cont'd.*)

that it sent forth a great Stench; and caused the Fishes to float on its Surface, and drove many of them onto the dry Land, at a considerable Distance, where they were taken up by the Negroes.

Many People were Witnesses of this uncommon Phænomenon, which could not be accounted for, from the known Cause of the Tides, nor from any other natural Cause, unless we supposed that an Earthquake was at some Distance in the Sea, as I then said: Though no Motion of the Earth was perceived here by any Person on the Land, or in the Ships in the Bay; neither was any Noise heard, either from the Earth, or in the Air.

But two Months after this, we received an Account of a most dreadful Earthquake, which happened on the same Day at *Lisbon* in *Portugal,* and destroyed the greatest Part of that populous rich City. We are told that the first Shock of the Earthquake there, happened at three Quarters of an Hour after nine o'Clock, and the second Shock which was much greater, and agitated the River and the Sea much more violently there, was at twenty Minutes after ten o'Clock before Noon: And the Sea at *Barbadoes* was agitated as above; first at twenty Minutes after two o'Clock in the Afternoon. The Distance between *Lisbon* and *Bridgetown* is near 3400 English Miles, and the Difference of Time is near three Hours and a Half, which makes seven Hours and a Half; and if the Sea was moved at *Barbadoes* by that Earthquake at *Lisbon,* as it is most probable that it was, then the vibrating Motion was communicated thro' so soft a Medium as the Body of Water is, 3400 Miles in seven Hours and a Half's Time, which is at the Rate of 450 Miles each Hour, or seven Miles and a Half in each Minute; which is a very swift Motion to be communicated by Percussion, through so soft a Medium as Water is.

Disease; and then it produced some different Symptoms, such as are peculiar to those Parts upon which it fell, when they are disordered, and consequently required some different Methods of Treatment: But as this was an inflammatory Fever, and appeared as such in all those different Shapes, with inflammatory Symptoms, they all required Bleeding and antiphlogistick Medicines, with variations *pro re nata.*

We had much Rain from the Beginning to the Middle of DECEMBER, accompanied with brisk cool Winds; but from the Middle to the End of the Month, it was more dry and cooler, than in most other Years. The Quantity of Rain which fell this Month, was equal to 8.91 cubic Inches deep. The lowest the Thermometer was in the Morning, was 72°F; the highest was 78°F; the lowest it was at Noon, was at 79°F; the highest at Noon was 82°F. The lowest the Barometer, was at 29.8 [inches of mercury]; the highest was at 29.9 [inches of mercury].

And the whole Quantity of Rain which fell in all this Year 1755, was equal to 57.29 cubical Inches deep.

Dysenteries continued to be epidemical in some Parts of the Island, though few in or near Town had it. We also had some inflammatory Fevers, and a few were seized with an Inflammation of the Bowels, but not many, neither was the Inflammation great or violent; though the Humours still continued to have an unusual Tendency and Afflux towards the Bowels. And Arthriticks, especially such as had weak Bowels, suffered much from the Gouty Humours turning that way: But in general it was tolerably healthful.

A.D. *1756*

THE MONTH of JANUARY was in general very dry, though we had a few small Showers at the Beginning of it. The Quantity of Rain which fell in it, was only equal to 0.45 Parts of a cubic Inch deep. The lowest the Thermometer was in the Morning, was at 71°F; the highest at 76°F; the lowest it was at Noon, was at 76°F; the highest at Noon was 80°F. The lowest the Barometer, was at 29.8 [inches of mercury]; the highest was at 29.9 [inches of mercury].

As the Weather was cool, pleasant, and dry, it was also in general pretty healthful; except that towards the North-east Part of the Island, they had some Dysenteries, which were attended with inflammatory Symptoms, and a Fever mali Moris, which was often followed with Aphthæ towards the latter End of the Disease: But Bleeding at the Beginning of the Disease pretty freely, a Dose of *Ipocacuan.* and *Rhubarb* and Opiates, *&c.*, and the Method hereafter mentioned, generally rendered it more moderate, and in a little time took it off. Though to some it was necessary to give the *Ipocacuanah* in small Doses after them, which generally was successful: Though several of them had taken the *Stibium Ceratum*, and repeated it several times before I saw them, without much or any Benefit from it; but they were not bled, or at least not sufficiently, and that Remedy seldom does succeed when an Inflammation attends the Disease, unless it first be taken off by suitable Evacuations.

We also had some Diarrhœas, which in general were more easily relieved.

FEBURARY continued to be very dry, and we had no Rain except a small Shower on the 12th, 13th, and 20th Nights. The Quantity [of rain] that fell in this Month, was only equal to 1.27 cubic Inch deep. The lowest the Thermometer was in the Morning, was 70°F; the highest 76°F; the lowest it was at Noon, was at 77°F; the highest was at 82°F. The lowest the Barometer, was at 29.8 [inches of mercury]; and the highest was at 30 [inches of mercury].

Though this Month was so dry, yet the Wind being generally in the N. E. Points, it was more cool than I ever observed it before; for I found *Fahrenheit's* Thermometer several Mornings as low as 70°F, which is the lowest that I ever saw it in *Barbadoes;*[†] neither did I ever see the Barometer as high as 30 [inches of mercury] before. And as it was thus cool, tho' dry, it was more than usually healthful, for we had no Diseases which were epidemical.

MARCH was also dry, the Quantity of Rain which fell, being only equal to 1.52 cubic Inch deep. The lowest the Thermometer was in the Morning, was at 73°F; the highest at 78°F; the lowest it was at Noon, was at 79°F; and the highest was at 83°F. The lowest the Barometer, was at 29.8½ [inches of mercury]; and the highest was at 29.9½ [inches of mercury].

This Month continued to be dry, and more than usually cool in this Climate, at this time of the Year; and it was pretty healthful.

But I observed that Arthriticks suffered pretty much in this dry cool Season; and several Persons were seized with the *Opisthotonos*[†] and the *Tetany,*[†] from seemingly very slight Causes.[16] And we had a few Catarrhs, and some few

---

16. *Query 13.* Did not this continued dry, cool Season, brace up the Solids, and render them more rigid, and diminish the Perspiration, and so affect the Arthriticks? And from this increased Rigidity of the Nerves, were not the *Opisthotonos* and *Tetany* more frequent, and more easily produced?

Quinseys; and some had Tumours about the Parotids, Fauces, and Neck: But in general it was pretty healthful.

APRIL was very dry, as well as the three preceding Months; but it was not only warmer than them, but it was warmer than usual at this time, especially towards the latter End of it. The Quantity of Rain which fell in this Month, being only equal to 0.37 Parts of a cubic Inch deep. The lowest the Thermometer was in the Morning, was at 75°F; the highest at 79°F; the lowest it was at Noon, was at 81°F; the highest at Noon was at 84°F. The lowest the Barometer, was at 29.8½ [inches of mercury]; the highest was at 29.9 [inches of mercury].

The first Part of this Month was in general pretty healthful, but towards the latter End of it, some were seized with a continued remitting Fever, which most commonly came on first with a Chilliness, not a Rigor, which was soon succeeded by a hot Fever, with great Pain in the Head and Back, a Sickness at the Stomach, and a frequent Reaching and Vomiting, so that some could retain little on their Stomachs, either Medicines or Nourishment; their Pulse was usually quick and full, in some a little hard and tense: Their Blood was florid, and of a soft loose Texture, but not so much dissolved as it usually is in the putrid bilious Fever, though something like it during the first two or three Days of the Fever, and very little Serum separated from the Crassamentum;[†] but as the Fever increased, it became more dense, and separated more Serum, though it still remained florid. They were very restless, almost continually tossing and tumbling, they got little Sleep, and that disturbed and without refreshing them; their Skin was generally hot and dry, though sometimes moist, and they in a fine breathing Sweat: Some had large cold clammy Sweats, especially on the extreme Parts, though very hot about the Præcordia. The Fever abated and remitted at some certain time, once in every twenty-four Hours, but still continued, and returned with great Heat, Vomiting, and all the same Symptoms at different times in the Day, in different Patients, but usually at the same time in the same Patient, and generally abated again in six, eight or ten Hours time; and thus returned once in every twenty-four Hours time, without being influenced or increased by the Heat of the Day, as most Fevers in this hot Climate are. Thus it continued to remit, and usually come to its Height, and began to abate a little between the fourth and fifth Days, and generally came to its Crisis on the ninth Day, and went off when it was properly treated.

Bleeding once at the Beginning of the Disease, and an Emetic after it, were

of great Service, and yet more so if a gentle antiphlogistick Purge, of Manna†
and Tamarinds† with a little Nitre, was given the next Day after it; or to those
who had a Diarrhœa, as some few had, a small Dose of Rhubarb after the
Vomit. In some plethoric Constitutions, Bleeding twice was necessary where
the Symptoms indicated it; but I observed that some Practitioners were too
hasty and too free of their Launcet at the Returns of the Fever, and that it was
prejudicial to the Sick. After these, the Use of soft smooth Antiphlogisticks,
and a Dose of the *Syr. e Meconio* at Nights (because I observed, that either
Tinct. vel Extract. Thebaic.† generally brought on a Delirium, or if present
before, increased it) most commonly greatly contributed to carry the Fever
regularly on, and brought it to a Crisis, and carried it off by a copious warm
critical Sweat on the ninth Day; some had a loose Stool or two also, after
which they soon recovered, and we had no other Diseases that were
epidemical.

MAY continued to be very dry, and also warmer than the last Month, till
near the latter End of it, when we had some Rain: The Quantity of Rain which
fell was but equal to 1.12 cubic Inch deep. The lowest the Thermometer was
in the Morning, was at 78°F; the highest was at 80°F; the lowest it was at
Noon, was at 83°F; and the highest at Noon was at 86°F. The lowest the
Barometer, was at 29.8 [inches of mercury]; and the highest was at 29.9 [inches
of mercury].

Upon the Increase of the Warmness of the Weather, the continued
remitting Fever became more frequent, and varied a little in its Symptoms:
The Vomiting was much less frequent, and the Head more affected, especially
with violent shooting darting Pain, mostly over the Eyes, particularly during
the Exacerbations and Returns of the Fever; and some had a comatous†
Stupor, others were delirious during that time: The Pulse was full and quick,
but generally soft, during the first two or three Days; but afterwards usually
became very variable, so that one seldom found the Pulse the same, in the
same Patient at different Times; sometimes it was very quick, fluttering,
irregular and small, at other times soft and full, then varying between these
almost every Hour; the Patient sometimes hot and dry, at other times in a
profuse Sweat, warm at one time, at other times cold: The Tongue mostly
furred over and white, sometimes brown; some were very thirsty, others
moderately so: They generally complained of a great Languor and Faintness;
their Urine was mostly high coloured, in some paler, and with a Cloud
suspended in it, never with a Sediment, not even when the Crisis came on,

nor even after it; and I have always observed, that a Sediment is very rarely seen in the Urine in this warm Climate, in any Fever; though it is frequently seen in England in most Fevers, upon the coming of the Crisis, and especially in this Fever, and is generally like Brick-dust:[17] So that little Judgment can be formed by inspecting the Urine in this Climate, though we frequently can in England.

Notwithstanding these Alterations, the Fever continued to come to its Height between the fourth and fifth Day, when properly treated, and Nature was assisted, and not hindered by improper Practice, and then gradually declined and came to its Crisis regularly on the ninth Day, as before, most commonly by a copious warm Sweat; in a chance one, by a few loose Stools: And I saw one Gentleman in whom it went off by a copious Discharge from the Glands of the Bronchia and Lungs, and probably some Part of the morbid Matter by the Salivary Glands, and was brought up by a frequent Coughing, and constant Expectorating and Spitting; as I have more than once seen in some other Fevers in England.

I observed that giving a Vomit in the Beginning of this Fever, when it was attended with so much Vomiting, in the last Month, was of great Service; but now when they vomited less, or not at all, and the Head was more affected, I found that an Emetic was of no Service, but rather hurtful: But that a gentle antiphlogistick Purge given the first or second Day of the Disease, was of very great Service, and generally rendered the Fever more mild and moderate, than when no such Purgative was given.

Except this Fever, and not many had it, we had no other Diseases which could be said to be epidemical; so that it was in general a pretty healthful Season.

The dry warm Weather continued to the Middle of JUNE, when a considerable Quantity of Rain fell, equal to 3.37 cubic Inches deep. The lowest the Thermometer was in the Morning, was at 79°F; the highest at 87°F; the lowest it was at Noon, was at 82°F; and the highest at Noon was at 87°F. The lowest the Barometer, was at 29.8½ [inches of mercury]; the highest was at 29.9½ [inches of mercury].

---

17. *Query 14*. Does not this proceed from the great Heat of the Climate, where Nature is constantly accustomed to a frequent and great Discharge of the animal Salts by Sweat, where the Sweat is always found to be much more salt than it is in colder Climates; which animal Salts are usually carried off by the Urine in all colder Countries?

Upon the falling of this Rain, the Weather became more cool and moist; and the continued remitting Fever totally disappeared, so that I did neither see, nor hear of any, except one that was seized with it after this Change. Some few had Catarrhs, and some were seized with Inflammations in the Breast, tho' not many; and upon the falling of this Rain the Season in general became healthful.

From the Middle of JUNE, to the End of JULY, we had frequent great Showers of Rain, and it was much cooler than the two preceding Months were, and more cool than usual in this Month in other Years. The Quantity of Rain which fell in this Month was equal to 6.75 cubical Inches deep. The lowest the Thermometer was in the Morning, was at 77°F; the highest was 80°F; the lowest it was at Noon, was at 82°F; the highest at Noon was at 86°F. The lowest the Barometer, was at 29.8½ [inches of mercury]; the highest was at 29.9½ [inches of mercury].

The Weather being in general much cooler, Catarrhs became more frequent, though not very bad; we had some Pleurisies and Peripneumonies, but not of a bad Kind; and they were commonly removed by Bleeding, and the usual antiphlogistick Method and Medicines. But Dysenteries, upon the falling of these Rains, became frequent, and some of them were of a bad malignant Kind: They usually came on gradually at the Beginning, and the Fever was very moderate on the two or three first Days, and sometimes scarce perceptible; but on the third, fourth or fifth Days, the Fever increased much, and sometimes to be violent, and the Purging also, with much griping Pain in the Bowels, and Sickness at the Stomach, and frequent Stools with much Blood and Brine-like Ichor, and much Mucus was discharged with them; the Pulse was very quick, sometimes full, but more frequently small, and often hard, but always very quick; they were often delirious, and their extreme Parts cold. Bleeding at the Beginning, and repeating it as the Fever, &c. indicated; *Ipocacuanha*, *Rhubarb*, and Opiates, with antiphlogistic Restringents and Opiates, were the most successful in general, with *Ipocacuan* in small Doses. But in some Cases, though these were given in the most cautious and judicious Manner, they did not give that Relief, nor answer as they usually do in other Years to some Patients, neither did the *Ipocacuanha* in small Doses; yet the Antiphlogisticks with subacid Restringents and Antispecticks† with small Doses of Opiates (and the Testacea† to some Children with Antiphlogisticks and gentle Anodynes) answered better, and often prevented a Mortification from coming on in some Patients; but in some few others, after four or five

Days more, though the Stools had been brought by these Methods to be more stercoraceous,[†] and they seemed to be something better, the Stools returned with more Violence, and the Pulse became more frequent, small, quick, and irregular, the extreme Parts grew cold, with cold clammy Sweats, the Delirium increased, a Coma came on, and nothing could prevent the fatal Period; and they died with all the Symptoms of a Mortification of the Bowels. This was the Case of a few; but others in general when bled and vomited at the first, and then giving the *Ipocacuanha* in small Doses, and Opiates, with Antiphlogisticks and subacid Restringents with gentle Opiates, generally recovered, tho' not without great Difficulty and Danger: But as this Disease continued, it became less malignant, and more moderate than it was at its first coming.

We had a considerable Quantity of Rain through all the MONTH of AUGUST, though but in Showers, and it was often clear and hot between them; and from the Middle of the Month to the End of it, it was very warm as we had but little Wind, and it was often calm. The Quantity of Rain which fell this Month, was equal to 3.89 cubic Inches deep. The lowest the Thermometer was in the Morning, was at 78°F; the highest was 80°F; the lowest it was at Noon, was at 82°F; and the highest at Noon was at 86°F. The lowest the Barometer, was at 29.8 [inches of mercury]; the highest was at 29.9 [inches of mercury].

The Dysentery continued, and became more frequent, especially among Children, but was not quite so malignant as in the last Month; for now by Bleeding once or twice, and in a chance-one thrice, a Dose of *Ipocacuan* and *Rhubarb* with an Opiate after it, and a few small Doses of the former after that, and antiphlogistick Subastringents with Opiates, they generally recovered. To Children, after Bleeding once or twice, a few small Doses of *Ipocacuan* from gr.i to gr.ij and a little *Rhubarb* with an Anodyne, then *Sal. Nitre, Coral. Rubr, vel Pulv. Bolo C.* equal Quantities, in the *Julep e Cret.*[†] or such like Mixture with an Anodyne, generally checked it, and took it off in four or five Day's time.

Ophthalmies were also frequent, but were generally carried off by Bleeding, and two or three cooling Purges, and a cooling repelling Collyrium:[†] And we had also a few Pleurisies and inflammatory Fevers.

The continued remitting Fever which we had in MAY and JUNE, and disappeared on the falling of the Rain towards the latter End of JUNE, and was not seen for near two Months, now returned about the Middle of this

Month, soon after the return of the hot Weather; but now differed in some of its Symptoms from what it was then: Now the Fever was continual during these three or four first Days, and then usually remitted regularly as it did before, but the Remissions were longer, and the Fever higher on its Return, which usually continued five or six Hours; the Pain in the Head was greater, not only during the first three Days, but in the Returns of the Paroxisms; the Pulse was usually quick and full at that time, in some it was attended with Vomiting, in few with loose Stools; and after five or six Hours the Fever abated, and the Pulse was lower, though often quick and small, and in some a little languid, and some seemed to have little or no Fever for several Hours, as if it would intermit, but it never did; neither would suitable Evacuations bring it to intermit, as they often do in England: The Thirst was great in all, even when the Fever was lowest; the Tongue was covered with a white or brownish Slough; their Sleep little, and that greatly disturbed; some had nervous Twitchings and slight Subsultus Tendinums, but these mostly in the Paroxisms; they generally were low and languid when the Fever abated, or was most remiss: And it usually now came to a Crisis on the fourteenth Day, when properly treated, and neither raised too high by too warm Medicines, nor brought too low by too great Evacuations, or over-cooling a Regimen, and was carried off by a general copious warm critical Sweat.

Those who had lax, weak or gross phlegmatic Constitutions, required Medicines that were a little warmer, and some Volatiles, to be given with the other; when those who were more plethoric, and had rigid tense Solids, required larger Bleeding and Antiphlogisticks, sometimes Emollients with some of the milder Volatiles, with suitable Variations *pro re nata.*

At this time several were afflicted with the Hæmorrhoids or Piles, both internal and external, which were attended with Inflammation and much Pain in those Parts; which were generally removed by the Use of proper sulphurous Medicines, Fomentations, *&c.*

The MONTH of SEPTEMBER was very warm, the Wind being mostly in the South, or in some of the southern Points, and often attended with Thunder and Lightning, and much Rain, and often calm, or very little Wind; so that it was very hot. The Quantity of Rain which fell in this Month, was equal to 7.69 cubic Inches deep. The lowest the Thermometer was in the Morning was at 78°F; the highest at 82°F; the lowest it was at Noon was at 82°F; and the highest at 85°F. The lowest the Barometer, was at 29.7½ [inches of mercury]; and the highest was at 29.9 [inches of mercury].

Dysenteries still continued to be frequent, and now were epidemical all over the Island, both among white and black people, and often of a bad Kind, and difficult to be cured, especially towards the latter End of the Disease; even after the Fever and its bad Symptoms were taken off, by Bleeding and antiphlogistick subastringent Medicines, it was difficult to corroborate and strengthen the great relaxed State of the Intestines, and divert the uncommon Afflux of the Humours from them.

Some few were seized with the continued remitting Fever still, though not many; the Symptoms were much the same as in the last Month.

And I saw several Patients who had both this Fever, and the Dysentery at the same time, which were evidently distinguishable from each other, by their peculiar Symptoms; [such] as a distinct Remission of the Fever, and its returning at or near the same time; and most commonly in the Evening, as that Fever now usually returned: When at the same time the Dysentery, with great Pain in the Bowels and griping bloody Stools, continued also; and this last was most commonly removed; and totally ceased or taken off, several Days before the other Fever came to its Crisis, which it usually did on the fourteenth Day, in this Case also, as well as when it was alone: And it has been observed by others that two different Diseases, when both were epidemical at the same time, frequently do partake of each other's Symptoms in the same Patient at the same time,[18] as I have also observed before.[19]

Several Children, and some few Adults, were seized with a Hæmorrhage from the Intestines, and voided considerable Quantities of Blood that Way, without any Fever, Sickness at their Stomach, and without Griping or much Pain, or much Excrement or Mucus, or any other Symptoms of the Dysentery; and soon were well again with only taking a little styptick Tincture: And I observed, that several Persons who seemed to be well, and walked about their Business, had unusual loose Stools, some for a longer, others for a shorter Time, and then ceased without taking any Medicines; kind Nature having thus discharged the infectious Matter that way, without any Assistance. And likewise, that those who were seized with Pleurisies, usually had a Purging during the three or four first Days of the Disease, which then ceased by a

18. Dris. Sydenhami. Dris. Rogers.
19. Hillary on the Small-Pox and epidemic Diseases.

Bleeding without any Medicines to restrain it.[20] I could not observe that we had any other epidemical Diseases at the time.

In the MONTH of OCTOBER we had frequent Showers of Rain, and sometimes much heavy Rain, both with and without Thunder, and often much Lightning without either of them; and the Weather was cooler than usual in other Years in this Month. The Quantity of Rain which fell in it, was equal to 5.44 cubical Inches deep. The lowest the Thermometer was in the Mornings, was at 75°F; the highest at 82°F; the lowest the Thermometer was at Noon, was at 78°F; and the highest was at 86°F. The lowest the Barometer, was at 29.8 [inches of mercury]; and the highest was at 29.9 [inches of mercury].

Upon the Weather being more cool, the continued remitting Fever totally ceased and disappeared; but the Dysentery still continued, with full as bad Symptoms, and was no less difficult to be cured than it was in the last Month.

We also had some Pleurisies and inflammatory Fevers, in several of which a Diarrhœa, and in some few a Vomiting, accompanied them during the two or three first Days, but was generally abated or totally stayed by Bleeding; as it arose from too great a Plethora, the Relaxation or Weakness of the Intestines, and the unusual Disposition of the Humours to flow towards the Bowels; after which Antiphlogisticks generally took off the Disease successfully. I also observed the same Disposition of the Humours towards the Bowels, in most other Diseases; and even where a Cathartic was given in any other Case, that a much less Dose would answer the Purpose, than usually did at other times: And Arthriticks also suffered much from this Disposition of the Humours.

During both this and the last Month several Persons had a Diarrhœa alba, or white Flux, in which their Stools were more white than usual in a Jaundice, though no Yellowishness appeared in their Skin or Eyes, neither had they Pain in the Region of the Liver, or in the biliary Ducts, nor any other icterical[†] Symptoms; neither had they any unusual Acidity in their Stomachs or Bowels that I could observe; yet their Stools were more white, than if their Diet had been only Milk, Bread and Flour, &c. and that in several Adults whose Dirt[†]

---

20. *Query 15.* Was not this uncommon Disposition and Afflux of the Humours to the Bowels, principally caused by the falling of so much Rain, and cooling [of] the Air, and thereby diminishing the Perspiration, and turning the perspirable Matter and Sweat too suddenly upon the Bowels? Especially as they had been so great before, and the Fluids much rarified by the preceding Warmness in the Months before?

was the reverse; neither were their Stools chilous,† as in a Lientery:† But these were generally pretty soon relieved by a Vomit, or a few small Doses of *Ipocacuanha*, and a little *Rhubarb* with an Opiate.

We had frequent Showers in NOVEMBER, though not quite so much Rain as in the last Month; and they both were more cool than they usually are in other Years. The Quantity of Rain which fell in this Month was only equal to 3.75 cubic Inches deep. The lowest that the Thermometer was in the Morning was at 74°F; the highest at 79°F; the lowest it was at Noon, was at 80°F; and the highest was at 83°F. The lowest the Barometer, was at 29.8 [inches of mercury]; and the highest was at 29.8½ [inches of mercury].

The Dysentery still continued, though not quite so frequent as it was in the two last Months, nor altogether so malignant, or difficult to be cured.

We had also a few inflammatory Fevers, and some Pleurisies, Peripneumonies, and Quinseys, towards the latter End of the Month, but not many; neither were they in general of a bad Kind, but were usually taken off by Bleeding, and the Use of proper antiphlogistick Medicines: And no other Diseases appeared which could be called epidemical.

DECEMBER was in general cool, and we had frequent Showers, and sometimes pretty heavy Rain; and on the 26th we had a Flood. The Quantity of Rain which fell in this Month, was equal to 5.44 cubic Inches deep. The lowest the Thermometer was in the Morning, was at 74°F; the highest at 76°F; the lowest it was at Noon, was at 76°F; and the highest was at 82°F. The lowest the Barometer, was at 29.7½ [inches of mercury]; and the highest was at 29.9 [inches of mercury].

The whole Quantity of Rain which fell in this Year, was but equal to 40.61 cubical Inches deep.

We still continued to have some Dysenteries, and a few Diarrhœas, though not many of either: We also had a few inflammatory Fevers, but they were all more mild and benign than they were in the preceding Months. Some had a Catarrh, and others a Choriza,† but in so moderate a Degree, that they were usually carried off in a few Days, by only drinking Sack-whey,† Tea, or other small Liquors warm.

A.D. *1757*

THE MONTH of JANUARY was in general cool and dry; but the Instrument with which the Quantity of Rain falling in each Month and Year being broke, and a new one not to be had here, my worthy Friend[†] could not carry on his Experiment any longer; so that I cannot give the exact Quantities this Year, but shall mention when we had any considerable Quantities of Rain; and how the Thermometer and Barometer stood, as I have done before.

The lowest the Thermometer was in the Morning, was at 70°F; the highest at 75°F; the lowest it was at Noon, was at 77°F; and the highest at Noon was at 80°F. The lowest the Barometer, was at 29.8 [inches of mercury]; and the highest at 29.9 [inches of mercury].

The Diseases we had in this Month were mostly of the inflammatory Kind, and chiefly those which affected the Head and Breast; though in the preceding Months, the Humours had an uncommon Afflux towards the Bowels, and lower Parts of the Body, during the wet Season; but it now being cool and dry, the Humours seemed to take a different Turn towards the superior Parts, and fell principally upon the Head and Breast, and produced Catarrhs, Chorizas, Quinseys, Peripneumonies, Pleurisies, and Paraphrenitises,[†] which are all Diseases of the inflammatory Kind; but the Pleurisies were most of them of the Nothous Kind, and so were some of the Peripneumonies, and did not require so large Bleeding, especially the first; after which it was usually carried off by the Use of antiphlogistick Pectorals with some Volatiles, and an antiphlogistick Purge or two; for these seldom expectorated any thing material, neither were expectorating Medicines of much Service, when they were given, as I observed in several where they were given before I was called to them. The other inflammatory Diseases were generally carried off by Bleeding, and a free use of Antiphlogisticks.

The MONTH of FEBRUARY was also cool and dry, except that on the 18th Day a considerable quantity of Rain fell.

The lowest the Thermometer was in the Morning, was 70°F; the highest at 75°F; the lowest it was at Noon, was at 76°F; and the highest was at 80°F. The lowest the Barometer was at 29.8 [inches of mercury]; the highest was at 29.9½ [inches of mercury].

This Month was cool and pleasant, and more healthful than any I can remember in the ten Years past; as we had no Diseases which could be said to be epidemical, except a Fever of the inflammatory Kind, which seized some Children and young People, and but very few Adults: It usually came on with a gentle Chilliness, not a Rigor, which seldom continued more than half an Hour, with a little Sickness at their Stomachs, after which a Fever came on, with a quick, and mostly a full Pulse, great Heat, and soon after a Pain in one Thigh, Leg, and Foot; in some in one Arm, not in both these, nor in both Legs, nor both Arms; and as the Fever increased, the Pain in the Leg, or in the Arm, increased and swelled and looked very red, like that of the scarlet Fever, or rather like that of the Elephantiasis, but it was not that Fever; in some the Fever was so high as to cause them to be delirious, in others to be comatose; in some a Cough came on, at the first, with it, in others the Cough did not come on till the third or fourth Day, and in some was very troublesome, in others it was much less so; after Bleeding once moderately, and giving some Antiphlogisticks, the Fever began to abate, and the Swelling and Inflammation in the Leg or Arm increased, and looked very red, and as that increased, the Fever abated, and gradually went off in six or seven Day's time; and the Swelling and inflamed Redness on the Leg or Arm also went off, with the Use of emollient, aperient Fomentations, and encouraging the Part to sweat after fomenting it, by keeping it warm in Flannel, in a few Day's time, and then the Cuticula peeled or scaled off; and they were well again.

When this Fever was treated with Alexipharmic Medicines,† or a hot Regimen, as some did, the Inflammation and Fever were increased, and it generally ended in an Abscess, which being opened, it discharged much Matter for a considerable time, and greatly reduced† the Sick; and did not relieve them near so soon, as when it was carried off by sweating the Part, as above, in the way which Nature indicated, neither did they recover near so soon. Others were so imprudent as to give the *Cortex Peruviana*, upon the abating of the Fever; which produced irremovable Obstructions, (as the great *Professor Boerhaave* says it will in such inflammatory Cases, as I have several times seen it, and sometimes predicted its doing so) which ended in a large Abscess, or Abscesses, from which, as they lay deep, the acrid Matter was absorbed, and produced a violent hectic Fever,† which, with the great Discharge from the Abscess, sunk the Patient in a short time.

Some People had only a troublesome Cough [for] a few Days, without any Fever, and a Swelling in the Hand or Arm came on; upon which the Cough abated, and went gradually off as that increased, as also did the Swelling in a few Days after that; so that this was something of the same Disease, but in a much easier Degree; and some had Abscesses, who neither had the Fever nor the Cough; Nature being thus disposed to cast off, whatever was thus injurious or offensive to her, whether it was from the Air, or from some kind of infectious Miasma, or from whatever other Cause it arose, by such an imperfect Crisis, in this manner.

We also had some inflammatory Rheumatisms, more than usual in this warm Climate; but they were generally carried off, by bleeding, a cooling Cathartic or two, and an Anodyne after them, as Dr *Sydenham* advises, and the Use of antiphlogistick Medicines.

The MONTH of MARCH continued to be very dry, and more cool than usual; tho' we had sometimes a few small Showers in the Nights.

The lowest the Thermometer was in the Morning, was at 73°F; the highest at 76°F; the lowest it was at Noon, was at 78°F; and the highest at Noon was at 81°F. The lowest the Barometer, was at 29.8½ [inches of mercury]; and the highest at 29.9½ [inches of mercury].

The State of Diseases continued to be much the same as in the last Month.

The MONTH of APRIL was also very dry, and likewise cool till near the latter End of it, when it began to be something† warmer, but dry. The lowest the Thermometer was in the Morning, was at 74°F; the highest at 76°F; the lowest it was at Noon was at 79°F; and the highest was at 82°F. The lowest the Barometer, was at 29.8½ [inches of mercury]; and the highest was at 29.9½ [inches of mercury].

These two Months continuing to be very dry and cool till near the latter End of the last, the Diseases that were epidemical, were chiefly of the inflammatory Kind, tho' they were not many; Coughs and Catarrhs were the most frequent, and we had a few Quinseys, Peripneumonies, and inflammatory Rheumatisms, and a few Paraphrenitises; but the depuratory Fever,† before mentioned, wherein the morbid Matter was cast upon the Leg or Arm, continued to be frequent in both these Months, and appeared with the same Symptoms as in the preceding Month; but as the Weather became more warm towards the latter End of this Month, the Coma attending it was more frequent, and something greater, so that the Patient usually lay as if asleep, and if awakened, he instantly dosed and slept again, and continued so till the Leg, or Arm became inflamed, and as that Inflammation increased, the Coma abated, and the Fever also, and both went off, and the Inflammation also after that, as before described.

Gentle cooling Diaphoretics, [such] as the saline Julep of *Sal. Absinth. Succ.*

Limon. &c. and Diluents,† were the most efficacious; tho' it was most commonly necessary to add Antiphlogisticks, especially to some to abate the too great Violence of the Fever, and also to bleed them; but to others who had lax, weak Constitutions, it was sometimes better to omit Bleeding, and most of the Antiphlogisticks, and only give the saline Mixture, or add *Acet. Camphorat, vel Spir. Mindereri,*† to assist Nature to carry off the morbid Matter in the way which she indicated.

The MONTH of MAY also continued to be very dry, and more warm, so that the Face of the Earth was burned brown; and scarce any thing appeared green, except the Trees, Shrubs, and some of the Sugar Canes; and most Ponds of Water were dried up; and we had very little Rain in this Month.

The lowest the Thermometer was in the Morning, was at 76°F; and the highest at 79°F; the lowest it was at Noon, was at 82°F; and the highest was at 85°F. The lowest the Barometer, was at 29.9 [inches of mercury]; and the highest was at 30 [inches of mercury].

This great Drought continuing, and it being more warm, inflammatory Diseases increased, and became much more frequent; [such] as Peripneumonies, Pleuroperipneumonies, and Pleurisies; in which the Fever was generally high, the Pulse quick, full, and most commonly hard; and their blood was sizzy and much inflamed. In the Peripneumonies, it appeared, from the Symptoms attending, that the Obstruction and Inflammation was more in the small Branches of the pulmonary Arteries, than in the Branches of the Bronchial Arteries; but it very often was in them both, which always renders the Disease much more dangerous, and often fatal, if not timely relieved by bleeding very largely, at the very first Appearance of its Symptoms: And this, with repeating it in some Cases, and a liberal Use of attenuating Antiphlogisticks, [such] as the *Sal. Ammoniac, Sal. Nitre, Spir. Mindereri, &c.* and diluting plentifully; also the Fumes or Streams of warm Water and Vinegar received into the Lungs by the Breath, with Fomentations to the Breast, were the most efficacious both in the Peripneumony, and Pleuroperipneumony, and if used plentifully, in time; were generally successful.

In some of these Patients, an erysipelatose† Eruption appeared about the Breast, and in others on several Parts of the Body, on the fifth or sixth Day of the Disease, which greatly relieved their Breathing, as the great *Hippocrates*, and also *Aræteus Capadox*,† both observe;[21] and I found that the Fever also,

---

21. Hippocrat. Aretæus Capadox. Cap. De Pluritid. et in Cap. de Pulmonar.

and all its Symptoms were considerably abated by and after that Eruption, especially when it was assisted by the above Antiphlogistick attenuating Medicines, and the Use of aperient sudorific Fomentations to the Breast, or Parts where it appeared, and also by bathing their Feet and Legs in the same Decoction, or Fomentation, as they all greatly contributed to revulse that erysipelatose Humour from the Lungs, to the external and remote Parts of the Body; agreeably to the Advice of the great *Hippocrates* in *Epidem*. Lib. vi. Sect 2.

Some few were seized with a Fever, which first came on with a Chilliness or gentle Rigor, which was succeeded by a hot Fever, in some the Heat was more intense, and more moderate in others, but in all with great Pain in the Head, Back, and Limbs; a little Sickness at their Stomachs; their Pulse was quick, full, and mostly hard; their Blood was generally of a florid red Colour, in some a little sizzy, but not so much as in those who had the Peripneumony.

Bleeding once, or those who were more plethoric, or had strong elastic Fibres, twice, in order to keep the Fever moderate; then giving the above antiphlogistic Medicines pretty freely, usually carried the Fever regularly on, and most commonly brought it to a Crisis on the seventh Day, when it went off by a copious warm critical Sweat.

Several Children, and some few Adults, were seized with a flushing Heat and great Redness in the Face and Head, both which swelled considerably, but no Blisters or erysipelatose Eruptions, like what is usually called St Anthony's Fire[†] appeared, with a little Pain in the Head; some were a little feverish, others had no Fever; this Swelling continued four or five Days, and then went gradually off by insensible Perspiration, without much Medicine. It was of the erysipelatose Kind, tho' no Eruption appeared, but the Humour passed off through the Pores without it; and the Humours continued during this dry warm Season, to have an unusual Tendency and Afflux towards the Head.

The MONTH of JUNE was mostly dry, tho' we sometimes had some small Showers of Rain, and some moderate cool Winds.

The lowest the Thermometer was in the Morning, was at 78°F; the highest at 80°F; the lowest it was at Noon, was at 80°F; and the highest was at 86°F. The lowest the Barometer, was at 29.8½ [inches of mercury]; and the highest was at 29.9½ [inches of mercury].

The before-mentioned depuratory Fever still continued, but was something less frequent than it was in the two last Months; and we still had some inflammatory Fevers, [such] as Peripneumonies, Pleuro-perioneumonies, and Quinseys; tho' not quite so many as we had in the two last Months; but the Inflammation and Fever in those who had them, were full as great, and their Blood when cold was covered with an inflammatory, sizzy, Buff-like Pellicle, and their Pulse was generally full, quick, and hard, and accompanied with great Pain in the Head, as well as in the Breast or Side. And these were not relieved, and the Disease taken off without bleeding largely, and that repeated several times in some Cases, and a liberal Use of Antiphlogisticks, given in large Doses, and that every two Hours, or oftener; by which the Inflammation and Fever were generally taken off, and they recovered much sooner.[22] And I must observe, that these antiphlogistick Medicines are usually given in such small trifling Doses, especially by some, in this Island, and I believe in most other Places, that they do but little Service, especially where the Inflammation is great, and the Fever violent; neither can they take off the Inflammation and conquer the Fever, unless they are given in much larger Doses, and much more frequently also in some Cases. I have seen a Pleurisy attended with a violent Inflammation and Fever, and very acute Pain, and the Patient's Blood sizzy like Buff, taken off by bleeding once to xxiv ℥, and giving *Sal. Nitri* j ℨ, *Sal. Ammoniac. Crud. depur.* gr xij, *vel* xiv in a Draught of *Decoct. Pectoral cum Spir Nitri Dul. Spir. Mindereri*† every Hour, in the first twelve Hours, and every two or three Hours after, till the Patient had taken sixteen or twenty Doses, in the Space of thirty-six Hours; whereas if they had been given in the small, or even in the usual, Doses, they could have had little Effect in that Case, even in a much longer time; tho' by thus giving them, the Pleurisy was taken off, and the Fever also, in the Space of thirty-six Hours time.

The Beginning of JULY was also dry, but we had frequent Showers after, and sometimes pretty heavy Rain, so that [on] the whole we had a good deal of Rain in this Month, and it was more cool than the last Month.

The lowest the Thermometer was in the Morning, was at 78°F; the highest at 79°F; the lowest it was at Noon, was at 80°F; and highest was at 84°F. The

---

22. *Query 16.* Were not these inflammatory Diseases caused or produced, by the long continued Dryness of the five preceding Months, by which the animal Fibres were so braced up as to be so tense and elastic, as to be ready to produce an Inflammation from the least accidental Cause, [such] as being too much heated by Exercise, or too suddenly taking cold, when hot, or being wet, or any other way stopping the Perspiration, and so increasing the Momentum of the Fluids?

lowest the Barometer, was at 29.8½ [inches of mercury]; and the highest was at 29.9½ [inches of mercury].

The depuratory Fever still continued in this Month, but after the falling of the Rain, it varied something in several of its Symptoms, from what they were in the preceding dry Months; it now came on with a moderate but greater Rigor, which usually continued about an Hour, and then was succeeded by a more hot Fever, with a full, quick, and most commonly a hard Pulse; great Thirst, and great Pain in the Head and Back, and in some in the Limbs, and some were delirious; some had a hot dry Skin, others sweated freely; their Blood was generally sizzy and covered with a Buff-like Pellicle. This continued in some but one Day, but most commonly four or five Days, and then Nature deposited the morbid Matter on the Thigh, Leg, or Arm, and very rarely on any Gland or glandulous Part, as sometimes happens in some other Fevers, where it now usually formed an Abscess, and did not go off by Sweating, as it did in the preceding Months; and as the Inflammation in the Thigh, Leg, or Arm increased, the Fever abated, and when the Tumour suppurated and the Abscess was formed and opened, the Fever went entirely off.

Towards the latter end of this Month,[23] after a considerable Quantity of Rain was fallen; some Dysenteries began to appear, but they were not attended with any Symptoms more than usual.

The MONTH of AUGUST was in general dry and warm, tho' we had some small Showers, and Lightning often, and sometimes some Thunder; on the 20th and 31st Days we had much Rain; and it was cooler.

The lowest the Thermometer was in the Morning, was at 76°F; the highest at 80°F; the lowest it was at Noon, was at 78°F; and the highest was at 85°F. The lowest the Barometer, was at 29.8 [inches of mercury]; and the highest was at 29.9 [inches of mercury].

---

23. On the 29th of this Month, we had an Earthquake in Barbadoes, which continued a little more than half a Minute: The Houses shook very much; but none fell, tho' some were expected to fall, and the Earth seemed to rise and fall as if some large Body had been rolled on under its Surface; and a grumbling Noise was heard in several Places, in the Earth, like the Noise of several Carriages passing on the Streets, or like a Drum, or Thunder at a Distance. The Motion caused many People to be giddy, and some to be sick and vomit, for some time after it was over. I could neither observe any sulphurious or other Smell to arise from the Earth, or to be in the Air, either during its Motion, or after it was over. Neither could I observe any Alteration in the Diseases then reigning, or in those that followed after it, which could be rationally ascribed to its Effects, or to be caused by it.

Upon the falling of this Rain, some Diarrhœas appeared, and the Dysentery became more frequent, especially among the Negroes; and I observed, that when the Dysentery got into an Estate among the Negroes, it generally became infectious and spread amongst them, so that many more were seized with it, and in several it was now attended with very bad Symptoms. And I have observed the same in some other Years, tho' not in all Years.

Bleeding once or twice, and vomiting, and a Dose of Rhubarb with an Anodyne; then giving some small Doses of Ipocacuanha, and Anodynes, with subacid Restringents after them, and some healing Balsamicks at the last, were generally successful.

Inflammatory Fevers were also frequent, [such] as Quinseys, Pleurisies, Peripneumonies, Pleuro-peripneumonies, and Rheumatic Fevers; in all which, their Blood was generally much inflamed; and they mostly required repeated Bleeding, and Antiphlogisticks to be given liberally, and when they were so given, they generally were successful.

The Depuratory Fever also continued to seize several People in this Month, and after it had continued one Day in some, in others two or three Days, the morbid Matter was cast upon some muscular or fleshy Part of the Body, and not upon any Gland as observed before, which is more usual in other Fevers, and in other Years, where it now formed a hard Tumour, which was difficult either to be suppurated, or to be dispersed; for it now often did not suppurate, but dispersed, but not easily, nor in a short time; which is something uncommon; however, as those Tumours rose, the Fever abated much, and as they suppurated, or dispersed, it went entirely off.

The Beginning of SEPTEMBER was hot and dry till the tenth Day, after which we had much Rain, almost every Day, and sometimes much Thunder and Lightning; and the Rain continued, at times, to the End of the Month, which rendered it more cool than this Month usually is in other Years.

The lowest the Thermometer was in the Morning, was at 77°F; the highest 80°F; the lowest it was at Noon, was at 76°F; and the highest was at 85°F. The lowest the Barometer, was at 29.8 [inches of mercury]; and the highest, was at 29.9 [inches of mercury].

As this Month continued to be wet, and more than usually cool, Dysenteries became more frequent, and were attended with some bad Symptoms, and were fatal to some Patients. We also had some Pleurisies, Peripneumonies, Pleuro-peripneumonies, and inflammatory Fevers; in which their Blood was most commonly much inflamed, and covered with a Starch-like, or Buff-like Pellicle. Some few were also seized with the before-mentioned Depuratory Fever; and the Tumours could now very rarely be brought to suppurate, and it often was a considerable time before they could be entirely dispersed, even tho' the Patient was recovered, and otherwise well.

Not long after the Rain began to fall, many were seized with a catarrhal Fever; in some it was moderate, and they only had a Cough, Hoarseness, and a Choriza, which went off in a few Days; but others were taken with a cold Rigor, which usually continued half an Hour or an Hour, and was succeeded by a hot Fever, with a great Defluxion of Rheum on the Bronchia and Lungs, and a violent Cough; they expectorated little the first two or three Days, but considerably more afterwards; it was frequently accompanied with a Peripneumony, or a Pleuro-peripneumony, in which the Bronchia and Lungs were much inflamed; and their Blood was covered with a Starch or Buff-like Pellicle. These required pretty large Bleeding, and a liberal Use of antiphlogistick Pectorals; and with which they were most commonly relieved.

Towards the latter end of the Month, some few Patients, in the North Part of this Island, were seized with a putrid Synochus Fever:† but it neither continued long amongst them; nor did it spread further into any other Parts of the Island.

We had a good deal of Rain in the MONTH of OCTOBER, and it was also more cool, in general, than is usual in this Month.

The lowest the Thermometer was in the Morning, was at 76°F; the highest at 80°F; the lowest it was at Noon, was at 78°F; and the highest at 84°F. The lowest the Barometer, was at 29.8 [inches of mercury]; and the highest at 29.9 [inches of mercury].

Dysenteries still continued, but were less frequent than they were in the two preceding Months. And the depuratory Fever which we had in the three or four last Months, now totally disappeared.

But the catarrhous Fever became more frequent, so that few escaped having either more or less of it, as in the last Month; tho' in some it only appeared as a common Cold, and went off in the same manner; but in some, the Catarrh with a Colluvies† of sharp serous Humour fell upon the Bronchia and Lungs, and produced a Peripneumomy with a violent Cough, great Inflammation, with great Difficulty of Breathing, and all the other Symptoms of that Disease. In some others it fell upon the Pleura, and produced a Pleurisy, with its Symptoms; and in some few, on the Mediastinum and Pericardium, and produced a Paraphrenitis: In all which the Inflammation was generally great, and their Blood much inflamed and more or less sizzy.

In some others the Inflammation was general, and did not fix upon any one Part of the Body; but they had a Fever with great Pain in the Head, and sometimes all over they Body, a quick full Pulse, and some were sometimes delirious, or comatous, for the Head was usually most affected; their Blood was inflamed, and very florid, but not sizzy as in the others above-mentioned. In these, after Bleeding once, and the Use of Antiphlogisticks, the Fever generally went off by a copious warm critical Sweat on the fifth Day. Some had this Fever in a much easier Degree; they only had a feverish Heat, with a flushing red Colour in their Face, a Pain in the Head, with a quick Pulse, which continued a few Hours, and then abated for a few Hours, and returned again in the same manner several times, and at last went off by a critical Sweat on the fifth Day, as in the others. But those who had the Peripueumony, Paraphrenitis, and the Pleurisy, required much larger Bleeding, and that very early in the Disease, and sometimes repeating it, and a more liberal and plentiful Use of the Antiphlogisticks, by which, if taken in time, they usually recovered.

The Dysentery became more frequent towards the latter end of the Month, than it was in the Beginning of it, and was now sometimes accompanied with the last-mentioned inflammatory catarrhous Fever, and usually had more Symptoms of that Fever in the first two or three Days; and then it all turned upon the Bowels, with a Purging, which did not carry that Fever off; but it increased and appeared with all the Symptoms of the Dysentery, accompanied with much griping Pain, and bloody Brine-like frequent Stools, &c. In these, Bleeding, and the Methods hereafter mentioned in the Treatise on that Disease, were usually successful.

The asthmatic and consumptive Patients suffered much from this catarrhous Fever, and it proved fatal to some of them.

Also the arthritic and rheumatic Patients, had more severe Attacks of those Diseases, than they usually had in other Years.

And I observed that, in general, the Inflammations attending all the inflammatory Diseases at this time, were more violent than usual, and their Blood was more sizzy, and covered with a thicker Buff-like Pellicle; and that they required more copious Bleeding before the Diseases could be taken off, than they did in other Years[24] in this warm Climate, at least since I came into this Country.[†]

The MONTH of NOVEMBER was, in general, warmer than the two

preceding Months, probably from the Wind's being often more southerly, though we had more Rain in it, especially towards the latter End of it, than we usually have in most other Years.

The lowest the Thermometer was in the Morning, was at 76°F; the highest at 78°F; the lowest it was at Noon, was at 79°F; and the highest was at 82°F. The lowest the Barometer, was at 29.7½[inches of mercury]; and the highest at 29.8½ [inches of mercury].

The Dysenteries, which began to increase towards the latter End of the last Month, continued to be more frequent most of this; but they began to abate again towards the latter End of this Month also. And the catarrhous Fever, which was so frequent in the preceding Months, continued to be so some Part of this; but it greatly abated, and became much less frequent towards the latter End of it, and totally disappeared and left us in the following Month.

Some few were seized with a Fever, which at the first usually appeared in a very irregular Manner, and sometimes with somewhat different Symptoms in one Patient, to what it did in others; but in general it seemed to be the nearest to what the Greeks call a ἡμιτριταῖον or semi-tertian Fever.† It most commonly appeared in all, like a continual Fever† during the first four, five, or six Days, and then seemed to remit like what the Greeks call a συνεχεῖς, or a continued remitting Fever, and in most continued so, with the usual Symptoms of that Fever for several Days, and much longer in some, especially if improperly treated. In others it had more of the Appearance and Symptoms of a semi-tertian Fever, but rarely or never came to intermit regularly; for intermitting Fevers are very seldom or never seen in this Island† now, unless they are brought from some of the other less cultivated Islands, or from some other Place; though it is said that they were more frequent before [this] Island

---

24. *Query 17.* Did not all these inflammatory Diseases arise from, or were much increased by, the long continued dry warm Weather, during the last six Months, which braced up the animal Fibres, and rendered them more rigid and elastic, and the Fluids more dense and dry, and consequently both more fit to produce inflammatory Diseases, tho' they did not much appear till after the falling of the Rain, which rendered the Air more cool and moist, and thereby contracted the perspiratory Pores, and considerably decreased that Excretion; did not these two Causes, thus acting the same way at the same time, the one to obstruct the Perspiration, and the other to increase the Momentum of the circulating Fluids, by thus jointly acting, produce all the above-mentioned inflammatory Diseases? And as these Causes were long continued, were not their Effects greater and the Inflammations in general much greater, and the Diseases more violent?

was cleared of its Woods, and cultivated. In this Fever their Pulse was quick and full, and sometimes a little hard; they had a great Pain in their Head, Back, and most commonly all over them, especially in their Knees and Joints; their Blood was florid and inflamed, but rarely covered with a sizzy inflammatory Pellicle.

Bleeding them once at the Beginning of the Disease, and the Use of attenuating Antiphlogisticks, generally brought the Fever either to remit regularly, or to appear as a regular semi-tertian Fever; and then they both were usually taken off by giving saline Draughts, or the following saline Mixture, which last I found to be the most efficacious.

Flor. Chamæmeli. Fol. Menthæ. ana. Mi. *Indfund. in Aq. Bull. q. s. ut Col. ℥xvi. Colaturæ adde Aq. Menthæ Spir. ℥iss. Sal. Absinth ℥ss. Syr. e Mecon. ℥iss. Elix. Vitrioli Acid q.s. ut reducet. Sal. Alkal. ad Stat. nutralem; misce, exhibe Colch. tria vel quatuor tertia quag; hora.*[†]

In some few the Fever remitted pretty regularly from the Beginning, but it never came to intermit; though some Evacuations were used to such to bring it to intermit, as they usually bring this fever to intermit in England, but would not do it in this warm Climate: But the above saline Mixture took the Fever quite off in all that I saw.

The MONTH of DECEMBER was more cool than the last Month, and it was often cloudy, and we had much more Rain than usual in this Month, in other Years; as also stronger or higher Winds, especially towards the latter End of it.

The lowest the Thermometer was in the Morning, was at 73°F; the highest was at 77°F; the lowest it was at Noon, was at 78°F; and the highest at Noon was at 82°F. The lowest the Barometer, was at 29.7½ [inches of mercury]; and the highest was at 29.8½ [inches of mercury].

Dysenteries, which were very frequent in the Beginning of the last Month, but began to abate towards the latter End of it, almost totally ceased in this.

Some few had the continued remitting Fever, as in the last Month; and in two or three Patients it now changed to a regular intermitting quotidian Fever:[†] And I saw two Patients who had an intermitting Quotidian [Fever], without having the remitting Fever before it; and these were the first regular intermitting Fevers that I have seen in this Island, except such as were brought hither from some other Places.

And the Bark[†] did not answer in any of these, so as to take the Fever off, as it usually does in England; or as it generally did in those intermitting Fevers which were brought hither, or as it is said to have done in those who had this Fever here formerly: Though various Things were now given with the Bark, in order to make it more effectual; [such] as *Elix. Vitrioli. Acid Camphor,*† the fixed alkaline and volatile salts, Allum, and Nutmeg, *&c.* and cold Bathing. Though the Fever was but moderate, the cold Fit continuing about half an Hour, and the hot Fit four or five Hours, and then it went off entirely by Sweating, as usual, and left the Patient free from any Fever for the Space of fifteen or sixteen Hours; yet the Bark would not answer, though very good: But the following Decoction took it off after giving a Vomit; though a Vomit had been given before the other Medicines also.

Rad. Serpent. Virg. ʒss. Sal. Absinth. ɟii. Misce, Coq. in Aq. pur. xx. ad ʒxii. et cola; Colaturæ adde Tinct. Terræ Japon. ʒi. Misce, Exhibe ʒii. singulis bihoris, vel tertia quaq; Hora absente Paroxismo.†

And I found this the most successful; and I added *Cortex Peruv. ʒi.* to this Decoction for some of them, but I did not find that it answered better than the other.

A.D. *1758*

JANUARY WAS MORE DRY, and also cooler than the last Month, though we had sometimes some small Showers of Rain in it.

The lowest the Thermometer was in the Morning, was at 72°F; the highest at 76°F; the lowest it was at Noon was 76°F; and the highest at Noon was at 81°F. The lowest the Barometer, was at 29.7½ [inches of mercury]; and the highest was at 29.9½ [inches of mercury].

The Dysentery, which began to abate in the last Month, now totally ceased and disappeared in this.

Several Children were seized with an uncommon Disorder in this Month, and we had it among Children here, about six or seven Years since; but I do not remember to have seen it in England, or elsewhere. It chiefly, if solely, seizes Children; for I never saw any but them have it, and none that were above seven or eight Years of Age: They seldom complain, or seem to be much uneasy or unwell, till after a great Number of small angry inflamed Eruptions, like little Boils appear on the Head, Neck and Face, but mostly on the Forehead and Head; and it is most frequent in those who have had a common sore Head, as Children sometimes have, for several Days or Weeks before these appear: Some chance one or two of these Boils suppurate tolerably well; but in general most of them do not, but contain a small tough white or yellowish Core, and not concocted Matter:† Upon, or a little before these Eruptions appear, the Humour which used to be discharged from the sore Head, suddenly dries up, or strikes in,† and the Boils turn to a livid or blackish Colour, and the Skin round them to a small Distance turns pale, and the Boils begin to gangrenesce;† and they now begin to be a little feverish, and have a small, quick Pulse, which is mostly low, and they have a great inward Heat, and Thirst, though not the last always; yet the external Heat is sometimes less than in Health, and sometimes the Extremities are cold, tho' the Pulse is quick, but small and low: In some the Feet and Hands begin to swell, and look pale as if œdematous or dropsical, or as sometimes comes on a Limb before it begins to mortify; a Stupor or Coma comes on, and the Scalp becomes more Livid, and a Mortification, or even a Sphacelus† down to the Cranium, if not on the Brain, comes on also, and they die.†

I have known some, who upon the Humour's striking in, have had all their Limbs become numb, like a slight Paraplegia,† but not a total Loss of either Sensation or Motion, as in a compleat Paraplegia, yet they were numb and in part paralytic: This is a very bad Symptom; but the Coma with a great Lividness of the Cranium, and the œdematous Swelling of the Hands and Feet, are worse, and almost certainly presage the Death of the little Patient, in thirty or forty Hours time, or sooner. I have been called to some in this State, when too late, and have found these Symptoms, and the Scalp down behind the Ears as low as the Neck, quite livid and almost black and mortified, if not sphacelated down to the Cranium; and from the Coma, great Stupor and Insensibility of the Patient, I judged that the Mortification extended to the Brain, or its Meninges.† In some the Fever is a little higher, the Pulse stronger and a little fuller, and the Heat greater, and more equally diffused all over the Body, and to the Extremities; and these [children], provided that the Fever is not very high, which rarely happens, are in less Danger, and if properly treated in time, most commonly recover.

The Intentions of Cure, are to keep the Vis Vitæ and the Fever moderate, neither too high, nor to let it sink too low (which is the greatest Danger) and bring on a Mortification, which, in that vital Part, must almost certainly end in Death. All the whole Tribe of the *Testacea* which are usually given to Children, and in some Cases are of great Service to them, here have no place, and are more hurtful than useful, as being Scepticks;† and the acrid

Antiscepticks are in general too acrid for their tender Stomachs: But as the great Disposition and Tendency to bring on a Mortification on the Parts affected, evidently indicate the best and strongest Antiscepticks to be given, provided that they are neither too acrid, nor too strong for such young tender Patients; [such] as a light Decoction or Infusion of the *Cortex. Peruv. Rad. Serpent. Virg. Croci Anglic. Vinum Croceum, Spir. Mindereri, Spir. Lavendul. C. &c.*† properly adapted to the Age and Strength of the Child, are the most suitable, and promise the best Success: And a warming Fotus† to the Head, made of aromatick antisceptick Herbs, [such] as *Fol. Piementi, Viburnii Salvae Rorismarin. Flor. Chamemel. Sambuc. &c.*† applyed warm three or four times a Day; and opening the Boils with a Launcet, as soon as they are ripe and fit to be opened, and dressing them with a warm Digestive,† [such] as *Liniment. Arcæi,*† *&c.* and then covering the Dressings and the whole Scalp, with the *Cataplasm. Maturans.*† I have found this Method, if taken in time, always to be the best and the most successful.

Towards the latter end of this Month, the exanthematous Eruption, commonly called the Chicken-pox, began to appear again in some Parts of the Town.

The MONTH of FEBRUARY was more dry than the last month, and continued to be cool and pleasant Weather, though we had some small Showers.

The lowest the Thermometer was in the Morning, was at 72°F; the highest at 74°F; the lowest it was at Noon, was at 76°F; and the highest was at 80°F. The lowest the Barometer, was at 29.8½ [inches of mercury]; and the highest was at 29.9½ [inches of mercury].

As this Month was in general very dry, and also moderately cool and pleasant Weather, it was also very healthful; so that we had not any Diseases which could be properly called epidemical, except the above-mentioned gangresescent Boils on the Heads of Children, which still continued, and were fatal to some; and the Chicken-pox.

MARCH continued to be very dry, rather more dry than the preceding Month, and likewise cool and pleasant Weather.

The lowest the Thermometer was in the Morning, was at 73°F; the highest at 76°F; the lowest it was at Noon, was at 78°F; and the highest at Noon, was at 81°F. The lowest the Barometer, was at 29.8½ [inches of mercury]; and the highest at 29.9½ [inches of mercury].

This Month was also no less pleasant and healthful than the last, for we had no Diseases that were epidemical in either of them, except the above-[mentioned] gangrenescent Boils, and the Chicken-pox; till after the Middle of the Month, when some few were seized with Coughs and Catarrhs, and a few had a Quinsey; but these were neither bad, nor many, neither did they continue long, for they as well as the gangrenescent Boils and sore Head, all disappeared before the End of the Month, and the Season became very healthful.

The MONTH of APRIL also continued to be very dry, though we sometimes had some Clouds, yet we had little or no Rain; and towards the latter End of the Month, the Weather grew very warm, as usual at this Time.

The lowest the Thermometer was in the Morning, was at 75°F; the highest at 79°F; the lowest it was at Noon, was at 78°F; and the highest was at 84°F. The lowest the Barometer, was at 29.8 [inches of mercury]; and the highest was at 29.9½ [inches of mercury].

The Season continued to be pretty healthful most of this Month, but the Weather begun to be warm towards the latter end of it; when some few inflammatory Diseases began to appear, [such] as a few Pleurisies, Peripneumonies, and some few Quinseys, but not many; but several Children were seized with a suffocating Catarrh,[†] in which the Glottis, Epiglottis, Bronchia, and sometimes the Lungs, were much inflamed, and they breathed with much Difficulty, though they could most commonly swallow Liquids tolerably well; their Pulse was quick, and mostly full and hard, their Blood was inflamed, florid, and dense, and generally sizzy soon after; their Skin was hot, and the Fever and Inflammation usually high. It generally seized Children of two or three Years old, and those that were younger; and when the Inflammation of the above-mentioned Parts was great, it soon suffocated them, if not speedily relieved by Bleeding, and the Use of Antiphlogisticks, &c. and several young Children died of it. Those who were elder, especially if almost grown to be young Men and Women, got more easily over it, and soon recovered by the following antiphlogistic Method of treating it.

Bleeding pretty largely *pro ratione Ætatis et Inflammationis*, at the first Beginning of the Disease, and giving antiphlogistic Pectorals freely, and keeping the Body open by cooling gentle eccoprotic[†] Catharticks, and Clysters (not strong or drastic Purgatives), Fomentations and emollient repelling Cataplasms to the Breast and Throat, were of the greatest Service, and the most successful.

The MONTH of MAY continued to be very dry, and also very warm, and very little Rain fell in all this Month, except a few small Showers.

The lowest the Thermometer was in the Morning was at 76°F; the highest at 80°F; the lowest it was at Noon, was at 82°F; and the highest at Noon was at 85°F. The lowest the Barometer, was at 29.8½ [inches of mercury]; and the highest was at 29.9½ [inches of mercury].

Tho' the Month of May continued to be very dry and warm, yet a great Part of it continued to be pretty healthful, and the Season did not begin to be more sickly, till after the hot Weather had continued three or four Weeks, when inflammatory Diseases began to increase and be more frequent; [such] as Ophthalmies, Quinseys, Peripneumonies, and Pleurisies, though we had not a great many of these during the Month: We also had some Vertigoes, and a few Apoplexies, and Palsies, and but few; so that it might be called a tolerable healthful Season.

On the thirtieth of this Month, I discontinued these Observations, and returned to England, and I now publish them for the benefit of the Inhabitants of that Island, and sincerely wish that they may be of Service to them and all theirs.

Part II

A TREATISE
ON SUCH DISEASES
AS ARE
The most frequent in, or are peculiar to, the
WEST-INDIA ISLANDS, or the TORRID-ZONE,
both Acute and Chronical.

Of the PUTRID BILIOUS FEVER, *commonly called the*
YELLOW FEVER

THIS DISEASE is most commonly known by the Name of the Yellow Fever, from a Yellowness like the Jaundice which diffuses itself all over the Body of the Sick, towards the latter end of the Disease. The French call it *La Maladie de Siam*, from its being frequent in the Kingdom of Siam† in the East-Indies, which is situated between the Tropicks,† near the same latitude as the West-India Islands: They also call it *La Fievre Matelotte*, because Strangers and Sea-faring People are the most obnoxious to† it: And the Spaniards call it *Vomito Preto*, or Black Vomiting, from one of its dangerous Symptoms. I shall not enter into any Dispute about the Name of this Fever, or the Propriety or Impropriety of calling it a Putrid Bilious Fever, (tho' some have objected to this),† as that is only a Dispute about Words. But as we have no Account of this Disease in the Ancients, not even in the *Arabian Writers*, who lived and practiced in the hot Climate; we must give it some Name, and I think this is the most suitable to the Nature of the Symptoms of the Disease.

From the best and most authentic Accounts that I can obtain, as also from the Nature and Symptoms of the Disease, it appears to be a Fever that is indigenous to the West-India Islands, and the Continent of America which is situated between, or near to the Tropicks, and most probably to all other Countries within the Torrid Zone. But I cannot conceive what were the Motives, which induced a late ingenious Author[†] to think that this Fever was first brought from Palestine to Marseilles, and from thence to Martinique, and so to Barbados, about thirty-seven Years since. A better Enquiry would have informed him, that this Fever had frequently appeared in this and the other West-India Islands, many Years before: for several judicious Practitioners, who were then and are now living here, whose Business was visiting the Sick, the greatest Part of their Life-time, some of them almost eighty Years of Age, remember to have seen this Fever frequently in this Island, not only many Years before that time, but many Years before that learned Gentleman came to it.[†]

That same Author supposes this Fever to be of the pestilential[†] kind; but his Reasons for it are chiefly founded on the same Supposition, that it proceeded from the Plague then raging in Marseilles. But a more strict Inquiry into the Nature of its Symptoms, and a better Examination of the State of the Blood of those who labour under it, would have sufficiently shewed him that it was a very different Fever: to which I may add, its not spreading and infecting others, as the Plague always does; for this Fever very rarely or never is infectious or contagious to others,[†] not even to those who attend the Sick, except a chance Time, when it is in its most putrid malignant State at the latter end of the Disease; or soon after the Death of the Patient, when the Season is very hot, and this Fever is accompanied with the Symptoms of some other malignant Fever which is then epidemical and contagious, as happened once at *Antigua*, and once or twice in this Island;[†] and the same may probably have happened in some other Places: but I never could observe any one Instance, where I could say that one Person was infected by, or received this Fever from, another Person who had it; neither have I even seen two People sick in this Fever in the same House at or near the same Time, unless they were brought into the same House when they had the Fever upon them before they came. From whence we may conclude, that it has nothing of a contagious or pestilential Nature in it: And that it is a very different Fever in all Respects, as will more fully appear hereafter.

It is remarkable that this Fever most commonly seizes Strangers, especially those who come from a colder, or more temperate Climate, to this much warmer; and most readily those who use vinous or spirituous Liquors too freely; and still more readily those who labour Hard, or use too violent Exercise, and are at the same time exposed to the Influence of the scorching Rays of the Sun in the Day-time, and soon after expose themselves too suddenly to the cool Dews and damp Air of the Night, and especially if they drink spirituous Liquors too freely at the same time: Hence the poor unthinking Sailors too frequently become a Prey to this too often fatal Disease.

It does not appear from the most accurate Observations of the Variations of the Weather, or any Difference of the Seasons, which I have been able to make for several Years past, that this fever is any way caused, or much influenced by them: For I have seen it at all Times, and in all Seasons of the Year, in the coolest, as well as in the hottest time of the Year: except that I have always observed that the Symptoms of this (as well as most other Fevers) are generally more acute, and the Fever usually higher, in a very hot Season, especially if it was preceded by warm, moist Weather, than it usually is when it is more cool.

This Fever most commonly seizes the Patient, at the first with a Faintness, then a Sickness at the Stomach, and mostly with a Giddiness in the Head, soon after with a small Chilliness and Horror,[†] very rarely with a Rigor, which is soon followed by a violent Heat, and high Fever, attended with acute darting Pains in the Head and Back; *a Flushing in the Face, with an inflamed Redness and a burning Heat in the Eyes; great Anxiety and Oppression about the Præcordia; these and the burning Heat and Pain in the Eyes are* the pathognomic[†] Symptoms of this Fever, especially when accompanied with *Sickness at the Stomach, with violent Reachings,[†] and bilious yellow Vomitings, and great Anxiety with frequent Sighing.* The Pulse is generally now very quick, high, soft, and sometimes throbbing, never hard; in some it is very quick, soft, low, and oppressed; a quick, full, and sometimes difficult Respiration: the Skin is very hot, and sometimes dry, tho' more frequently moist. Blood taken from the Patient, even at the first Beginning of the Disease, is often of an exceeding florid red Colour, much rarefied and thin, and without the least Appearance of Sizeness,[†] and the Crassamentum, when it has stood till it is cold, will scarce cohere, but fluctuates; the Serum is very yellow: most of the above-mentioned

Symptoms continually increase, and are much aggravated; the Reaching and Vomiting become almost incessant, the Anxiety great, and Sighing frequent, great Restlessness, continual Tossing, no Ease in any Posture, little or no Sleep, and that disturbed, uneasy, and without any Refreshment to the Sick: And when they are fainting they turn yellow about the Face and Neck instead of turning pale, and as the Fainting goes off, they recover their natural Colour again. These Symptoms generally continue to the third Day, tho' sometimes not longer than the first or second Day, in others to the end of the fourth Day; the first shews the quicker Dissolution of the Blood, and greater Malignity of the Disease, but the last contrary, or the less Degree of it; which the improper Manner of treating the Disease sometimes hastens and increases, or the proper Method retards. This may be called the first Stadium[†] of the Disease, and most commonly ends on the third Day.

Blood taken from the Sick on the second or third Day, is much more dissolved,[†] the Serum more yellow, and the Crassamentum florid, loose, scarce cohering, but undulates like sizzy Water when shaken, and sometimes has dark blackish Spots on its Surface, shewing a strong gangrenescent Diathesis.

About the third Day, the Pulse, which was quick and full before, now generally sinks greatly, and becomes very low,[†] tho' sometimes it remains very quick, yet in others it is not much quicker than when the Patient is in Health, but is always low; the Vomiting grows porraceous,[†] and almost incessant, if not so before, and the Patient begins to be comatous, attended with interrupted Deliria.[†] The Thirst in some great, in others not much; the Pulse still low and quick, attended with cold clammy Sweats, and sometimes with Deliquia.[†] The Eyes, which were inflamed and red[†] before, and began to be of a more duskish[†] Colour, now turn yellow; this Yellowness also soon appears round the Mouth, Eyes, Temples and Neck, and soon diffuses itself all over the Body. This total Yellowness is so far from being always an encouraging Prognostic,[†] as Dr *Town*[†] says, that it most commonly, on the contrary, proves a mortal Symptom; as it, when it comes on, shews a greater Coagulation and Dissolution of the Blood, and a gangrenescent State of the Fluids. I grant that this yellow suffusion[†] of Bile upon the Surface of the Body has, at a chance time (tho' very seldom), proved critical;[†] but then it did not come on till the eighth or ninth Day, nor appear till the Coma, and all the other bad Symptoms began to abate, and as the Yellowness increases, they all decrease; but this very rarely happens. But this Yellowness is most commonly quite the reverse, especially when it comes soon on, and is not only symptomatical, as it arises from the colliquated,† putrid, dissolved and gangrenescent State of the Blood; but it too often ushers in all the last and most fatal Symptoms of the Disease, *viz.* a deep Coma, a low vermicular† and intermitting Pulse, great Hæmorrhages from various Parts of the Body, a Delirium, with a laborious and interrupted Respiration, great Anxiety, deep Sighing, great Restlessness, a Subsultus Tendinium, great Coldness of the extreme Parts first and then all over the Body, a Faltering of the Speech, Tremors, Convulsions and Death. So that from the first Appearance of this symptomatical Yellowness, we may say, the Patient is in the last Stage of the Disease, how soon soever it may come on; tho' in some it has not come on till the eighth or ninth Day, and then is usually critical, but this very rarely happens.

It has also been observed, that in some sanguine strong Constitutions, when they have not been bled to a sufficient Quantity in the first, second, or third Days of the Disease, to restrain its Violence, the Pulse has continued full, strong, and rapid, but never hard, the Face flushed, Eyes inflamed, the Tongue dry, with great Thirst and Heat, till the second or last Stage of the Fever is come on, when the Pulse has suddenly sunk, and Death has soon after ensued: Yet in others, who seemed to have plethorick Habits, the Tongue has been moist all along, tho' they have been delirious most of the time, and the Heat of their Skin, and the Strength and Quickness of their Pulse has continued, after the first Stage of the Disease was over, pretty near to that of their natural State of Health, till within a few Hours of their Death; and when they have had a Coma on them, one who is not well acquainted with this Fever, would from their Pulse, Heat, Breathing, and other Symptoms, have taken them to be in a natural Sleep. Others, when the Pulse has begun to sink, and the fatal Period seemed to be just approaching, to the great Surprise of all present, the Patient has recovered his Senses, sat up, and talked pretty cheerfully for an Hour or two, and in the midst of this seeming Security, has been suddenly seized with strong Convulsions, and died immediately.†

I mentioned Hæmorrhages before, for in the latter Stage of this Fever, the Blood is so attenuated and dissolved, that we frequently see it flowing, not only out of the Nose and Mouth, but from the Eyes, and even through the very Pores of the Skin; and also great Quantities of black half-baked, or half-mortified Blood is frequently voided, both by Vomiting and by Stool, with great Quantities of yellow and blackish putrid Bile by the same ways; and the Urine, which was before of a high ictericious† Colour, is now almost black, and is frequently mixed with a considerable Quantity of half-dissolved Blood.

The Pulse, which was much sunk before, now becomes very low, unequal and intermitting; the Breathing difficult and laborious; and the Anxiety becomes inexpressible, and an Oppression with a burning Heat about the Præcordia comes on, tho' the Extremities are cold, and often covered with cold clammy Sweats; a constant Delirium, and then a total Loss of Reason and the outward Senses, with livid Spots in many Parts of the Body, especially about the Præcordia, and sometimes Gangrenes in other Parts of the Body, which are soon followed by Death.

And soon after Death the Body appears much fuller of livid large blackish mortified Spots, particularly about the Præcordia and Hypoconders,[†] especially the Right; which Parts seem even from the first Seizure, to be the principal Seat of this terrible Disease. And upon opening the Bodies of those who die of it, we generally find the Gall-Bladder and Biliary Ducts turgid, and filled with a putrid blackish Bile; and the Liver, and Stomach, and adjoining Parts, full of livid blackish mortified Spots, and sometimes Gangrenes, in those, as also in several other Parts of the Body. And the whole Corpse soon putrefies after Death, and can but be kept a few Hours above Ground.

From an attentive Consideration of all the Symptoms which attend this Disease, and a strict Examination of the putrid State, and dissolved gangrenescent Condition in which we find the Blood of those who labour under it; as well as the half-putrefied and mortified State in which the Body is found immediately after their Death: Whether this Fever proceeds from infectious Miasmata, or it arises from the great Heat of the Air, and Water, and the Putrefaction of our Fluids, &c. from thence, and is thereby *indigenous* to those Countries which are situated within the Torrid Zone; or whatever is its *procatarctic Cause*; it evidently appears from all the Symptoms that attend it, as well as from their putrid Effects, that a bilious putrefying Diathesis, is actually introduced into the Blood and all the circulating Fluids of the Body, whereby not only the first and second Concoctions,[†] or the Chylification[†] and Sanguification[†] of the Blood are so disturbed, altered and changed, that all the Humours, and particularly the Bile, are by the rapid Motion of the Blood and greatly increased Heat of the Body, so inquinated[†] with a putrid bilious Acrimony,[†] which in a little time so attenuates and dissolves the Texture of the Blood, that it runs off by the various excretory Passages, and the Pores, but also *Errores Loci Fluidorum* are produced, whence the Brain is affected, and all animal Functions so disturbed and altered, and the Texture of the

Blood is so dissolved, that all the Humours of the Body are almost changed into a putrescent lethiferous† Ichor,† (if not timely prevented) which must inevitably end in Death.

That the Bile has a great, if not much the greatest Share in producing this Fever, and this putrid gangrenescent State of the Blood, I think is too evident to be doubted; notwithstanding what a late ingenious Author† has said to the contrary: For it is well known, that the Bile will putrefy much sooner, and to a much higher Degree of Acrimony, than any other Humour in all the human Body, and also will dissolve the Texture of the Blood much sooner: And we not only observe that a great Quantity of deep yellow and almost black, putrescent, acrid Bile, is constantly discharged both upwards and downwards,† even from the first Beginning of this Disease; and the Suffusion of it all over the Body afterwards, confirms the same; and we also find upon opening the Bodies of those who die of it, that the Gall-bladder, and its Ducts, are always found turgid with a porraceous, blackish, putrescent Bile; and we likewise observe, that the Hypochonders, especially the Right, and the adjoining Præcordia, are the most affected throughout the whole time of the Disease, which is the Seat of the Liver and Gall-bladder; insomuch, that the same Author says, "it seems to be the Seat and Throne of the Disease". And I have always observed, that the Sick cannot bear the least Pressure of one's Hand, upon the Parts where the Gall-bladder and biliary Ducts and the Liver are situated.

No doubt but when the Blood is once inquinated by this putrescent bilious Humour, that the great Relaxation of the Solids, and the great Diminution of the Momentum of the Fluids, subsequent to and arising from thence, and which generally comes on in the third Day, or soon after, with the second State of the Disease, does greatly contribute to produce the putrescent Diathesis, and increase the gangrenescent Disposition of the Fluids and Solids, which always attends the latter Stage of the Disease.

From all the above-mentioned Symptoms, and from the Nature, Disposition, and State of the Humours, which are consequential to them, we must endeavour to deduce our Indications and Intentions of Cure; since we have none of the Ancients to follow, or to direct us, nor yet to appeal to; as none of them has ever mentioned, or probably ever seen, this Disease; neither have I seen any modern Author, except the above-quoted Author, from whom I must beg Leave to dissent, because I cannot think as he does; wherefore I drew up the following Intentions of Cure, which are:

Firstly: *To moderate the too great and rapid Motion of the Fluids, and abate the too great Heat and Violence of the Fever, in the two first Days of the Disease, as safely and as much as we can.*

Secondly: *To evacuate and carry out of the Body, as much of that putrid Bile and those putrid Humours, as expeditiously and as safely as possibly we can.*

And thirdly: *To put a Stop to the putrescent Disposition of the Fluids, and prevent the Gangrenes from coming on, by suitable Antiscepticks.*

For it is observed, that most, if not all, who die of this Disease, generally have, and die of, Mortifications, either internally or externally, or both.

And as this Fever and most of its Symptoms, are generally great and violent, and the Pulse very quick and full, the Heat of the Patient is most commonly very great; since Heat, or Fire, is always collected in proportion to the Quantity of Matter, multiplied by its Quantity of Motion, or as the Momentum of the circulating Fluids is; and this being very great, consequently the first Intention of Cure, *viz., To moderate the too great and rapid Motion of the Fluids, and abate the Heat and Violence of the Fever, in the two first Days of the Disease*, is indicated, and is absolutely necessary: And as it is well known to Physicians, and may be demonstrated by hydraulic Laws, that by lessening the Quantity of the Blood, we diminish its Motion, and consequently abate the Violence of the Heat and Fever: Wherefore Bleeding, in the Beginning of the first Stage of this Fever, either to a greater or less Quantity, accordingly as the following Symptoms and Circumstances indicate, is always absolutely necessary: And the Quantity to be taken away should always be as the Age and Strength of the Patient, the Degree of the Plethora, and the greater or less elastic State of his Solids, the Fullness of his Pulse, and the Violence of the Fever and its Symptoms. For which Reasons, when I have been called in time (which is too seldom the Case) I generally order 12, 14, 16, 18, or 20 Ounces of Blood† to be taken away, on the first or second Day; but always as the above-mentioned Symptoms and Rules indicate and direct: And if the Patient's Pulse rises after the first Bleeding, or if the Fever continue to be still high and the Pulse full (for it is never hard in this Fever), I repeat the Bleeding once, in the first or second Day of the Disease, if the above-mentioned Symptoms indicate it: but Bleeding a third time is seldom or never required, neither is Bleeding on the third Day almost ever required; and when it is performed on that Day, it ought not to be advised without great Caution and Judgment; neither should a Vein be opened after the third Day in this Fever, unless some very extraordinary Symptoms and Circumstances require it, which very rarely or never happen: Because the Pulse generally sinks to be low on that Day, or very soon after it, when Bleeding must be greatly prejudicial, as the Blood is then in a dissolved State, and the Pulse sunk low, which it now must sink lower, by diminishing the Momentum of the Fluids, and consequently increase their gangrenescent Disposition, and so bring on a Mortification and Death. These probably were the Reasons why the before-mentioned Author advised not to bleed at all in this Fever; but as the Pulse is generally so exceeding quick and full, and the Heat and Violence of the Fever so great in the two or three first Days of it, it is absolutely necessary to abate and moderate them, by taking some Blood away in those Days, otherwise that violent Heat and rapid Motion of the Blood, arising from that putrescent bilious Acrimony, so attenuates and dissolves it, that it brings on more fatal Consequences much sooner, as I have more than once or twice observed; and I have always found that taking away a moderate, but sufficient Quantity of Blood on the first or second Days has rendered the Fever more moderate, and abated the putrescent Diathesis afterwards: But as to the Quantity of Blood to be taken away in this Case, either the first or second time, or on the first or second Days, it is impossible to ascertain it, since that must be different in different Patients; because some Constitutions can better bear the loss of fifty Ounces of Blood, than others can the Loss of eight or ten; therefore the only Rules that can be given, are those laid down before.[†]

After Bleeding, we come to the second Intention of Cure; which is, *to evacuate and carry off as much of the bilious putrid Humours, as soon and as safely as we can.*

The great Irritation of the Stomach, by the putrid bilious Humours which constantly attend this Fever, with almost continual Reachings and violent Vomitings, seem to indicate giving an Emetic; but the Coats of the Stomach, I have always observed, are here so violently stimulated and irritated, and most commonly inflamed by the Acrimony of the putrescent Bile, that any Emetic, even the most gentle, and mild, and small Dose, generally brings on such an incessant Vomiting, that it continues in spite of all Remedies, till an Inflammation and Mortification of the Stomach comes on, which soon ends in Death; as I have too often observed, when called in after they have been given: Neither could I ever find that Antiemeticks, Fomentations, or any other Methods would very seldom avail and prevent it. Wherefore I have always strictly forbid giving any Emeticks whatever.

But as the carrying off [of] those putrid bilious Humours, before their putrid Acrimony is too much increased by the Heat of the Fever, or is carried into the Blood, is so absolutely necessary; I usually order the Patients to drink large Draughts of warm Water,† to which I sometimes add a little simple Oximel,† or a little small green Tea, in order to carry off those putrid Humours; and they are most commonly very copiously discharged by this Means, and the Patient much relieved thereby, as I have often with Pleasure observed. For here no additional Stimulus to the Coats of the Stomach, is necessary to excite Vomiting, that being already too great; and the warm Water, being a smooth Emollient, acts as a Fotus to the Stomach, and so contributes to prevent those bad Consequences before-mentioned from coming on.

And after the Patient has by this Means vomited seven, eight, or nine times, and discharged a good deal of yellow and blackish bilious Matter, as they generally do, and the Stomach is very well cleansed; in order to gain a Truce and some Respite from their Anxiety, and almost continual Reaching, Vomiting, and Sickness, which are not increased, but somewhat relieved by drinking the warm Water, I usually give *Extract. Thebaic*, *gr. i vel gr. iss*,† and order them to take nothing into their Stomachs for two Hours after it, that they may retain it; and it being in so small a Compass,† they scarce ever reject it: By this Method, the poor distressed Patient gets some Rest and Respite, and all the Symptoms are generally considerably abated, the Reaching and Vomiting either totally cease, or do but seldom return; so that other Medicines may be given and retained on the Stomach, which it could not retain before; such as cooling acid Juleps, or other antiphlogistick and antiseptick Medicines; but neither *Nitre*, nor any Preparations of it, will rarely either agree with or stay on their Stomachs, or if they or the common saline Draughts, though esteemed Antiemeticks, do by chance stay with them, which they seldom do, yet as Attenuants they ought rather to be ranked among the *Ledentia*† in this Disease, however useful they may be, and often are, in most inflammatory and some other Diseases.

And if the Patient has not a Stool or two after drinking the warm Water and Vomiting, it is necessary to give a gentle purging Clyster soon after the Vomiting, and before the Opiate begins to affect the Patient, to evacuate the Excrement, and as much of the bilious putrid Humours as we can: And after six or eight Hours' Rest and Respite, I order a gentle antiphlogistick and antiseptick Purge to be given; in order to carry as much more of those putrid bilious Humours off as we possibly can. Or if the Patient has a Purging before, which sometimes tho' very seldom happens, I order a gentle Dose of toasted Rhubarb to be given, and an antiseptick Anodyne after it has operated, to abate and check the too much purging, but not to stop it; as I have always observed it to be of Service in this Case, provided that it is moderate and not too violent: And I observed that all those who had this Purging, generally did well with it, if the Patient's Strength was but properly supported with suitable Nourishment, and proper antiseptick Medicines; which last are always absolutely necessary in this Fever.

And tho' Purging in many other Fevers, except the second Fever of Small-pox, in the Pleuritis and Peripneumonia Notha,[†] and in a few other Fevers, may be deemed bad Practice; yet in this Fever, as Nature indicated it, I have always found it of singular Service, and the Patient not only greatly relieved by it, but the Disease always rendered more moderate and manageable afterwards: Wherefore whenever a painful burning Heat in the Hypochonders, or about the Præcodia, comes on, I generally give a little Manna and Tamarinds, which seldom or never fails to carry off a good deal of putrid bilious Matter, and that burning pain which causes it, with it; wherefore I generally repeat this Purging, whenever that burning Pain returns and indicates it, and with all the Success we can desire.

I have observed before, that this Fever greatly abates, the Pulse sinks very much and becomes low, and the Heat of the Body becomes moderate on the third Day; tho' the other bad Symptoms continue, and sometimes grow worse, and a Coma comes on, with a great Yellowness diffused all over the Skin, which with the before-mentioned Symptoms, are the distinguishing Characteristicks of this Disease. This extraordinary Change in the Fever, from being very hot and high, and the Pulse very rapid and full, though soft, to become very small and low, and the Patient's Skin which was burning hot before, to become little warmer than when in Health, and sometimes colder, with a Coma and all the other bad Symptoms as above, at the same time, is such a Change, as requires a very different Method of Treatment from what it did in the first two or three Days of the Disease.

For now every Symptom and Circumstance evidently shew, that a Dissolution of the Globules and Texture of the Blood, and a putrescent, colliquative,[†] gangrenescent State of the Fluids, now hasten on apace, with all their fatal Symptoms. Hence the third and last Intention of Cure evidently appears, *viz.*, *To put a Stop to the putrescent Diathesis of the Fluids, and prevent the Gangrenes from coming on.*

In these Circumstances it is absolutely necessary, that the Vis Vitæ, and the Momentum of the circulating Fluids, be increased and kept up in a moderate brisk State; and the most effectual Antisepticks given, to put a Stop to the putrescent Disposition of the Fluids, or Gangrenes will come on.

In these Circumstances the *Cortex. Peruv.* may be thought to be the best, and most likely Medicine to succeed: I grant that its well known Efficacy, in preventing or putting a Stop to Mortifications, promises much; but the Misfortune is, that this Drug is so disagreeable to most Palates, and the Stomachs of the Sick in this Disease are so much affected, and so weak and so subject to reject every thing, even the most pleasant and innocent, that they can very rarely take it in any Shape, and still much fewer can retain it when they have got it down; so that no Stress or Dependence can be laid on it: And the only way that I could get a Patient to take and retain two Doses of the Bark in this Case, was the Extract[†] of it, with a Spoonful or two of Milk and Water, and even thus they could not retain a third Dose of it; wherefore I soon laid aside all future Attempts to give it, foreseeing that it would be in vain, and that we should thereby only lose Time, not to be recovered, and our Patients also, when we might probably save them by another Method; and I am told that several others have tried to give the Bark in this Case, but with no better Success.

The *Radix Serpentaria Virginiana*, is the next best *Antiseptick*, whose extraordinary Effects in stopping the Progress of Gangrenes, has been known for many Years; wherefore I tried it mixed with some others in the following Manner, and with much better Success than I could hope for, or durst[†] expect: For I found that a light Infusion[†] of this Root, not only sat easily on their Stomachs, but it moderately raised the Pulse and Fever, which were now sunk too low, and kept them in an equal moderate State, if prudently given, which is a thing of the greatest Importance at this time of the Fever, as on that chiefly depends the Recovery of the Patient, [and] therefore should be diligently attended to by the attending Physician; and as soon as ever he perceives that the Pulse begins to abate and sink lower, either on the third Day, or sooner, he must immediately begin to give the antiseptick and warmer Medicines, to support the Vis Vitæ. I have found the following Form both the most agreeable to their weak Stomachs, and the most powerful Antiseptick, and indeed the most successful Medicine.

℞ *Rad. Serpent. Virg. ℨij. Croci Angl. ℨss. m. et infund. Vase clauso in Aq. Bul. q.s. per Horam unam ut Col. ℥vi. adde Aq. Menthæ Simp. ℥ij. Vini*

Manderiens. ʒiv. Syr. Croci vel Syr. e Mecon. ʒi. Elix. Vitrioli Acid. gut. q.s. ad gratum acidor. Saporem; m. exhibe Colchl. Duo vel tria singulis horis vel bihoris, vel sæpius pro re nata.[†]

This very rarely fails to sit light and easily on their Stomachs, even when the saline antiemetic Mixtures will not; and often when every thing else is rejected. By the Use of this and proper Nourishment, taken in small quantities, and often, (for when it is given in larger Quantities, the Stomach too often rejects it, and the Patients sink for want of Support); and their Food or Whey should now be made a little stronger of the Wine than before, or than usual in other Fevers: By this Method the Pulse is raised, and usually kept up, and the fever rendered moderate, and the Coma and other bad Symptoms greatly abated, and the Patient usually goes on well. But if after taking this a little while, we find that the Pulse does not rise, and the Heat becomes equal all over the Body, and moderate; but on the contrary, a Coldness of the extreme Parts comes on, and increases, these Medicines must be made more warming, either by increasing the Quantity of the *Rad. Serpent.*[†] and Saffron, or by adding *Vinum Croceum,*[†] or *Confec. Cardiac.*[†] or some such like Medicines, till the Pulse is raised, and the Heat equally expanded all over the Body; and then the Fever may be kept in a moderate State, by giving the before-mentioned antiseptic Julep, or such like Medicine: But not by the Use of *volatile alkaline Salts, or Spirits, [such] as Sal. et Spir. C.C. Salis Ammoniac. Vol. Spir. Vol. Aromat &c.* which dissolve and increase the putrescent State of the animal Fluids, as is well known both by Observation and Experiments, not made on Pieces of dead Flesh, or dead stagnating animal Fluids; but by giving these alkaline volatile Salts and Spirits to the Living, which when they are taken into and mixed with the circulating Blood, do greatly attenuate and dissolve it, and with the Heat of the Body, do bring on a putrescent Diathesis, and a putrid Colliquation of the Fluids, and consequently must be greatly prejudicial in this Fever, which arises from a putrescent bilious Acrimony, and wherein the Fluids are already really in a dissolved putrid gangrenescent State: Whereas the *Rad. Serpent. Crocus, & Elix. Vitrioli*[†] are very powerful Antisepticks, and prevent the Dissolution and Putrefaction of the Blood; and consequently prevent or stop the Hæmorrhages also, which usually come on in this second Stage of the Disease.

It may be expected that the low Pulse, Coma, Delirium, and the Coldness of the extreme Parts, with the Tremors and convulsive Spasms, &c. should induce me to think that Vesicatories are indicated, and that I should both use and advise them. I allow that they seem at the first View to be indicated, but a further Enquiry into the Cause and Nature of these Symptoms, and a due Consideration of the dissolved colliquative State which the Fluids are in, in this Fever; and an Examination into the Effects of the alkaline Salts of the Cantharides,[†] when carried into our Blood, will clearly demonstrate and sufficiently convince us of the contrary: For this Coma, low Pulse, Coldness of the extreme Parts, Delirium, Tremors, and the other bad Symptoms attending this Fever, do not proceed from a Lentor[†] and Viscidity of the circulating Fluids, as in some other Fevers, [such] as the slow nervous Fever, and some others; but from a Dissolution of the red Globules of the Blood, and their being carried into such small Vessels as do not naturally admit them, whence an *Error loci fluidorum in Cerebro, &c.* is produced, and a due Secretion of the nervous and other fine Fluids, or animal Spirits in the Brain, is obstructed or hindered, and a diminished Momentum of the Blood, the Consequence of the former, at the same time: The Application of Vesicatories must increase all these, and render very bad, much worse. But in other Fevers, where these Symptoms arise from a Lentor and Viscidity of the Fluids, which retard and hinder their free Circulation, and due Secretion; Blisters being applied, the Salts of the Cantharides pass into the circulating Fluids, as the Stranguries and increased Motion of the Blood demonstrate, and attenuate, and dissolve the Lentor and Viscidity, and so remove the Cause of those Symptoms, and produce almost surprising good Effects, as we often see when they are judiciously applied, in such Cases. For the same Reasons, the Application of Vesicatories in this Fever, must dissolve the Blood more, which was in a dissolved putrid State before, and render the Disease and all its Symptoms worse.

The Truth of this is confirmed by Observation and Experience; but such is the unreasonable fondness of Blisters, in this Island, and in some other Countries also, almost in every Case where Pain and a Fever seize, that they are too often applied even in Dysenteries, and in the Beginning of inflammatory Fevers, and much too often in this Fever, even in the last State of it, to the great Prejudice of their Patients: There are some few who practice there who know better, but in general from the want of reading such Authors as would inform them better, they ignorantly follow the Practice of their Fathers and Masters, who read very little; and themselves read less, and follow Custom, which has rendered the Use of Blistering almost sacred, and the Fear of Reproach for not using them almost unavoidable, if the Practitioners have not Fortitude and Judgment sufficient to oppose this their unwarrantable and pernicious Use.

This has but too often given me an Opportunity of seeing their bad Effects, especially in this Fever; where I have observed that the Coma, Tremors, Subsultus Tendinum, the Coldness of the extreme Parts, and the low Pulse (tho' this sometimes has been rendered a little quicker, but not more full), have not only not been relieved by their Application, but have been increased thereby, and the Hæmorrhage, which usually attends this Fever, has been hastened on, or if come on before, has been increased by their Application: And I have seen a Vesicatory, which I ordered to be taken off, as I usually do as soon as I come in this Fever, that the Part where it laid was turned black and perfectly sphacelated,† and if the Spine and Ends of the Ribs had not hindered, a large square Passage into the Cavity of the Thorax would have been opened, if the Patient had lived a few Hours after it, but he died two Hours after I came. And the Reflection, that I have never ordered any Vesicatories to be applied in this Fever, and have always strictly forbidden their Application in it, I must say, gives me great Satisfaction.

But let us return to that Method of treating this Disease, which not only seems to be the most rational, but has been found to be the most successful; tho' it may be almost of as much Service to remark the *Ledentia*, as to mention the *Adjuvantia*.† As the Disease advances, the putrescent State of the Fluids increases, if not prevented by the Use of antisceptick Medicines, and observing carefully to keep the Fever in a moderate State, and that it neither rise too high, as it often does in the two or three first Days of the Disease, nor on the contrary sink too low, as it frequently is very subject to be, in the second State of the Disease, and in which there is the greatest Danger: Wherefore, whenever the Fever begins to sink too low, we must endeavour to keep it up in a moderate State; by giving something of the Nature of the before-mentioned antiseptick Julep, which may be made more warming when necessary. And if the Anxiety, with the burning Pain and Tenseness of the Præcordia and Hypochonder return, either alone, or with the Coma, or a Delirium accompanying it, as is too often the Case, and always arises from an Increase or Collection of those putrid bilious Humours, they must be carried off by repeating the antiseptick Purge, as before; and the following Form is what I have always found to agree the best with most Patients, and seldom fails to remove these bad Symptoms.

℞ *Mannæ Calab.* ℥iss. *vel* ℥ii. *Tamerind. Cond.* ℥i. *Tart. Vitriolat. gr. x. M.*

Solv. in Seri Lactis Vino Maderiens. præparat ʒvi. et Cola, Adde Tinct. Senæ. ʒss. Misce, Dividet. in tres vel quatuor Partes, de quibus capiat Æger unam omni hora, donec incipiat purgare.†

This may be made stronger or weaker, as the Strength of the Sick requires; and it seldom fails to carry off a Quantity of yellow and blackish putrid bilious Matter, by which the Patient is much relieved, and the above-mentioned bad Symptoms are either much abated, or totally removed.

And I most commonly find it necessary to repeat this purging every second or third Day, for two or three times; and sometimes, when the Symptoms are very bad, and have not much abated upon taking the first and second Purge, and the Patient has not been treated in the Method before described, or I have not been called in, till late in the Disease, I have found it necessary to repeat the gentle Purging every Day, for four or five Days successively, and with the desired success too. But when I have been called in at the Beginning of the Disease, and treated the Patient in the Method before described, the Repetition of the Purging, is very seldom required more than twice or three times at most, in the whole Course of the Disease; especially if the antiseptick Medicines have been sufficiently taken in the Intervals between the Purging during the whole time of the second State of the Disease; this Method rarely fails to succeed.

This Method has been, and may probably be thought by some others, too simple and easy, to conquer so violent and formidable a Disease: What! only bleed once or twice, and give a little warm Water, and two or three simple Purges, and this simple Julep, to subdue such a terrible Disease! without any fine Boluses,† cordial Volatiles, and Vesicatories! But I must tell such Persons, that the more simple a Method is, if it be but judiciously and fitly adapted to the Nature and Cause of the Disease, it is so much the better, because, *Contraria contrariis medentur.*† And I flatter myself that the Learned and Judicious, will think so with me, especially when they duly consider, that the first and principal Seat of the Disease, is in the Hypochonders, especially the Right, where the Liver and biliary Ducts are seated; and that the Bile, of all the Humours in the Body, does most readily putresce, and that to the highest Degree of Acrimony; and that this putrid acrimonious Bile is, at least some Part of it, carried into the Blood; where its putrescent Acrimony is greatly increased, by the great Heat of the Fever; and as the Bile is a liquid animal Soap, whose Property is to dissolve all such Bodies as are soluble by it, especially the animal Fluids, and this dissolving Property being now greatly heightened and increased by its putrid Acrimony, more readily dissolves the red Globules of the Blood, if not those of the Serum and the finer Fluids also: And the Blood being thus dissolved; and that Dissolution being still heightened and increased by the Heat of the Air, and the Fever, the whole Mass of the Cruor[†] is soon brought into a putrid, colliquative, gangrenescent State, and the dissolved red Globules are carried into such small ferous,[†] lymphatic, or still smaller Vessels, as do not naturally admit them, whence the Brain is affected, and the Coma, Tremors, Convulsions, and all the other Symptoms attending this Disease are produced, as also the Hæmorrhages, and the Blood flowing thro' all or most of the excretory Ducts, from its being so dissolved; also a deep Yellowness suffused all over the Body, with many livid Spots, and Mortifications in various Parts of it; all which arise from the putrescent Bile, and are produced in this manner.

This being the Cause, and this the Manner of producing this Fever, and all its Symptoms; a just Method of reasoning from them makes it evidently appear, that this Method of moderate Bleeding and giving cooling Acids, in the two or three first Days of the Fever, to prevent its being too violent, as it often is, yet being careful not to bleed too much, lest it sink the Patient and his Pulse too much after in the second State of it; and evacuating and carrying off as much of the putrid bilious Humours, both by the warm Water at the first, and by purging after; and then giving the best antiseptick Medicines that the Patients can take, in a liberal manner, as before-mentioned, to prevent the Hæmorrhages and Gangrenes from coming on; not only appeared to be the most rational, and the most judicious, but I found this Method to be much more successful, than more pompous Medicines, or the Methods generally used.

For as I found that all the Methods of treating this Fever, which had been used both in this, and the other Islands, were very uncertain, and too often unsuccessful; it induced me carefully to observe, and attentively to enquire into the Cause and Nature of this Fever, and all its Symptoms, and the above Method of Reasoning first dictated to me this Method of treating it, not long after I came here, and induced me to try it, the first Opportunity I should have, as it appeared to be more rational than any of the others. And an Opportunity soon offered, which I shall beg the Reader's Patience, to relate, as it proved so successful.

A young Man about twenty-four Years of Age, Surgeon to a Guinea Ship,[†] was brought into a House where I was visiting a Patient; he was of a sanguine, robust Constitution, and a Lover of spirituous Liquors, and had been drunk three Days and Nights successively, and in that Condition had run several Races on the hot Sea-shore, near Noon, with the Sailors, in the Heat of the Sun, and to compleat his Folly, laid the last Night after that exercise, in the open Air under a Tamarind-Tree all the Night, where he was seized in the Morning with all the Symptoms of this Fever, in the most violent manner that I have ever seen any one; in this Condition he was brought to the House where I was: His Reaching and Vomiting were so incessant, that he could not get Time to say Yes, or No, to the Questions which I asked, without waiting some time for it, each time; his Eyes were red and inflamed, attended with a burning Heat, as usual in the Beginning of this Fever, and he had all the other Symptoms which attend the first Attack of this Fever, in the most violent manner, which I need not repeat. I ordered [16 ounces] of Blood to be taken from him, which was very florid, thin, and much dissolved, and then directed him to drink warm Water freely, and to vomit eight or ten times; and after that to take *Extract. Thebaic.* [1½ grains], and take nothing for two Hours after it; but I being gone, and he finding that he vomited with more Ease, less Sickness and Reaching, with the warm Water than he did before, and being much alarmed at his having this Fever, he drank three Gallons of the Water, and brought up great Quantities of yellow and blackish bilious Matter with it, and washed his Stomach effectually. He then took the *Extr. Thebaic.* and slept three or four Hours after it; and the Vomiting ceased: he took some Panada,[†] and four Hours after that, the Purge of Manna and Tamarinds, &c. which gave him eight stools, and carried a good deal more of the putrid bilious Matter off downwards; and got some Rest after it: He then took of an antiseptick Julep often, and light Nourishment a little acid, at the Intervals; and repeated the Purge on the third Day, as directed. I being called out of the Town, I did not see him till the fourth Morning after; he said, that he had followed my Directions, and I found him free from the Fever and all its Symptoms, but weak and low, and his Skin a little Yellow, but much less so than usual, unless when the bilious Matter is thus carried off. I ordered him to take *Elix. Vitrioli Acid. Gut.* [9 drops] three or four times a Day for a few Days, in an infusion of Mint Leaves with a little Snake-root, made as Tea, which he did; and soon recovered perfectly well, in seven or eight Day's time.[†]

This Patient being seized in so violent a manner, and recovering in so short a time, and so near to the Rule which the elegant *Celsus*[†] recommends, *Citò, tutò, et jucundè*,† not only confirmed the above manner of Reasoning on the Cause and Nature of this Disease to be right, but made me determine to follow the same Method as near as I possibly could ever since, and I must add, with the same good Success also, when I am called so early on in the Disease that I can strictly pursue it: which is too seldom the Case; for in general the Physician is not called in till the fourth or fifth Day, or after, when the putrid acrid bilious Matter is, a great Part of it, carried into the Blood, which it has so dissolved and brought its whole Mass into a colliquated, putrid, gangrenescent State, that the best of Methods, and the most efficacious Medicines, however judiciously timed and applied, are precarious and uncertain; or sometimes it is so far advanced, that the ablest Physician can do no more than tell the Relations of the Sick, that it is too late, and that they can live but a few Hours: For I know no Disease in which the Recovery of the Patient, so much depends upon the right or wrong Method of treating it, at the very first Attack or Beginning of the Disease, as this Fever does: For by thus discharging and carrying the putrid, acrimonious, bilious Matter, out of the Body, before much of it is carried into the Blood, not only most of the bad Symptoms which attend the second State of the Fever are prevented from coming [on], but the Hæmorrhages, and the Yellowness of the Skin, &c. also, and the Fever soon taken off too; for I have never seen any Hæmorrhage come on, and but little Yellowness, or in some none, when they were thus treated.

And when the last Stage of the Fever is come on before we are called in, provided that it is not at the very latter End of it, I have always found that this Method of gentle Purging, whenever the before-mentioned Symptoms indicate it, and a liberal Use of the antispetick Medicines in the Intervals, has been so successful, that I have seen but two Patients that have died in this Fever during the eight Years past, in which I treated it in this manner; and one of them was so weak that he could not take a Spoonful of any thing, and so near his End, that he died about two Hours after without taking any Medicine; and the other killed himself by drinking a Gallon of cold Water in less than three Hours' time (after taking half an ounce of Manna in the Morning), which struck such a Coldness into his whole Body that he died; tho' I have visited several every Year, and in some Years a great many: therefore I take the Liberty of recommending this Method to others, and wish it to be as successful to all.

I have said little of the dietetic Part of Cure in this Disease, tho' it is necessary to say something, especially as their Stomachs are generally so very weak, and so much irritated by the acrid Bile, that they almost reject every thing, and can but often retain very little. It may be said that their Diet must be thin, light, and little; but these Qualities alone are not sufficient in this Disease, for it must be made as pleasant and as palatable as possible, in the three first Days of it; and as much antiseptick as possible to be made also agreeable, or otherwise they will neither be able to take or retain it. As,

℞ *Panis bene. Fermentati leviter cocti ʒiv. Coq. in Aq. Pur. per horam, tum tere diu, dein preme per linteum densissimum ut sit Liquoris sic parati ℔ iss. cui immisce Limonii maturi talcolatim scissi ʒi. Nucis Moscat. in Polinem triti ʒi. Servetur usui; Sumat Æger omni bi-hori ʒii vel ʒiii. tempore usus admiscendo Vini Maderiensis ô et Sacchari quantum placet Palato Ægri.*†

Or Pearl Barley† may be boiled, and mixed in the same manner; also Madeira, or Rhenish Wine-whey,† and given often, and in small Quantities, during the two or three first Days of the Fever. But after the third Day, when the Pulse begins to sink, and the Fever is too low, it is absolutely necessary that both the Food and Drink should be made more antiseptick, and more generous and warming by increasing the Quantity of Wine in the Panada, and the Whey, especially if the Patient's Pulse and the Fever are too low; and if he has been accustomed to drink Wine pretty freely; or if the Fever be very low, and the Patient be faint, I sometimes order him a Glass of old Hock,† or old Madeira Wine, alone, or sometimes mixed with a little Water; and I find them to be much better Cordials, than the hot spirituous compound Waters of the Shops are, in this Fever; and sometimes I order a Beverage of Water, Lemon-juice, Sugar, and Madeira Wine, of which they drink a little and often, to assist the antiseptick Medicines to raise the Pulse, and keep the Fever in a moderate State.

And we must now carefully avoid giving any thing, either as Nourishment or in Medicine, that is of a septic Nature, or that has the least Tendency to putresce; but on the contrary both Diet and Medicines should be as much of the antiseptick Nature as they can be made, so as to make them suitable in all other Respects; and that not only in this Case, but in all other Diseases the Physician ought to take care that the Diet of the Sick be of the same Disposition, and have the same Tendency, as the Medicines which he prescribes for them have; for if they are of contrary Natures, and have opposite Effects, they will do little Service, and seldom be attended with Success, how good and efficacious soever the Medicines may be; since the Quantity of the first taken into the Body, and mixed with our circulating Fluids, in all Cases so far exceeds the Quantity of the last, that if they are of opposite and contrary Natures, they must at best only destroy each other, and consequently the Medicines can have but little Effect. This, I think, is a material thing, which I think is but too much neglected in Practice, at least by some, wherefore I take the liberty to mention it here.

Of the DRY GRIPES, or DRY BELLY-ACHE

THIS COLIC is most commonly called the Dry-gripes, and dry Belly-ache, and is a most painful Disease, which frequently seizes the Inhabitants of the West-India Islands, and the Continent of America, and especially the Strangers who come to reside there; and sometimes, though very rarely, some of the Inhabitants in England, and some other Parts of Europe: For I have seen several Patients in this Disease, when I resided at Bath, who never had been out of England, as also did Dr *Sydenham* long before. I think that *Riverius*[†] is the first that mentions it, and calls it Colica Pictonum, the Colic of Poictiers, a Province in France, where it was first taken notice of.[†]

Those who have thin dry Constitutions, and are much emaciated by excessive Perspiration and Sweating, or labour under great Anxiety and Affliction of Mind, or are immoderate drinkers of spirituous Liquors, especially such as are fiery and new; or those who are very irregular in the Use of the six Non-naturals, and especially those who live in America, and the West-India Islands, are the most subject to this cruel Disease; to which Countries it seems to be endemial.

It generally seizes the Patient with an acute Pain at the Pit of the Stomach, which extends itself down with griping Pains to the Bowels, which are soon after much distended with Wind, with frequent Reachings to vomit, which sometimes bring up small Quantities of Bile and Phlegm. An obstinate Costiveness, yet sometimes attended with a Tenesmus, and the Bowels seem to the Patient as if they were drawn up towards the Back, at other times they are drawn into hard Lumps, or hard Rolls, which are plainly perceptible to the Hand on the Belly, by strong convulsive Spasms: And sometimes the Coats of the Intestines seem to be contracted and drawn up from the Anus, and down from the Pylorus, towards the Part first and most affected near the Navel, as to the Centre of their Misery: The Fæces, when they are discharged afterwards, are in little hard dry Lumps like Bullets; the Belly usually continues most obstinately costive, and the Patient discharges but little Urine, and that often with Pain and much Difficulty. The Pulse is generally low, though often a little quicker from the acute Pain, but no Fever, nor any Symptoms of an Inflammation of the Parts affected, either perceptible by the Pulse, or any other Symptoms; though one Year I saw two or three Patients in this Disease, who had some inflammatory Symptoms, and their Blood was a little sizzy, when inflammatory Fevers were epidemical, and they probably had got a little Cold just before; but this rarely happens.[1] The extreme Parts of the Body are often cold, and sometimes the violence of the pain causes cold clammy Sweats, and Faintings: Their Mind is generally much affected, and their Spirits sunk very low. And when this Distemper has been improperly treated, this State of Costiveness, Pain, and Misery has continued twenty or thirty Days, and sometimes longer; for I remember a Case which being thus treated in a wrong Manner, the Patient continued, with some small Intervals of being something easier, in this painful Condition for six Months, or more, and then recovered by a different Method of treatment, in one Week's time. When the Sick fall into the Hands of those who treat them in this wrong Manner, the pain continues to be very violent, and at times almost intolerable, and that for a long time; and then the Patient's Breath commonly acquires a strong, fœtid, stercoraceous Smell, like Excrements, from a long Retention of the Fæces, and an Absorption of the putrid Effluvia from them into the Lacteals,[†] by the strong convulsive Contractions of the Guts: And when the Pain in the Bowels has continued long, and at last begins to abate, a Pain in the Shoulder-points, and adjoining Muscles, comes on, with an unusual Sensation and Tingling along the spinal Marrow;[†] which soon after extends itself from thence to the Nerves of the Arms and Legs, and they become weak, and that Weakness increases till those extreme Parts become paralytic, with a total Loss of Motion, though a benumbed Sensation often remains.

The subtle Cause of this Disease, is sometimes carried by a sudden Metastasis[†] of it to the Brain, and produces a Stupor, or a Delirium; and soon after the whole nervous System is so affected, as to produce strong Convulsions, which are too often followed by Death. At other times, the Violence of the Pain reverts[†] the peristaltic Motion of the Intestines, and violent Vomitings, and all the Symptoms of a *Misereri mei*[†] are produced, and

---

1. See the foregoing *Observations on the Air, and Epidemical Diseases.*

the Patient being exceedingly reduced by the long Continuance of the violent Pain, it is too frequently followed by the same Fate.

The Cause of this Disease will often lay still in the Legs and Arms, without giving the least Sensation of Pain, and sometimes is very suddenly translated from them to the Bowels, or Head; where it instantly produces the most violent Pain, and often fatal Effects: And as this Metastasis is so very sudden, it shews that the Humour, or cause, is exceedingly subtle, as I have often observed; and I will beg Leave to relate a remarkable Case, which I saw in a Gentleman when I lived at Bath.

He had laboured under this painful Disease some Years in Maryland, which at last rendered his Hands and Arms paralytic; and they had continued in that useless State two Years, without any Pain in them all that Time; he had no Strength, and little Motion, but a tolerable Degree of numb Sensation in them: And during these two Years, he was pretty free from any Pain in his Bowels. He came to Bath, drank the Waters, and bathed in them; and I suppose took proper Medicines with them three or four Months, and returned to London without any Relief. The next Spring he came to Bath again, and sent for me, and informed me how he had proceeded the Season before; and then was so exceedingly uneasy at the Loss of the Use of his Hands, and his not being able to write to his Family, that he said he was determined to have the Use of them restored if possible, how dangerous soever the Attempt might be: I told him, that if the Cause or Humour could be removed from his Hands, it probably would return to his Bowels with the same violent Pain as before; or it might possibly be carried to his Brain, with more fatal Effects: He thought that was not possible, as it gave him no Pain in his Hands; and said he was resolved that if I would not try to remove it, some other Person should attempt it; who he was pleased to say, probably could not give him that Assistance as he thought I could, if it did so; and insisted so strongly on my attempting to remove it from his Hands; that at last I unwillingly assented to try: Accordingly he had his Hands and Arms pumped† at the Hot-pump, then anointed with *Liniment Saponac.*† mixed with some chemical Oils, then wrapped up in Flannel, in order to continue their Sweating, and if possible to carry the morbid matter off that way; and to assist which, he took a Draught with *Bals. Peruv. gut.* xxx† immediately after it: He slept well that Night without any Alteration, and repeated all the same Method the Night following, slept, and was easy till towards Morning, when he awakened with the most excruciating Pain in his Bowels, and his hands perfectly restored to their Use and Motion, as well as ever before. The Pain in his Bowels was now so violent, that he desired the Attendants to shoot him, or put an end to his Misery any way. Tho' the morbid Matter had laid in his Hands, tho' on their Nerves, for two Years before, without giving the least Sensation of Pain; yet now being removed to his Bowels, it gave him as great Pain as ever before. In this Condition I came to him, and presently gave him a Draught with *Bals. Peruv. gut* xl *Philon. Londin.* ℈i[†] and in less than five Minutes time, the Pain was entirely removed from his Bowels, and his Hands became paralytic as before, in less than a Minute's time, but without any pain in them. This Metastasis was therefore produced by the *Bals. Peruv.* before the Opiate could act; and as the morbid Matter was thus put into Motion, I told him that we would try to carry it off, by only bathing his Hands and Arms in the warm Bath-water[†] every Night, and sweating them in warm Flannel after it, (without either pumping it on them, or using the Liniment) and taking the *Bals. Peruv.* with a corroborating[†] Bitter,[†] in the Bath-water, which he did, and recovered the perfect Use of his Hands, without any Return of the Pain in his Bowels, or elsewhere, in two or three Week's' [*sic*] time.

Various Methods of Cure have been attempted and used in these Parts of the World. As they were so costive, strong Purgatives and Clysters were much used, from the first Appearance of this Disease, almost down to this Time; but all the strong drastic Catharticks, (and the weaker were thought insufficient, as the stronger did not operate) do so irritate the Stomach and intestines, and thereby increase the Pain and the convulsive Contractions and Spasms of the Guts, and rendered them more obstinate and worse; so that these Medicines were generally either sooner or later rejected, almost without ever passing, and the Clysters were mostly returned without having any Effect, but that of increasing the Spasms and Pain: And if they chanced to pass, they so much increased the Pain and convulsive Spasms, that they either inverted the peristaltic Motion of the Intestines, and brought on a *Misereri mei*, or cast the morbid Matter upon the Brain, and produced strong Convulsions; both which most commonly ended in Death: Or if the poor Patient escaped with Life, he lost the Use of his Limbs, and generally dragged on a miserable helpless Life to the End of his Days. This Method was therefore justly exploded[†] several Years since, though I have known it proposed by a Physician of some considerable Practice; tho' in general the Disease and its Nature and Cause, are now better known.

The honest and worthy Dr *Sydenham* treated this Disease (which is some chance times seen in England) with giving *Bals. Peruv. a gut.* xx *ad gut.* xl *bis vel ter in die in pauco Sacchari,*[†] and with much better Success than the Method above, for this is a valuable Medicine in this Case.

The ingenious Dr *Warren* advises a Method of treating this Disease,[†] which is more judicious, and better adapted to the Nature and Cure of it than either of them; and I think that some considerable Improvements in the Knowledge of this Disease, have been made both in its Theory, as also in the Practice, or Manner of treating it, since his Time.

From the Nature and Symptoms of this Disease, the strong convulsive Contractions and Spasms which attend it, without an Inflammation or Fever; and the sudden [metastases] of its Cause, from one Part of the Body to another, which sometimes happens; it plainly appears, that it proceeds from a very subtle Cause, which irritates, and chiefly affects the Nerves; those of the Stomach and Bowels first, whence those painful, strong, convulsive Spasms in them; and sometimes the Brain and whole System of the Nerves, whence the Convulsions; and lastly those of the hands and Feet, whence the Loss of their Motion: And the Disease and its Symptoms being increased and aggravated by such things as irritate and stimulate those Parts, which confirm this Opinion, and at the same time indicate to us the proper Intentions of Cure of it; and they are these,

Firstly. *To abate the Pain, and take off the Irritation of the Nerves, from whence the convulsive Spasms arise.*

Secondly. *To procure a free Passage through the Bowels, and so carry off the morbid Matter that Way, without increasing the Irritation.*

As this Disease proceeds from something which greatly stimulates and irritates the nervous Coats of the Stomach and Intestines, and thereby produces those painful convulsive Contractions and Spasms, which always attend it; it is evident that whatever will abate and take off that Irritation, must take off the convulsive Contractions also, and abate the Pain; and whatever will increase the Irritation, must increase them and the Pain also: And as all Emetics and strong drastic Purgatives, are well known to operate by their stimulating and irritating Quality, so they are found always to increase the convulsive Spasms and Pain, which attend this Disease. And on the contrary, as it is as well known that Opium takes off all Irritation and Pain the most effectually, especially where the Nerves are principally affected; as in this, and the *Opisthotonos*[†] and *Tetany*, and some few other Diseases; wherefore Opium is in this Case a principal Remedy, and often repeated Experience has fully confirmed this: And we have found the following Method of treating this Disease, to be the most safe, expeditious, and successful; and therefore recommend it to others, at least till they can find a better.

When I have been called in, and found the Patient was seized with this Disease, and that the Pain at the Pit of the Stomach, and in the Bowels, was very great, as it generally is; in order to abate that Pain and take off the Irritation and Spasms, I always first give an Anodyne; and have generally found some of the following Forms to answer the best, with Variations *pro re nata*.

℞ *Extracti Thebaic. gr.* ij. *vel* iij. *fi. Pilul.*[†]

Vel ℞ *Philon. Londin.* ℈i. *Extract. Thebaic. gr.* i. *vel.* ij. *Bals. Peruv. gut.* x. *m. fi. Bolus.*[†]

Vel ℞ *Aq. Menthæ Simp.* ℥iss. *Extract. Thebaic. gr.* ij *vel* iij. *Bals. Peruv. gut* xx. *Syr. e Mecon.* ℥ss. *m. fi. Haut. statim sumend.*[†]

By taking one of these, the patient generally finds his Pain much abated, the Irritation is taken off, and the convulsive Contractions of the Intestines also; so that their peristaltic Motion is restored, and the progressive Motion of their contained Fæces is more easily assisted by a soft lenient Eccoprotic,[†] (for most other purgatives increase it,) which must be given as soon as he finds himself tolerably easy: But if the Pain does not cease, or if it returns again, one of the above Opiates, or a somewhat smaller Dose of it, must be repeated till the Patient finds himself tolerably easy: These may be thought too large Doses of the Opium, but I must observe, that small Doses will not answer in this Case, and the Tetany, &c, and they may be given very safely.

But if the Vomiting be so violent (as it sometimes happens) that the patient cannot retain any of these on his Stomach, not even the *Extr. Theb.* which is in so small a Compass,[†] I have found the following most commonly to stay, and take the Vomiting off also.

℞ *Tart. Vitriolat. gr.* x. *Ol. Cinnam. gut.* i. *vel Menthæ gut.* i. *m. exhibe in Cochl.* i. *Aq. Menthæ Simp. et repatur omni hora donec cessant Vomitiones, deinde exhibe Extr. Thebiac. gr.* ij. *vel* iij. *quam primum.*[†]

This most commonly stays the Vomiting, even when the saline anti-emetic Draughts will not, and the Opiate abates the Pain and convulsive Spasms.

But if the Patient be plethoric, and any Symptoms of Inflammation attend, which very rarely happens, ten or twelve Ounces of Blood may be taken away, and his Stomach may be fomented with a proper emollient Fotus, and then these Powders may be given, and the Opiate.

And as soon as the Patient finds himself tolerably easy, I usually begin to give something of the following kind, every two or three Hours, till three or four Stools are obtained.

℞ *Cremor. Tartari. Pulv.* ℥iij. *Tart. Solubil.* ℥iss. *Tart. Vitriolat.* ℈ij. *Ol. Cinnam. vel Menthæ gut.* iij. *mis. fi. Pulv. in Dos.* vi. *divid. de quibus capiat Æger unam secunda vel tertia quaq; hora in vehicul. quovis idon.*[†]

I usually give them in a small Draught of Wine-whey, Mint-tea, Posset-drink,[†] or an Infusion of Bread toasted brown, and infused in boiling water.

After taking these Powders thirty or forty Hours, the Pain which was at the Pit of the Stomach, removes down towards the lower Part of the Belly, where a Sense of Weight is usually observed by the Patient, and presages Stools to follow soon, and generally carries both the Disease and its Cause quite off, sometimes in twenty-four Hours' time, but seldom fails to do it in three Days time: But if Stools are not thus procured, or that Sense of Weight perceived in the lower Part of the Belly, by the Beginning of the third Day, I usually add *Rad. Jalapii. gr.* v. *vel* vi.[†] to each Paper[†] of the Powder, and give *Bals. Peruv. gut.* xv.[†] mixed with a little Sugar, and give it in the Whey with the Powders, which I think never fails to give Stools on or before the fourth Day; for I can truly say, that ever since I treated this Disease in this Manner, which is now above ten Years, I have never met with any Case, where the Patients would take their Medicines regularly, but Stools were procured on the third, or the beginning of the fourth Day at the longest, and often sooner; and the Disease with all its Symptoms were carried off thus with them. But I must observe, that the Opiate must be repeated whenever the pain returns, and as often as it returns, whilst they take these Powders.

And if from some particular Circumstances of the Patient's Constitution, or his not taking the Medicines, or his Stomach not retaining them when taken, the Pain still remains, or returns, and no Stools are obtained; the Opiate must be repeated till the Pain and the Spasms are taken off, or greatly abated, that the other Medicines may take effect; to which purpose, fomenting the Region of the Stomach and all the Abdomen, with an emollient anodyne Fomentation, every six Hours, will be of great Service: Some have recommended a Semicupium,[†] but often without success, as I have more than once observed; and I have always found that fomenting as above, has been of much more Service; as,

℞ *Fol. Altheæ (vel Alcæ)* Miij. *Menthæ Flor. Sambuci Chamemeli ana* Mij. *Sem. Lini.* ℥i. *Sapon. Venet.* ℥i. *Misce: Coq. in Aq.* lbviij. *diende adde Theriac. Androm.* ℥i. *Pisellii Barbadens.* ℥ij. *Spir. Sacchari* lbss. *Misce, fi. Fotus, quo foveant Regionem Ventriculi et Abdom. pannis laneis in fotu tepide intinct, sexta quaq; hora, donec cessant Dolores.*[†]

And a Clyster of the following kind, may be given immediately after the Use of the Fomentation; and I sometimes order an anodyne emollient Liniment to be applied to the Abdomen, after use of the Fotus: As,

℞ *Decotc. Fotu sine Addit.* ʒviij. *Sapon. Venet.* ʒi. *Piselii Barbad.* ʒss. *Bals. Peruv.* ʒi. *Ol. Ricini Americani vel Ol. Palmæ Christi* ʒiss. *m. fi. Enema.*[†]

℞ *Ung. Dialtheæ, Ol. Palmæ Christ. ana* ʒi. *Opii Camphor. Bals. Peruv. ana* ʒi. *Ol. Macis per Express.* ʒss. *Misce, fi. Liniment. ut supra utend.*[†]

And if the Patient's Stomach cannot take or retain the Powders when taken, the same Powders may be dissolved in a little boiling Water over the Fire, and a little *Aq. Menthæ, Bals. Peruv.* mixed with Sugar, and made agreeable to the Patient's Palate, and given in the same Quantity every two or three Hours, till they pass and give two or three Stools; which they usually do, much sooner than any other stronger Cathartics, as these last usually stimulate and increase the Disorder.

If from the Violence of the pain, and great Irritation of the Nerves, strong Convulsions come on, as it sometimes happens, I usually give Musk with the Opium, which seldom fails to take the Convulsions off; and then the above mentioned Powders, or a Solution of them, must be continued till some Stools are obtained. As:

℞ *Moschi Orient. gr.* x. *Extr. Thebaic. gr.* ii. *vel* iii. *vel* iv. *Bals. Peruv. q. s. M. fi. Pil.* iv. *vel* fi. *Bol. cum Bals. Peruv. q. s.*[†]

This seldom fails to take off the Convulsions and the Pain, if they can be removed. But no stimulating volatile Salts, or Spirits, nor any Medicines usually called Nervous,[†] that will irritate; neither Vesicatories, nor Cathartics, that will stimulate; for all these must be avoided and forbidden, as they increase the Convulsions; and the last will increase the convulsive Contractions of the Bowels, and at last produce a Palsy of the Legs or Hands, or both: But the above Powders, or their Solutions, must be continued till they pass downwards, which they scarce ever fail to do, in three Day's time at the longest, and relieve the Patient from his Misery; and if they do not pass so soon as expected, it is better to repeat the Dose of Musk and Opium, and wait a few Hours longer with Patience, in the Use of the above Powders, which will in a little time bring certain Relief.

It is possible that there may be some other particular Symptoms and Circumstances, which may attend some peculiar Patients and Constitutions, which I have not mentioned here; but the judicious Physician will readily know from what is already said, how to make all such Alterations in the Medicines as may be necessary, and how to remove those Symptoms.

And tho' the Patient generally finds himself quite easy and well, after these Medicines have procured for him a few Stools; yet it is most commonly necessary to keep the Body open for a few Days after, by giving something of the following Nature, once or twice a Day, in a little Whey or Gruel for a few Days. As:

℞ *Crem. Tart.* ʒi. *Tartar. Solubil.* ʒss. *Tart. Vitriolat.* Ʒss. *Ol. Cinnam. gut.* i. *Misce, fi. pulv. primo mane sumend. in haustu seri lactis.*†

But the Custom of giving Calomel, or any other mercurial Preparation, or any drastic Cathartic, either at this or any other time of this Disease, as recommended by a late ingenious and learned Author,[2] and is too often given here, I can by no means approve of; because it is well known that Mercurials have too great a Disposition or Tendency to bring on a Palsy, as also to increase it; and that all stimulating drastic Cathartics, are as bad or worse, as is well known; both from Observation and Experience, as also from what has been said before; but there are likewise other sufficient Reasons for our not giving them at this time of the Disease: because the Patient is now generally reduced pretty low, and his Bowels at this time are too tender and sore, by the preceding convulsive Spasms and long continued Pain, to bear the Irritation of such strong Purgatives.

As to the Diet of the Sick in this Disease, it is almost unnecessary to say that all their Aliments must be thin, light, and of easy Digestion, as in all other acute Cases: because they can generally take nothing but what is so; but I must observe, that some are preferable and much more suitable than some others that are equally light; and I have always found from repeated Observation, that Wine Posset-drink, and Wine-whey, and Polenta† made of Bread toasted brown and infused in boiling Water, till it is the Colour of old Wine or Malt-liquor,† agree much the best with, and sit the lightest and easiest on, their weak Stomachs, and that often when no other Food or Drinkables will stay with them; and they are sufficiently nourishing in so painful a Disease, especially for four or five Days, as it is now most commonly got over in that time, when it is treated in the manner above described: tho' they used formerly to continue as many Weeks, and sometimes as many Months in this State of

2. Dr Town on the *Diseases of the West-Indies.*

Misery, and then too often came off with the Loss of the Use of their Limbs, or died.

Light Food, of easy Digestion, should be continued for a Week or two, and sometimes longer, after the Pain is quite over, and they begin to recover; because the Stomach and Bowels, are generally now very sore and tender, from the Violence of the Pain which they have so long endured in them; and they often continue to be very sore several Days after the Pain is quite over, till they recover their proper Tone and Strength again. To assist which I have always found that easy moderate Riding on Horseback, and taking something of the following kind, has both contributed much to their present Recovery, and also to strengthen their Bowels, and prevent any Relapse. As:

℞ *Cort. Peruv. grosso modo pulv.* ʒi. *Cort. Aurant.* iii. *Rad. Cassumunar. Rhabarb. opt. ana* ʒiss. *Bals. Peruv.* ʒii. *Vini Maderiens* lbii. *m. Digere loco calid. S. A. et Cola, Colatur. capiat Æger Cochl. tria bis vel ter de die Ventriculo.*†

The Palsy, which formerly very frequently seized their Hands and Feet, and sometimes now also, and deprives them of their proper Use and Motion; at the going off of this Disease, as before-mentioned, generally proceeds either from giving some strong drastic purging Medicines, or from some other wrong Treatment of the Disease; and when it is once fixed in their Limbs, is exceeding difficult to be removed and cured; especially when the Patient has continued a long time in that lame helpless State. Drinking of the Waters of some of the warm chalybeate† and sulphurous Baths, and Pumping the paralytic Limbs, or Bathing them (not the whole Body) in the same hot Waters, as those of Bath in England, Aix la Chapelle in Germany, Barages in the Pyrenean Mountains, or those of Portugal, and most probably those in Jamaica, Nevis, and Carolina, if they were properly examined, and suitable Conveniences were made there, may answer as well: These, with a little *Bals. Peruv. Camphor and Extract. Valerian Sylvest.*† given in proper Quantities with those Waters, twice a Day for some time, with daily repeated Frictions on the Spine of the Back and the paralytic Limbs, are most likely, and have sometimes succeeded and restored to them the Use of their Limbs.

But it is much more easy to prevent this Palsy from coming on, or seizing the Patient, by treating the Disease in a proper manner as before recommended; than it is to cure it, when it has seized and taken away the Use of the Patient's Limbs.†

Of the DYSENTERY

THE DISEASES of the Intestines are rather more frequent in this warm Climate, than they usually are in Europe, especially the *Dysentery*, and the *Colica Pictonum*, or Dry Belly-ache, both which we too frequently meet with; of the last I have already treated before. We also usually have a *Cholera Morbus*, especially towards the latter End of the hot Months, as we usually have in England, and the other Parts of Europe; but it is seldom so severe and violent here, as it often is there, tho' this Island is so much warmer; and we too often meet with Inflammations of the Bowels, and sometimes with the *bilious Colic*, the *flatulent Colic*, and the *hysteric Colic*, tho' the last is not near so frequent here as it is in England: We have also at times, all the different kinds of *Diarrhœas*, [such] as *Diarrhœa Febrilis*, a *Diarrhœa Colliquativa*,† and the *Fluxus Hepaticus*,† all which are very different Diseases from each other, tho' they all affect the same Parts, and should be treated with as different Methods and Medicines, according to their different Natures and causes; but all much in the same manner as they usually are treated in England, when they are treated in a rational and proper manner, with some Allowances for the Warmth of the Climate. But as these last are all judiciously treated on by several learned and able Physicians in Europe, it is not necessary to say any thing on them here, since they should be treated here, much in the same manner as they are there; save that a more liberal Use of the *Antiseptics*, especially in the colliquative Diarrhœa and the hepatic Flux, is necessary, because all the Humours usually putresce more readily, and to a higher Degree in this warm Climate, than they usually do in the colder Climates.

But *Dysenteries* are so frequent in this warm Climate, that they may be truly said to be endemial, and more or less epidemical every Year; especially during the rainy Seasons. For after two or three of the hotter Months are passed over, and are succeeded by the usual rainy Months of August and September, in which considerable great Quantities of Rain usually fall, sometimes for several Days successively together, which are often followed by two or three or more clear and very hot Days, and then Rain again, and often so by Turns: the falling of the Rains, especially when in great Quantities, renders the Air cooler, moist, and damp, for many Hours, and sometimes Days, when it is very cloudy, which being succeeded by clear and very hot dry Days, as is often the Case, insomuch that the Months of August, September, and October are generally called the hottest Months of the Year; these great and often sudden Changes of the Air, almost constantly produce Dysenteries, which usually become frequent and epidemical, especially among the Negroes, who are usually little clothed, and more exposed to the Inclemencies of the Weather, and among the White people also; and when the above Changes of the Air are sudden and great, they too often become malignant or mali moris also.

For I have always found from the best Observations that I could make on the Variations of the Air and Weather, in this Island, that if the Months of May, June, July, and August were very hot and dry, and the following Months of September, October, and November were accompanied with much Rain, so that the Air was rendered cool, moist, and damp, and if the intermediate Days between the rainy Days, were very hot, I always observed that the Dysenteries were very frequent and epidemical, and generally were more or less malignant, as the above-mentioned Changes of the Weather were greater or less, more sudden or more gradual, and shorter, or longer Continuation.

Hence must we not conclude, that this great Dryness and Heat of the Air, especially when it continues long, so acts on our Bodies, as gradually to change their animal Oil and Salts, from their neutral, soft, bland, smooth, semi-ammoniacal State, to a semi-rancid and semi-volatile acrid State, whereby they become unfit to perform the Functions of animal Life; and by their Acrimony so stimulate and irritate the most sensible Parts of the Body, as greatly to disturb and oppress Nature? and as she always endeavours to discharge and carry off whatever is so oppressive and offensive to her, by some of the excretory Glands and Pores, and in this Case it is most probable that she first endeavours it by exciting a free Perspiration and Sweating, as these Evacuations are the most assisted by the great Heat. But the sudden falling of the Rain, changing the Air so as to render it cool, moist, and damp, which as suddenly checks and stops that free Perspiration and Sweating, and the discharge of those acrid Humours by those ways being thus hindered, they are turned upon the Bowels, which they constantly stimulate and irritate; and so produce a continual Secretion and Discharge of the mucous Matter of the intestinal Glands, and probably some of the acrid Humours with it. This still continuing, increases the Afflux of the Humours to those Glands, where they produce an Inflammation of those Glands, and the Heat and Fever are again increased by that Inflammation, and the Humours still rendered more acrid by that Heat and Fever; and the Momentum of the Blood being thus increased, its red Globules are forced and discharged, with the mucous Matter of those Glands, into the Intestines, and so carried off by Stool. And the Acrimony of the Humours being still increased by the Heat of the Fever, and the Fever again increased by the Acrimony, and the thinnest Parts of the circulating Fluids being continually carried off, the remaining Fluids are in time rendered too thick to pass thro' the smaller Vessels, which still increases the Inflammation, and produces a Tenesmus, and violent Pain, with all the other bad Symptoms attending this Disease; which if not speedily relieved, soon form Obstructions, and a total Suffocation of the sanguiferous Vessels,† which soon produces a Mortification of the Intestines, that soon ends in Death.

As we have Dysenteries constantly returning every Year in the West-India Islands, with those Rains at that time of the Year, which are always epidemical, tho' not always equally malignant, no more than the seasons are equally alike; may we not justly conclude, that the Dysentery is most commonly produced from these Causes, especially as these Causes are sufficient to produce it?

Tho' it is also probable that it may be sometimes produced by *infectious Miasmata* also; which were exhaled from diseased Bodies and are floating in the Air, and received into the Mouth with it when we breathe, and there stick to the Saliva, and are carried with it down into the Stomach and Intestines, where they produce all the above-mentioned Symptoms and Effects, when they meet with a Constitution fitted by the above-mentioned Causes to receive these infectious Effluvia, and produce the Disease. However, I think, that we are certain from Observation, that this Disease, when it is thus produced in the manner as above, from the aforesaid Causes, it often happens that after it has continued a considerable time, and many are seized with it at or near the same time, that the Humours are in time rendered so acrid, semi-volatile, and putrid, that they become infectious, and being exhaled from their Bodies, but more especially from the putrid offensive Stools of the Sick, into the Air, are carried with it, and often infect those who were well and sound before; and thus it becomes both epidemical and contagious, tho' it was not the latter at its first Invasion or seizing [of] the first Patient. This I have often observed, especially when great Numbers have laboured under it at the same time, as often happens among the Negroes; wherefore I have constantly ordered that the Close-stools† should always be emptied immediately after they are used, and not suffered to remain in the same Room with the Sick: so that no more infectious putrid Effluvia might be either conveyed to the Sick, or to the Attendants; and I think it is a very necessary Precaution.

I have always observed, that all those Diseases, which are epidemical, generally seize the Negroes first: Is it not because they are little or thin clothed, and often poorly fed, and much more exposed to all the Variations of the Air, and Inclemencies of the Weather?

This Disease does not always seize the Patients in the same manner: Sometimes it seizes them with a Diarrhœa, which is moderate the first Day or Two, but it gradually increases in all its Symptoms, till it becomes a perfect Dysentery, with all its Symptoms. At other times it seizes them with an Oppression and Sickness at their Stomachs, a gentle Rigor, with Pain in the Head, and sometimes all over the Body, which are soon followed by a Fever, with griping Pain in the Bowels, and frequent griping Stools. The Sickness at the Stomach increases, and is often attended with a Reaching to vomit, or with Vomiting: The fever increases; the Pulse becomes very quick, and generally tense and hard, and sometimes full, though rarely so full as it is in most other Fevers, neither is the external heat of the Body usually so great as it is in many other Fevers, though the internal Heat be greater. The Stools become more frequent, the griping Pain increases, and the Excrement discharged is mixed with much Mucus of the Guts, and considerable Quantities of Blood; and sometimes nothing but Blood and Mucus is discharged by stool; at other times a bloody Sanies,† or Ichor,† like bloody Beef-brine, and a Tenesmus comes on, with a continual painful Neediness or Desire of going to Stool. All these Symptoms continue and increase, if not timely relieved by proper Remedies: The Fever increases, the Pulse is very quick, the Thirst and internal Heat great, though the external Heat continues to be less than in most other Fevers, as all the Humours have so great an Afflux towards the Bowels, which too often deceives the injudicious or incautious Practitioner. Now the Patient's Strength sinks, he grows delirious, his extreme Parts cold, accompanied with cold clammy Sweats; his Pulse becomes irregular, unequal, and often intermits;† the Stools sometimes run from the Patient insensibly; the Coldness of the Extremities and the cold Sweats increase, and all the other Symptoms are worse, the Patient grows very faint, and a Mortification seizes the Bowels, which soon ends in Death.

From the Nature of the preceding Causes, their Manner of acting, and the Symptoms which attend this Disease, we must take our Intentions of Cure, which are these:

First: *To carry off those acrid, putrid, and infectious Humours, as soon and as safely as we can; and to abate and take off the Fever.*

Secondly: *To stay the Purging, heal the inflamed and abraded Intestines; and then corroborate† and restore their Tone and proper Action.*

As we always observe, that this Disease is constantly attended with a Fever, in a greater or less Degree; it is always necessary to take away some Blood, more or less as the Nature of the Fever, the Strength, Quickness and Fullness of the Pulse do indicate, and the Strength and other Circumstances of the Patient will permit; in order to abate the Fever and Inflammation as well as the increase of Heat, Putrefaction, and Acrimony of the Humours.

And as there is such an Afflux of the Humours to the Stomach and Bowels, attended with a Sickness, Reaching, and sometimes Vomiting, an *Emetic* is clearly indicated; and the sooner it is given, the better, both to carry off those Humours, and as much of the infectious Matter as we can, as also to revulse† them from the Bowels, and clear the Stomach, that the Medicines to be given after may have the better Effect; and it is well known that the *Ipocacuanha* in Powder is the best in this Case, as it operates the safest, and somewhat restringes† the Bowels after: and in order to answer the first Intention of Cure, and carry off as much of those putrid Humours as we can, in the Beginning of the Disease, it is necessary to give a Dose of *torrified Rhubarb* mixed with an *Opiate*, to procure the distressed patient some Respite and Ease, and abate the Flux; and I have found something of this Nature the best:

℞ *Rad. Rhei. tor. pulv.* ℈i. *Electar. e Scord.* ℨss. *Extract. Thebaic. gr.* iss. *vel* ii. *Ol. Cinnam. gut.* i. *Syr. e Mecon. q. s. m. fi. Bol. hora post Emet. operat. sumendus.*†

If the Fever and Purging are considerably abated by these Medicines, as they sometimes are, when given early at the Beginning of the Disease; giving something of the following Nature, sometimes takes the remaining Fever off, stays the Flux, and heals the Bowels, and sometimes effects the Cure, or at least greatly abates them, if a proper Regimen is prescribed, and strictly followed by the Patient.

℞ *Cort. Restring. Barbad.* (Bastard Locus dict.) *Visci Arboris Limonifer.* (Misleto of the Lemon-tree dict.) *ana* ℥i. *Cort. Granator. Cinnamomi.* ℨiss. Misce. *Coq. in Aq font.* lbii. *ad* lbiss. *et sub finem coction. adde Electar. e Scord.* ℥i. *Coq. partum et Cola* lbiss. *Colaturæ adde Tinct. Terræ Japon* ℥i. *Sp. Nitri Dul.* ℥ss. *Sal. Nitri. purif.* ℥ss. *Syr. e Mecon.* ℥i. *m. fi. Decoc. cujus capiat Æger Cochl. tria vel quatuor tertia quaq; hora vel post singulam alvi dejectionem liquidam.*†

The Quantity of the Sal Nitre, and also of the Opiate here, may be increased or diminished as the Physician sees it necessary. I have here ordered the *Cortex Restring. Barbad.* and the *Viscus Arbor Liminofer*, because they can be easily gotten in Barbadoes, and are the most efficacious cooling Restringents in this and some other Cases. The first is the Bark of a non-descript Tree; and makes a fine Extract, which, as well as the Bark, both greatly restringe and strengthen without Heating, and both may be brought to England; and I wish we had them here† for the Benefit of the Profession, and the Good of Mankind: and the Misleto of the Lemon-tree, on which and the Lime-trees it only grows, and is a fine subacid cooling Restringent, and was used as a Secret in the Cure of this Disease for many Years, but I fear will not retain its Virtues when brought to England, neither will it be got to grow here; but both may be tried: I have often experienced the good Use of both this and the above Bark and Extract, and wish we had them here.

As I write on this Disease, as well as on most of the other Diseases in this Book, principally for the Use and Benefit of the Inhabitants and Practitioners in Barbadoes, and the other West-India islands, who in general have too little Learning, I have been more explicit and copious in the Theory and Reasoning on those Diseases, than would have been necessary if I had only written for the Use of the Learned, which I hope the last will excuse, and pardon this and the preceding Digression.

Giving Sal Nitre also in this Case, where such a violent Purging attends, may be thought by those who are not able to see the Reasons for giving it, not only a *new*, but an injudicious Practice, as it is known that Nitre will sometimes gently loosen the Belly. But I must observe to such, that it rarely or never happens that the Purging, though violent, takes the Patient off, but the Violence of the Fever, and the Inflammation of the Intestines, which ends in a Mortification, especially in this hot Climate, and kills him. And that it is both injudicious, and bad Practice to stop the Purging, by strong Restringents and hot alexipharmic Medicines, before the fever and Inflammation are abated or taken off: And if they can stop the Purging by such Medicines, the Fever will be thereby so increased, as to bring on a Train of fatal Symptoms, which will soon put an end to his Life. Wherefore the Physician's greatest Care should be to take off the Fever and Inflammation, by Bleeding *&c.* and a proper Use of *Antiphlogisticks*, given with gentle cooling Restringents, and suitable *Anodynes* to abate the Irritation of the Bowels. And in this Case I have always found Nitre thus given, or mixed with a little *Elect. e Scord.*† or *Bals. Locotel.*† to be the best *Antiphlogistick*.

And even to Children, when the bloody Stools have been frequent, and with much Pain, that after *Bleeding*, an *Emetic*, and a little *torrefied Rhubarb*, giving *Nitre* mixed with a little red Coral, in an anodyne testaceous Julep, has in a short time, both taken the Fever and Inflammation off, and the Purging also soon ceased, and they soon recovered, being taken at the first beginning of the Disease. For if we can but take off the Fever and Inflammation, the Purging generally soon stops, as its Cause is removed: Or if by reason of too great a Laxness and Weakness of the Bowels, the Purging continues, it may be soon stayed by a moderate restringent Anodyne and a Clyster.

But if the Fever still continues, or the Inflammation remains, after Bleeding, and the Use of the above-mentioned Medicines, and the bloody Stools with much Pain are not abated, as too often it happens, Bleeding must be repeated on the second or third Day after the first Bleeding; and in some Cases more than once, especially where the Quickness, Hardness, and Fullness of the Pulse indicates it; and that to such a Quantity as the Urgency of the Symptoms require, and the Strength of the Patient will bear: After which, it will soon be necessary to give the *Ipocacuanah* in small Doses, from gr. ij to gr. v. mixed with ʒi of *Theriac. Androm.* twice a Day, and an Anodyne, after it has vomited the Patient once or twice, for three or four Days, and the antiphlogistick anodyne restringent Decoction as before, in the intermediate times of taking the *Ipocacuanah*, which may also be given after, if the Stools still continue; these seldom fail to give Relief, and take off the Disease.

But if the Fever and Inflammation are considerably abated, or taken off, and yet the bloody or Brine-like Stools continue, and are frequent; giving a Dose or two, and sometimes a third Dose of the *Stibium Ceratum*, at proper Distances after each other, and a suitable Opiate a little time after the last, has been of great Service: But I must observe that this Medicine, how much it may be recommended and extolled by some Persons, though it may be a good Medicine when properly timed; yet as it is frequently and promiscuously given at all times of this Disease, and in all Circumstances, by some Persons, it cannot succeed; for if the Fever and Inflammation are not first taken off, or considerably abated, it seldom or never answers their Expectations: But these being taken off, or greatly abated, it sometimes proves to be a good Medicine, though I think I have seen the *Ipocacuanah* in small Doses answer much better even then, when it would not.

But when we find that the Fever and Inflammation still continue, after all the repeated Evacuations of Bleeding and Vomiting, &c. and the Patient is reduced so low, that he cannot bear any further Evacuations, and yet the Fever continues, with a very quick, low, weak Pulse, and is delirious, his Skin hot and dry, and the Stools frequent and bloody, or Brine-like; I have with great Pleasure seen, that giving the *Ipocacuan.* in small Doses, viz. gr. iij and repeating it every three Hours, till the Patient had taken four Doses, and increasing the last Dose to six or seven Grains, it has, after giving a gentle Puke or two, almost surprisingly restrained the Flux, and brought on a fine free Diaphoresis all over the Body, which was continued for some Hours, by being properly encouraged by drinking small warm Liquids; and the Delirium, Tremors, and all the other bad Symptoms went off, and the Patient has from that time soon recovered, by only giving a few Doses of a restringent diaphoretic Opiate, as before; and was thus as it were snatched from the Jaws of Death.

But we cannot always expect to meet with such happy Success, in every Patient and Case; yet in these Circumstances, I have more than twice seen this Method succeed; so that the Fever and all its bad Symptoms have been either taken off, or so much abated, that by giving something of the Nature of the above-mentioned restringent anodyne Decoction, or such like Medicines for a few Days, and a few proper Clysters, with a suitable Regimen, the Fever has been entirely taken off, and the Purging also, and they recovered; at least I have always found this method the most successful, even after all other Methods have failed.

There is another painful Circumstance which frequently attends this Disease, which is a painful Griping accompanied with a great Soreness in the Bowels; and most commonly arises from the great Heat and Acrimony of the Humours, and their continual Motion downwards, and the fine soft Mucus which lines and defends the Intestines being carried off by the so much Purging, those acrid Humours irritate and inflame, and sometimes almost corrode the *Tunica Villosa* of the Guts, so that they are in part excoriated; and sometimes large Portions of that fine Membrane [have] been known to come away several Inches long, by which the Intestines become exceeding sore and painful. When this Pain and Soreness is found to be pretty high up in the Guts; *Bals. Locotelli,* or the following Electuary, and the *Wax Emulsion,* are found to be the most effectual Remedies: [such] as:

℞ *Electar. e Scord. Bals. Locotel. ana ʒi. Sperm. Ceti, Pulv. e Bolo cum Opio ana ʒiss. Syr. Balsamic. q.s. Misce, fi Elect. cujus capiat Æger q. Nuc. Mosc. quarta, quinta vel sexta quaq; hora superbib. Emuls. cum Cer præprat Cochl. tria.†*

But when the Pain and Soreness are found to be lower down in the Belly, it most commonly arises from an Excoriation, or from little small Ulcerations of the *Rectum* or *Secum,*† which the acrid Humours irritate, and produce a painful Tenesmus; in which Case, not only the above-mentioned healing Medicines are necessary, but soft balsamic healing Clysters must be frequently injected also; which may be made of fat Broth, or Milk, mixed with *Bals. Locotel. Wax, Sperm, Ceti,*† and an Anodyne; [such] as, *Elect. e. Scordio, Theriac. Androm.* or *Tinct. Thebiac.*

But this Tenesmus, especially when the Disease has been severe, and has continued a considerable long time, and is situated low down in the Belly, most frequently arises from the indurated Fæces; which are often formed into hard round Lumps like Balls, by the convulsive Spasms of the Guts, and are almost half baked by the Heat and Fever attending the Disease, and often are pretty large and very hard, as I have often observed them to come away at the latter End of it, that it is almost surprising to think how these hard Lumps should remain in the Guts so long, and such a violent liquid Purging continue all that time, and they not be carried off with it; as is almost incredible, if they did not so frequently come away at the last: And so long as these Lumps continue in the Intestines, they must very much irritate and stimulate them, as they are in that tender sore excoriated State, and so long will the Tenesmus remain. In this Case, a proper Purgative and suitable Clysters, must be given to carry those Lumps off; but I must observe, that I cannot approve of giving *Senna*† in any shape, or at any time in this Disease, notwithstanding that the great and honest Dr *Sydenham* (to whom all possessing the medical Art are much obliged, for the many useful Observations and Discoveries which he made) frequently used and recommends it; because it is observed that this Drug always increases either more or less, any Inflammation; but this probably was not known at his time: and as some Degree of Inflammation, more or less on the Intestines, always attends this Disease; giving *Senna* must consequently increase it, and render the Evil worse: But I have always found that giving a little *Manna* and *Rhubarb*, with a little *Sal. Polychrestum*† and *Oil*, seldom fail to carry these hard Lumps quite off; and it may be assisted if necessary with a Clyster of warm Water, a little Honey and Oil, and a small Quantity of Soap to dissolve those Lumps, and render the Guts more slippery, and their Exit more easy; which Method seldom fails. And when these Lumps are thus carried off, the Patient usually soon recovers with the Use of the above-mentioned balsamic healing Medicines, and a Clyster or two of the same kind; with a suitable soft, healing, and nourishing Diet, at the same time.†

I am very sensible that there are, and often may be, some other Circumstances, and considerable Variations in the Symptoms which at times do attend this Disease, either arising from the different epidemical Constitution of different Years, or from the different Constitutions of the Patients, which may require some Variations in the Method of treating them, as well as in the Medicines to be given: But it is neither possible nor necessary to describe or mention them all here; since every judicious Physician will be able to observe them, and to make such Alterations both in the Method of Cure, and such Variations in the Medicines, as may be necessary: And these are sufficient, and I hope may be of Service to some in the Practice; wherefore I communicate them to the Public, and sincerely wish that they may be as useful to others, as some of the Observations have been to me.

Of the OPISTHOTONOS and TETANY

THIS IS A MOST PAINFUL and dangerous Disease, which was well known, and is often mentioned by the great *Hippocrates*, and the other *Greek Physicians*, though they most commonly speak of it as the Consequence and Effect of Wounds made by Darts, or other Weapons, and have not so accurately described it as it could be desired; and few of the Moderns have done any more than cursorily mentioning it, not even *Bontius*,† who lived some time in the East Indies, has but very imperfectly described it; though it is probable that he saw it often, although it is so very seldom seen in England, and the other cold northern Countries, yet it is so frequently seen in the West-India Islands, and the neighbouring warm Countries; that it may be justly said to be indigenous, or at least endemial in those Countries which are within or near the Torrid Zone; hence it might be more frequent in *Greece* than it is in England, as the Island of *Coos*† and adjacent Countries, where the great *Father of Physic* lived and made his Observations, are much warmer.

The Greeks distinguished this Disease by these three Names, as they express the primary Effects it has on the Body, ἐπροσθότονος, ὀπισθότονος, τετύνος, which the Latins called by one Name, *Rigor Nervorum*, and we a *Tetany* or *Convulsion*. When the Body was bowed and bended down forward, the Greeks called it an *Emprosthotonos*; and when it was bended backwards in a Curve, and immoveable, they called it an *Opisthotonos*; and when the Body was fixed in an erect, rigid, immoveable Posture, like a Statue, or when a Limb was so fixed, they called it a *Tetanus*. The first is very seldom seen, tho' the last two are very frequent in the warm Climates.

This Disease, though distinguished by these three Names, may most properly be called but one Disease; as they generally all three arise from the same Causes, and only differ from each other, as they reduce the Body into the three different Positions before-mentioned. And all these, or this one Disease, in general arises from three Causes, which are very different from each other; though in some particular Cases and Constitutions there may be some other concurring Causes: The first is from a slight small Puncture with a Pin, Needle, or small Bone of a Fish, a Nail, or small Splinter of Wood, accidentally run into the Foot, Hand, Finger or Toe, the Head, or some other nervous Parts of the Body; or from a small Wound with a sharp Edge of a Stone, often not much more than Skin deep, and too often from the Ligatures on the Arteries (probably with a Nerve,) after the Amputation of a Limb: It is difficult to conceive how such a small slight Puncture or Wound, and such a trifling Cause as a small Puncture with a Pin, a small Bone of a Fish, or a Nail, or a small slight Cut with a sharp Stone, but little more than Skin deep, in such remote parts of the Body, should produce such violent Symptoms, and so fatal a Disease; nay it is almost incredible to those who have never seen such Cases, yet it is but too certainly true, as both I and many others have but too often seen them.

Secondly, it often arises from taking a Cold, by suddenly exposing the Body to a Current of cool Air, when warm and sweating, or being suddenly wet when warm; or going into cold Water when sweating. And lastly, young Children are frequently seized with this Disease, from a Retention of Meconium, or from a cheesy Matter, or something which is acrid, taken into the Stomach and Bowels.

These Causes are all too often followed by an Opisthotonos and Tetany, and when from the first mentioned Causes, it most commonly comes on between the tenth and fourteenth Day after such a slight Puncture or Wound is made, and sometimes (though very rarely) sooner than the tenth Day, and often when the small Wound has given the Patient little Pain or Uneasiness, and has had no bad Appearance, but has digested† and looked well, and often when the Puncture or Wound has been perfectly healed up by some common Plaster, and has been well for several Days before the Convulsions have come on, and that without any Fever, or other Symptoms but as hereafter mentioned.

But when this Disease proceeds from the second mentioned Causes, *viz.* from suddenly taking Cold, it usually comes on much sooner, though they have only had the common Symptoms of catching Cold, with little or no Fever, till the fourth or fifth Day after the convulsive Symptoms have seized the Patient, when a Fever of the inflammatory Kind usually comes on.

In Children, from the above-mentioned Causes, it usually still comes on sooner.

The Patient usually first complains of an uneasy Sensation, and small Tenderness about the Præcordia, and a Stiffness in his Jaws, which gradually increases, and brings on a Difficulty in Swallowing, but no Swelling either internally or externally appears in the Throat; and a Pain all along the Spine of the Back, with a Contraction and Stiffness of the dorsal Muscles, and those of the Neck soon follow, and gradually increase for a Day or two; and the Head, Neck, and Back-bone, are gradually and strongly bended backwards, and the Body is fixed and retained in that retro-curved Posture, and the Jaws are now close locked and immovably fixed, and most commonly an Impossibility of Swallowing any thing, from the Muscles serving for Deglutition being fixed in a rigid State, now comes on; if any thing that is Liquid can be got into the Mouth, which is usually about the third or fourth Day, and sometimes sooner; now frequent strong convulsive Spasms come on, first under the Sternum and on the Diaphragm, and quickly extend themselves to the Jaws, Neck, and the whole Spine of the Back, with such Violence and Force, as well as dreadful Pain, as often raise the Body with a sudden Jerk, quite up from the Bed, or Place on which it lays, to a considerable Height; at other Times only so that his Occiput and Heels only touch them, the Body forming Part of an Arch, if the Patient lays on his Back, which is the easier Posture of the two, or almost a Circle, by his Head and Heels being brought so near together if he lays on his Belly, which they rarely can bear to do, tho' sometimes the Head, Neck, and Back, are only retro-curved, and the Legs strongly and rigidly extended. As the Disease advances, these strong convulsive Spasms become more frequent, and also more violent, and now return every, ten, fifteen, or twenty Minutes; which reduces the poor Patient to the most distressed Condition, both from the Violence of the Pain which he continually feels, and the Dread of the frequent Returns of those violent convulsive Spasms, which greatly increases it, and he commonly expects; and now the Disease is become a perfect Tetany, and in the Intervals between those Spasms, he lays in a rigid immovable State; except that they most commonly can move their Tongue and speak, as also their Fingers, but not their Arms. When the Disease proceeds from a Puncture or Wound, I never yet saw or observed any Fever attend it; the Pulse is generally small, regular, and rather slower, but usually a little harder, as well as the Heat of the Body, no greater than when in Health; and they usually breathe freely and well, as when well, except during the time of, and a little after the Spasms, when the Pulse is often small, fluttering, and irregular, for a short time, and the Breathing quick as if violently exercised, but the Spasm being over, they both soon become calm, slow, and regular again; but the Body is sometimes covered with Sweat, from the Violence of the Agonies, yet no feverish Heat attends; neither is the Thirst great, or the Tongue foul, though it is often stiff and attended with a Torpor, arising from the Contraction of its Muscles; the Urine not much altered, only a little higher coloured and less in Quantity, as they can drink little, and sometimes none: The Belly is generally costive, and drawn inward and flat, and all the abdominal Muscles are tense, rigid, and contracted, as are most of the Muscles of the Body after *Tetany* comes on. They seldom can sleep, they only get some short Slumbers, from which they are soon roused by the convulsive Spasms, especially towards the latter End of the Disease, when they can seldom get any: The Countenance is mostly pale and contracted, and strongly expresses great Anxiety and Distress. Thus the convulsive Spasms continue to return more frequently and with greater Violence, till at last a general strong Convulsion puts an end to their Misery; and in this Case they most commonly retain all their Senses to the last Moment.

They usually continue in this State, with these violent Symptoms, gradually increasing to the fifth or seventh, and sometimes to the tenth or eleventh Day; but when the Disease comes on with more Violence at the first, and its Symptoms increase more quickly in their Violence, and return more frequently also; they often put a Period to Life on the third or fourth Day, if the Violence of the Symptoms are not abated by suitable Medicines; at other times when less violent it continues longer, and usually for some Weeks before they perfectly recover the proper Tone of the Nerves and Muscles again; but if they survive the ninth or eleventh Day, they most commonly recover in three or four Week's time; though not the perfect Tone of the Nerves, and the Use of the Muscles, in less than five or six Week's time, and sometimes longer.

When the *Opisthotonos* and *Tetany* arise from taking Cold, [they are] attended with all the same Symptoms, and they usually come sooner on after taking the Cold, than when from a Puncture or Wound, though not usually with more Violence, and without a Fever in the first three or four Days, tho' the Pulse is usually a little more full, and a little harder, though seldom quicker during those first Days, but most commonly about the fourth or fifth Day, the Pulse begins to be both more full, and more quick and hard, and a Fever come on with some inflammatory Symptoms, which indicate Bleeding, and some are a little delirious at times, and their Blood is now a little more florid and more dense, than it usually is in the former, where it usually is more lax and of a looser Texture, and somewhat less florid, and sometimes mixed with darker Spots: But in all other Respects, except that the Thirst is greater, the Symptoms and Progress of the Disease are the same as in the other, as also its fatal Effects rather more so, if not timely relieved by proper Remedies.

Infants likewise, who are seized with this Disease, usually have the Symptoms and the Convulsions, as also the *Tetany* coming on sooner, and generally more or less of a Fever with them; and the *Insultus Epilepticus*, as Dr *Sydenham* calls it, if it continues any time, is in this hot Climate changed into a Tetany in them.

It is generally observed that the Negroes are more subject to this Disease, than the white People usually are; and it must be allowed, that the Negroes are seized with it much more frequently than the white People are: But I apprehend that this only proceeds from the Negroes going barefoot, and thereby being more exposed to such Injuries, and their being worse clothed, and accustomed to Labour with, or in such work as renders them more liable to get such Wounds, and a Custom which many of them have of going into the cold Water when they are Sweating on the Road, &c. which [renders] them more liable to this Disease; but the white People are much more subject to this Disease in this hot Climate, than they are in the colder Countries.

As this Disease so frequently proceeds from such slight Causes, it is extremely difficult to account for it, in a rational and satisfactory Manner: To say that it is effected by the Consent† of the Nerves, one small Nerve being lacerated or wounded, gives great Pain, and that is communicated to, and affects the whole nervous System: This may be plausible, and may satisfy some People, but it is far from being clear and satisfactory, to an exact Enquirer; for the Pain is generally ceased in the wounded Part, and the small Wound often perfectly healed up and well, several Days before either the Convulsions, or their preceding Symptoms come on: And how such a Cause, which has nothing acrid in its Nature, when the small Instrument which made the Wound is removed, should lay still, and often without Pain, for ten Days or more, and then produce such terrible Effects; at present only serves to shew us how imperfectly we are acquainted with the Structure and Nature of the Nerves and their contained Fluid, and how they act so as to produce their various and wonderful Effects; and also shews us how much a further Knowledge of them is wanting, and ought to be enquired into, and obtained if possible.

I think we may say, that all we know at present of this Matter, is, that we know by Observation, that these slight Causes, do actually produce those terrible Effects. And we also observe that the *Will* or *Thought*, which is not *Matter*, can act on the Body which is Matter, and give it Motion, *&c.* but how either of these act, so as to produce their peculiar Effects, we know almost as little of the one, as we do of the other: Tho' there may be some more Probability of obtaining some Knowledge of the former, than we can hope for of the latter; and that if it ever be obtained, it must be by accurate Observation, and just inductive Reasoning.

But till further Discoveries are made of the Nature and Action of the Nerves, we must be content with such Observations as we have, and such Reasonings as we can justly draw from them, and endeavour to keep as near to Truth, as we possibly can.

We know then from Observation, that there is such a thing as Consent of Parts, or that one Part of the Body being irritated or hurt, another Part of it will be affected in the same manner, though not hurt; as a Moat† falling into one Eye, considerably affects both Eyes; and an Inflammation, or a Stone, in one Kidney, greatly affects them both, and the Stomach also, as it receives a Branch from the same Nerve;† and the same is observed of some other Parts of the Body. We have an Account in the *Philosophical Transactions*, by Dr *Short,*³ of a small sharp Bone which closely adhered to a Branch of the crural Nerve,† which being irritated by certain Motions of the Leg in which it was, it so irritated and affected the whole nervous System, as to bring on strong epileptic Fits, and greatly affect the whole Body with strong convulsive Motions. And there seems to be a great Analogy between this Case, and what

---

3. Philos. Transact. Abridg. Vol. 7.

happens in this Disease, both as to the Cause and the Cure; for that Bone being taken out, the Patient was freed from his epileptic Fits: and in this Case, the lacerated Nerve being entirely divided above the Wound, I have found it abate the convulsive Spasms, and contribute much towards the Cure, wherefore I have made dividing the Nerve near to, and above the Wound, one of the first Intentions of Cure in this Disease, when it arises from a Puncture or Wound.

The Causes of this dreadful Disease, may be most properly divided into three, (tho' in some particular Cases, there may sometimes be some other concurring Causes) which are very different from each other: First a small Puncture or Wound in the Feet or Hands, or sometimes in the Head, or in other Parts of the Body; tho' most commonly in the two first, which are most exposed to such Injuries, especially in the Negroes who go barefoot, and thence are more subject to this Disease. Secondly, catching Cold suddenly, when very warm and Sweating with Exercise, Labour, or otherwise; and especially if any Part of the Body, which is more nervous and sensible, was any way contused before. And, Thirdly, in young Children from a retention and insufficient Discharge of the Meconium, or from an acrid cheesy Matter generated and retained in their tender Stomachs, or from any acrid, acid Humour which is retained in, and irritates their tender Bowels: For the *Insultus Epilepticus* as usual in Children in England, if it continues any time in this warm Climate, is frequently changed in them into a Tetany, and often proves fatal.

These being the causes of this Disease, the proper Intentions of Cure, evidently appear to be: First, *To remove and take away the irritating Cause which affects the Nerves; and then to diminish and take off the Stimulation and Irritation of the Nerves.* And Secondly, *To relax the rigid Tenseness and Contraction of the Nerves, Tendons, and Muscles, of the Parts affected.* For the old Adage, *Tolle causam et cessabit effectum,*† is as justly applicable in this, as it is in all other Cases.

Wherefore, when we are first called, and find that either the *Opisthotonos,* or *Tetany,* or their presaging Symptoms, have seized the Patient, and that they proceed from such a Puncture, or small Wound, as before-mentioned, it is necessary to call in a *Surgeon* to examine the Puncture or Wound very carefully, that if any Part of the Splinter, Fish-bone, Needle, or Nail remain in the Wound, he may take it away. Then in order to take off the Sense of the Irritation of the wounded or lacerated Nerve, and prevent its being conveyed to the other Nerves, let the *Surgeon* make an Incision near to, and a little above the Puncture or Wound, so deep as totally to cut the lacerated Nerve in two,† which conveys the Sense of the Irritation from the Puncture or the wounded Part; then dress both the Wounds with a mild Digestive† mixed with a little Opium, to lessen the Irritation and Pain more.

This being done, I generally give an Opiate [such] as, the following Bolus, Draught, or Pills as soon as I can, which most commonly takes off the nervous Spasms, and greatly abates the convulsive Contractions and Tetany also.

℞ *Moschi Oriental. gr.* xii. *Extracti Thebaici gr.* ii *vel* iii. *Theriac. Androm.* Ʒi. *Bals. Peruv. q.s.* Misce, *fi. Bolus. statim sumend.*†

Vel. ℞ *Aq Alex Simp* ʒjss. *Spir. Lavend. Comp.* Ʒj. *Sp. C. C. ver. gut.* xxx. *Moschi. Orient. gr.* viii. *Extracti Thebaic. gr.* ij. *Bals. Peruv. gut.* xx. *Syr. e. Mecon.* ʒss. *M. fi. Haust. quam prim. sumendus.*†

Vel, ℞ *Extract. Thebaic. gr.* ij *vel* iij. *Moschi Orient. gr.* x. *Bals, Peruv. q.s.* Misce, *fi. Pil.* iv *statim sumend.*†

And one of these must be repeated, every twelve, ten, eight or six Hours, accordingly as the convulsive Spasms are more or less violent and strong, and return the oftener; and sometimes I have found it necessary to repeat them oftener than every six Hours, where the Spasms were very great, and returned very often, or where the Tetany was violent; neither need we fear any bad Consequences to attend the giving such large Doses of the Opiates,† or the repeating of them so often, where the convulsive Spasms are so violent, or return so frequently, tho' to Persons who are not accustomed to take Opium in any Shape; nor have I ever seen that the giving such large and frequent Doses of the Opiates in this Case, have ever produced any Stupor, or great Disposition to Sleep, tho' I have ordered sixteen or twenty Grains of *Extr. Thebaic.* to be given in the Space of twenty-four Hours, where the Spasms were violent, yet they seldom procured more than two or three Hours' Sleep, and seldom more than one Hour at a Time without being awakened by the Spasms, and rarely more than three Hours' Sleep in twenty-four Hours time, and that most commonly without any Stupor, or heavy sleepy Disposition; yet I have observed that the Opiates have always greatly abated the convulsive Spasms, and the *Opisthotonos* and *Tetany* also; and when they are given with *Musk*, I think, that I have sufficient Reasons from Observation, to say that they both more effectually remove, and sooner take off this much dreaded Disease. And as the convulsive Spasms abate and return less frequently, the Intervals between giving the Doses of *Musk* and *Opium* may be made longer, and longer, till the

Spasms entirely cease, and the Patient can begin to move and help himself, and at last the Spasms entirely cease, when these Medicines may be entirely left off, tho' it will not be proper to leave them off entirely till then.

But in order to remove these painful Symptoms the sooner, and relax the rigid tense Contraction of the Nerves, Tendons, and Muscles of the Parts affected, it is necessary to foment the Præcordia, Jaws, Neck, and Spine, with an emollient relaxing Fomentation, four or five times a Day; and I have found that something of the following Nature has succeeded the best:

℞ *Fol. Althæ vel Alcæ.* M. iv. *Salvæ, Flor Sambuci, ana* M ij. *Sem. Lini contus.* ʒij. *Sapon. Venet.* ʒij. *Sal Ammon. Crud.* ʒj. M. *Coq. in Aq. Cong.* j. *deinde adde, Pisselii Barbadoens.* ʒiij. *in Spir. Sacchar. Com.* lbss. *Solut. Theriac Androm.* ʒij. *Misce, fi. Fotus, cum quo foveant Region. Præcord, Faucium et Spinæ Dorsi, tepide ope Pannis laneis s.a. Sexta quaq; hora.*[†]

After which let the same Parts affected be anointed with the following Ointment, each time, and then be covered with Flannel.

℞ *Liniment. Saponac. Volatil. Nervin. Pisselii Indic. ana* ʒj. *Bals. Peruv.* ʒij. *Ol. Lavendul. Roismar. ana gut.* xx. *Opii* ʒj. *Misce, fi Liniment ut supra utend.*[†]

Some have strongly recommended the Use of the *Semicupium* in this Case; and I have known it used several times, and its Use seems to be both very reasonable and promising; but I have always observed that the Patients have received more Benefit from the Use of emollient Fomentations and anointing the Parts affected, as above, than ever I could observe from [use of] the warm Bath; and I have more than once known the Patient die immediately after being taken out of the warm Bath, tho' the Bath was not made too warm, being only about ninety-five Degrees in *Fahrenheit's* Scale, and they said he had not stayed more than twenty Minutes in the Bath: for which Reasons, I have constantly made use of the Fomentations and Liniment, and omitted Bathing, and I may add, with the desired Success in general.

In this Case the Pulse is generally small, languid and slow, only during the Continuance of the convulsive Spasms, and a Minute after them, it is often small, quick, and irregular, but soon becomes slow again, and the Patient is usually rather cool than warm, especially his extreme Parts, which are usually cold, and often covered with a cold clammy Sweat; wherefore some warming cordial Medicines are necessary to increase and keep up the Momentum of the circulating Fluids; [such] as a little soft warm Wine and Water given several times a Day, or something of the following Nature when sick or faint:

℞ *Aq. Menthæ Simp. Alexit. Simp. ana* ℥iv. *Vini Maderiens. vel Canar.* ℥iiij. *Spir. Lavend. C.* ℥ss. *Tinct. Cast. Spir. Aromat. vol. ana* ʒij. *Syr. e Mecon.* ʒj. *Misce, Dentur Cochl. duo vel tria in Spir. languorib.*†

For it is necessary to support the Patient with these, and the Use of a cordial vinous Diet, if they can get them swallowed, which in this Case is often done with Difficulty, as their Jaws are close locked together, and swallowing even Liquids is very painful and difficult; [such] as Gruel with Wine, and Wine-whey made pretty strong of the Wine; as it is absolutely necessary in this Case, to keep up a moderate equal Warmth all over the Body, and a moderate warm breathing Sweat† also, for I have always observed that where this can be done, and kept up, they generally recover; and where this equal Warmth and moderate Perspiration cannot be obtained, but the extreme Parts remain cold, and covered with cold Sweats, they most commonly die.

In this Disease, the Sick are generally costive, which is generally rendered more so, by giving such large and frequent Doses of Opiates, yet without which they can neither live nor recover; wherefore an emollient relaxing Clyster must be injected every other Day, or oftener if necessary. [Such] as:

℞ *Decoct. Emol. pro Clys.* ℥viij. *Elect. Lenitiv, Ol. Palmæ Christi, ana* ʒj. *Bals. Peruv.* ʒj. *Pisselii Indic.* ʒj. *Misce, fi. Enema.*†

But neither Purging, Bleeding, nor any other Evacuations are of any Service, but on the contrary are rather hurtful; except in a chance Case, where the Patient is of a plethoric Constitution, as I once saw one who was so, and had been treated with very hot Medicines, which had brought on some inflammatory Symptoms, with pleuretic Pains, and his Blood was become sizzy by taking such hot inflaming Medicines; but by bleeding him once, and the Use of antiphlogistic Medicines, with the Musk and Opium at proper Intervals, the Fever and Inflammation were taken off, and the Convulsions also, and the Person soon recovered. But Bleeding in this Case, when from a Puncture as this was, should be advised with great Caution and Judgment.

When the *Opisthotonos* and *Tetany* proceed from taking Cold, as before-mentioned, the Patient is usually seized with all the same Symptoms, as when they arise from a Puncture or Wound, and they usually come on in the same manner, first a Pain in the Head with a Stiffness in the Jaws, which after some time become close locked together and immovable, then spasmodic Contractions with acute Pain at the Scrobiculum Cordis, or where the Diaphragm, Mediastinum, Pleura, and Peritoneum meet and unite, these gradually extend to the Muscles of the Neck, and the Spine, and so produce the *Opisthotonos*, and lastly to all the anterior as well as posterior Muscles, and those of the whole Body, and produce a perfect *Tetany*, so that the *locked Jaw*, the *Opisthotonos*, and the *Tetany*, may be said to be the same Disease, only more or less extended, and the *Tetany* may be esteemed only a greater and more universal extended Degree of the former. But I must observe that when this Disease proceeds from taking Cold, it generally comes on sooner, *viz.* in three, four, or five Days after taking Cold, and sometimes sooner, even the next Night or Day; but when from a Puncture or Wound, it usually comes on after the tenth Day, rarely sooner, sometimes not before the fourteenth Day. And tho' the Symptoms are the same, and usually come on in the same manner in both Cases; yet when it proceeds from taking Cold, they not only come on sooner, but most commonly a small Fever usually begins to appear about the third or fourth Day after the locked Jaw has appeared, and in some, increases and appears with some inflammatory Symptoms in a few Days more, which indicate and require Bleeding; tho' their Blood in this Case is generally more florid, yet I never saw it covered with an inflammatory sizzy Pellicle.

The Indications and Intentions of Cure are the same in this Case as they are in the preceding, when from a Puncture or Wound; excepting the Incision, and what relates to the Wound, which cannot be necessary nor used here; as also are the same Methods and Medicines, [such] as the *Musk* and *Opiates*, fomenting and anointing the rigid and contracted Parts, as, the Præcordia, the Articulation of the Jaws, Neck, and Spina Dorsi, four or five times a Day, and the Use of all the other before-mentioned Medicines. But as this arises from taking Cold suddenly, by which the Perspiration is obstructed and diminished, and the Quantity of the Fluids is increased, whereby more or less of a Fever is produced, which is most commonly attended with some inflammatory Symptoms, which render it necessary to take some Blood from the Patient, more or less, accordingly as the Symptoms indicate; and sometimes to give some antiphlogistick Medicines, with the *Opiates* and *Musk* as before.

This Method I have found to be the most successful, and it generally answers our Expectations, when taken in time, and these Medicines are suitably given; but when they are too long deferred, it most commonly proves mortal, as well as the former: And when the Patient does recover, the Danger is usually over in six or eight Day's time; yet the Stiffness of his Neck and back generally continues for two or three Weeks, and sometimes longer, before it goes entirely off.

The *Opisthotonos* and *Tetany*, which seize young Children in this warm

Climate, arise from the same Causes, which usually produce the *Insultus Epilepticus*, or Convulsions, in them in England, *viz.* a Retention of the Meconium, or first Excrement after the Birth; or from a glutinous Matter which is too often found in the Intestines of young Children, soon after the other is discharged; or from a cheesy Matter from the Coagulation of the Milk by an Acid in the Stomach; or from hard Excrements; or from something taken in by the Mouth which is over acrid, or too hard to digest, which irritates their tender Bowels, and so produces Startings and convulsive Spasms, with all the other Symptoms which precede and accompany Convulsions in young Children in England; and shews how much more readily and easily the Nerves are affected and irritated in that warm Climate, and the *Tetany* produced from a much less Cause there, than it is in England, where it is but seldom seen: But these Causes not being timely removed, their Acrimony is increased, partly by the Heat of the Climate, and partly by the Fever which they produce, which still renders them more acrid, and so increases the Irritation of their Bowels, that it first brings on Startings, then convulsive Spasms, and regular Convulsion-fits, which, if not soon removed, usually end in a perfect *Tetany* there, and is but seldom cured in such young Children, when [the disease] arrives at that State: For when the Child lays in this miserable, rigid, immovable Condition, upon moving its Hands or Feet in the most gentle Manner, or softly touching any Part of its Body, or giving it the least Motion, even feeling its Pulse in the most gentle, tender Manner, or the least Noise, or even touching its Cloaths,[†] will bring on the convulsive Spasms, and cause it to be strongly convulsed backwards, or drawn into a rigid strait Line, strongly extended and immovable like a Statue, and will so remain immovable out of either of those Postures, for a considerable time, a Minute or two; and when the Disease is arrived at this Degree, I think it is never cured. But if the Physician is called in time, before the *Tetany* has seized the Child, (which is too seldom the Case there), though he finds strong convulsive Spasms have seized the Child, or that it has had a convulsive fit or two, provided that the *Tetany* is not come on, it may most commonly be relieved, and the coming of the *Tetany* be prevented, and the Life of the Babe be saved; as I have more than once seen, by removing and carrying off the irritating Cause, which stimulates and irritates their tender Bowels, by such gentle Evacuations as are suitable to their tender Age; and then quieting and composing the Irritation of their Nerves with suitable Anodynes, and correcting the remaining Acrimony of the nutritious Juices, in the *Primæ Viæ*.

To answer which Intentions, I have found the following Method, with Variations *pro re nata et pro ratione Ætatis*,[†] as the Cause is different, to answer the desired Effect the best. [Such] as:

℞ *Seri Lactis* ℥ij. *Sapon. Venet.* ℈j. *Manæ Chalab.* ℥ij vel iij. *Ol. Amigd. Dul.* ℥ss. *Fæniculi Dul. gut* ij. *Bals. Peruv. gut* v. *Misce, fi Enema quam primum injicienda.*[†]

And if the Symptoms of the approaching *Tetany* will permit, I usually give something of the following Nature to assist the Operation of the Clyster, and to carry off the Acrimony the sooner:

℞ *Aq. Sem. Fæniculi* ℥iij. *Magnes. Albæ* ℥ss. *Ocul. Cancr. præp.* ℈j. *Syr. e Cichor. cum Rheo, Rosar. Solut. ana* ℥iij. *Misce.*

Vel, ℞ *Aq. Sem. Fæniculi* ℥iij. *Sapon. Amigdal.* ℥ss. *Magnes. Albæ* ℥ss. *Syr. e Cichor. cum Rheo, Mannæ opt. ana* ℥ij. *Ol. Amigd. Dul.* ℥iij. *Misce, Exhibe Cochl. parv. vel duo pro ratione Ætatis omni semihora, vel omni hora, donec respond. Alvus.*[†]

Two or three Stools being obtained by these, I generally give something of the following Nature, in order to abate the convulsive Twitchings, and prevent the *Tetany* from coming on:

℞ *Aq. Sem. Fæniculi* ℥iij. *Magnes. Albæ.* ℥ss. *Ocul. Cancr. præp.* ℈j. *Moschi. Orient. gr* iij. *Spir. C.C. ver. gut.* xv. *Syr. e Mecon.* ℥ss. *Misce, Exhibe Cochl. Parv. (a Child's Spoonful dict) ter quaterve de die, vel sæpius, urgent. Convuls. vel Spasm.*[†]

But if the Symptoms shew that the *Tetany* is more immediately coming on, so that we have not time to wait till the Operation of the Clyster and opening Laxative be over, something of the following Nature must be immediately given; or the *Tetany* will come on, and most commonly proves fatal to such tender Babes.

℞ *Aq. Sem. Fæniculi* ℥iiij. *Moschi. Orient. gr.* j. *Tinct. Thebaic. gut.* iiij. *Syr. e Mecon.* ℥ij. *Misce pro duobus Dos. de quibus exhibe unam quam primum, et alter fi Convul. Spasm. redeunt.*[†]

This may be thought a bold Attempt, to give *Tinct. Thebaica* to such a tender young Infant; but as we are but too certain that it will die if the *Tetany* seize it, and that it will come on if this do not prevent it; and I have known a bold ignorant old Midwife give four or five Drops of that Tincture to a very young Infant without any Prejudice, more than its dosing three or four Hours, though not in this Case, but in one much less violent; and we ought not to think it below us, to gather Good from Evil, or Knowledge from the Bold and Ignorant, when we can, for the Good of Mankind in any Case, as it is neither unbecoming a good Man, or a Philosopher.

The Clyster may be given at the same time, and the opening Laxative not long after it, [and] though it may retard the Operation of that, for some time, yet it operates soon after, and gives Relief; after which the other Medicines, and fomenting the Body and anointing it, as before, may be used, if the Physician finds it necessary; also a little of the laxative Mixture may be given once or twice a Day, if the above Julep does not answer that Intention of keeping the Child's Body open for a few Days afterwards, which in this Case I have generally found it necessary to observe.

These Methods and Medicines may be varied accordingly as the Causes of the Convulsions differ, and the other concomitant Circumstances of the Patient may require, as the attending Physician sees it necessary; for neither the same Method, nor [the] same Medicines, will answer in all Cases, though the Disease be the same, but they must be changed as the causes differ, or the Constitution of the Sick, or the Time of the Disease, or as some other Circumstances may require; which is a thing of great Importance, not only in this, but in the Cure of most other Diseases; wherefore I mention it here, chiefly to caution the Practitioners in the West-Indies.

And when proper Medicines are thus timely and judiciously given in this Case, they seldom fail to carry off the irritating Cause, and quieten and ease the Nerves, and remove the Convulsions and Spasms, and consequently prevent the *Tetany's* coming on, and the Death of the Patient.

But if calling in the Physician be deferred, till the *Tetany* has already strongly seized the Child, as is too often the Case here, neither warm Bathing, Fomenting, nor these Methods and Medicines, nor any others whatever, as far as I have been able to observe, will remove it, or its Causes,† nor save the Life of the little tender Patient.

Of the RABIES CANINA, *or* MADNESS *from the Bite of mad Animals.*

THOUGH THIS DISEASE is neither new, nor endemial or epidemical to Mankind; yet it is so frequently seen in most hot Countries, and especially in the West-India Islands,† that it may be said to be endemial to the Dog-kind, and their bite infectious to Mankind; and as the Method of treating it, which is intended to be communicated here, has hitherto been found to be always successful, I hope it will be a sufficient Apology for my troubling the World with it here now, after so many learned Authors, in various Nations, have written so learnedly upon it.[†]

The great Professor *Boerhaave* has already treated so judiciously and learnedly on its Theory, that I have nothing new to add to it. *See his Aphorisms,* §1128 *&c.* or *his* Lectures on them, taken in short-hand and published by the learned *Baron Van Swieten.*[†] What I have to add here, chiefly relates to the *Prophylactic* and *Therapeutic* Methods of Cure.

The *Rabies Canina*, so called from the savage Madness, which is caused by the Bite of Mad-dogs, hence also called canine Madness; and from its most terrible Symptom of dreading Water, it is also called *Hydrophobia*, and by some *Hygrophobia*.

This Disease, tho' indigenous in warm Climates to the Dog-kind; always proceeds from a poisonous Contagion[†] taken into the Blood of Men, by the Wounds made by the Bite of some Animal which was mad before. As of Dogs, Wolves, Foxes, Cats, Apes, Horses, Asses, Mules, Oxen, Sheep, Swine or Fowls, which are mad; as also from Men labouring under this Disease, when they bite and wound those who attend upon them. But it appears from History, that Dogs, Foxes, and Wolves, (which are all of the Dog-kind) are subject to this Disease from immediate internal Causes, without being bitten or infected by other Animals; which most commonly arises from the long continued great Heat of the Climate, and great Dryness of the Country, a Want of Water, and being ill fed, or from their feeding upon putrid, fœtid, maggoty Meats, and sometimes from Worms bred in the Kidneys, Intestines, and Brains or high up in the Nostrils of those Animals.

And as great Heats and Dryness frequently continue long in these Islands, and are sometimes attended with a Scarcity of Water, and that the Dogs are often much starved and ill fed, and frequently get putrid and maggoty Flesh of dead Animals, it is no wonder that those poor creatures frequently run mad, and then bite other Dogs, and other Animals as well, as well as Men, which soon after become mad also; and thus this dreadful Disease is too often fatally propagated.[†]

Wherefore I shall here carefully describe the Symptoms or Signs, which generally seize those Animals, especially the Dogs, when they have been bitten, or are otherwise become mad, that their Owners may take proper care of, or destroy them, before they bite and infect others, and so propagate the Disease.

Not long after these Animals, especially the Dogs, have been bitten, by a mad Dog, they first begin to look dull and sad, and endeavour to hide themselves, or seek a Solitude in some dark or bye[†] Place; seldom or never bark, yet will grumble and be angry with, or fly at, Strangers, but yet know and will fawn upon their Owners; they begin to refuse their Meat and Drink, or just slightly taste them; they droop and hang down their Ears and Tails, look very dull and sleepy, and often lay down; this is the first Degree of the Disease, and their Bite is now dangerous, but not always infectious. Soon after this, they begin to breathe quick and heavily, [then] gape and shut out their Tongues, and discharge much Slaver and Froth from their Mouths, and looking as if half asleep they suddenly fly at the By-standers, then run forward, not in a straight but in a crooked line; these Symptoms increase, and they begin not to know their Owners; their Eyes look exceeding dull and dusty, and much Water runs from their Eyes like Tears; their Tongues are of a Lead-colour, they grow weak and often fall down, then rise and attempt to fly at something, grow mad and furious: This is the second and last Degree of the Disease, which seldom continues above thirty Hours before they die. Their bite, during the second State of the Disease, is commonly said to be incurable, and the longer it has continued, the more furious their Madness; and the nearer they are to their Deaths, the more dangerous and more fatal their Bite, and the sooner it produces its Symptoms and direful effects.

Scarce any Poison known, is so infectious, or so easily and readily communicated by so many and various ways as this of a mad Dog is; for the slightest Bite, only tearing the Skin, without drawing Blood, or the smallest Quantity of the Slaver of the mad Animal, either fresh, or dried for some time, taken upon the Tongue or Lips,[4] or rending a Person's Cloaths and leaving the Slaver on them to dry, has produced this Disease; as a Woman[5] had her Coat torn by a mad Dog, which she a considerable time after sowed up, and bit off the Thread with her Teeth, and some time after died rabid from biting off that Thread. Also a Man only kissing his Children to take his leave of them, when he had the Rabies upon him, they all soon after died rabid.[6] Kissing a favourite Dog that was mad, had the same Effect; and a small Wound received from a Sword which had killed a mad Dog a considerable

---

4. Celius Aurelian. de Morb. Acut. lib. Iii.
5. F. Hildanus Obs. Chirurg. Cent. I.
6. Palmarius de morb. Contagios. p. 266 et Schenkii, Obs. Med. p. 848.

long time before has produced this most fatal Disease. Hence we see that we cannot be too cautious in avoiding this infectious Poison; nor too careful in burning such infected or torn Garments, or in carefully cleaning such Knife, Sword, or Instruments as were used to kill such mad Animals; neither in using the utmost Care to avoid getting any the least Particle of such infectious Saliva into or near our Mouths, or on any excoriated or wounded Parts of our Bodies, though ever so slight, and immediately to wash them in salt Water and Vinegar.

However, we do not find from any History that this Poison infects us through [intact] Skin;[7] but it may be prudent to wash such a Part with salt Water and Vinegar, to take the Slaver off.

Neither do we know any Poison or Infection, which produces such terrible Effects, in so short a Space of time, as this has been known to do, and at other times to lay so long dormant or hid in the Body, without any Pain till it was brought into Action, and then produced its most dreadful Effects, as this Poison is said to have done: for History informs us, that some have been seized with its dreadful Symptoms in a very short Time after they have been bitten,[8] others have continued well for twenty Years,[9] and were then seized with them, and died hydrophobous;† and others again have been seized with it at all the intermediate Times between these.[10] Hence we see that this Poison sometimes enters into Action very speedily, and on the contrary that at other times it lies dormant many Years, and then proves suddenly destructive, when it is once roused into Action.

I shall first describe the Symptoms of it, when it seizes Men. A Person in perfect Health, being seized with this canine Contagion, is sooner or later seized with the following Symptoms, and in the following Order: First, the Part which was wounded, or where the contagious Poison was first fixed or given, begins to be painful, then wandering Pains gradually spread round it, and so to other Parts of the Body; a Weariness, Heaviness, and Inaptitude to Motion through all the Muscles follows; their Sleep is disturbed with frightful Dreams, accompanied with great Startings and convulsive Spasms; great Restlessness, and continual Tossings of the Body, Sighing, Sorrowfulness, and

---

7. Paul. Æginet. Lib. v. Ch. 3. Ætius, Tetrabit. Lib, vi. Ch. 24. Sauvages fur la Rage, p. 5.
8. Stalpart Van der Weilen Observ. Rarior. p. 413.
9. Du Choicels de la Rage.
10. Schmid. in Miscel. Curios. Dec. 1. Ann. 9. p. 119.

a Desire of Solitude; these Symptoms usually attend the first Beginning of the Disease, and continue to the End of the first Stage of it: Blood now being taken from a Vein, has all the Signs of Health in it. This State continues in some a longer, in others a shorter Time, and then they enter upon the second Stage of the Disease, in which all the above Symptoms are increased, with the Addition of a violent Oppression at the Præcordia, a great Difficulty of Breathing, with Sighing; great Horror and Dread of Mind; which is increased upon the Sight of Water or other Liquors, or the Face of a Looking-glass, as it resembles Water, with great Tremors: A Loss of Appetite, yet they generally can swallow soft, solid Food or Medicines; but touching any kind of Liquids gives them intolerable Anxiety, with great Tremors and Convulsions, and often throws them into raving Madness: They vomit a glutinous, brownish, bilious Matter, or a porraceous Bile; a Fever, with great inward Heat and Thirst comes on, attended with continual Watchings, and sometimes with a Priapism;† very disturbed and unusual rambling Thoughts, and sometimes Ravings; and thus continues and ends the second Stage of this Disease. But after this, all the above-mentioned Symptoms are continually aggravated and increased, the Tongue becomes dry and rough, and is often thrust out of the Mouth; the Voice becomes hoarse, and the Thirst almost inexpressibly great, yet [they] cannot drink anything, because now on the Sight of, or attempting to touch any Liquor, they are strongly convulsed and thrown into a raving Madness: A great Quantity of frothy Saliva is collected in their Mouths, which they cannot swallow, but endeavour to spit out upon the By-standers, even against their Inclinations when they are more sensible; with a Desire of biting those they can come at, though often contrary to all the Force of their Will; they rage and foam at [the] Mouth; their Pulse sinks, and their Breathing fails; cold clammy Sweats come on; they are raving mad, yet have Intervals in which they are rational and speak prudently, and are fearful of hurting others who are present. And thus most commonly, Death with a suffocating Breathing and Convulsions, puts an end to their miserable Life, within the fourth Day from the first Stage of the Disease.

Having thus plainly described this Disease, and its most remarkable Symptoms, by which it may certainly be known, both when it seizes Dogs, that they may be destroyed; and also when it seizes Men, when they have the Misfortune to be bitten by any mad Animal, and are seized with it, so that it may be known to be this dreadful Disease, and that they may apply to proper Assistance before it be too late; I shall not enter any farther into the Theory of this Disease, than is absolutely necessary to explain my Reasons for proposing what I may hereafter recommend: As that is already done by a more able Hand.[11] Neither shall I say any thing more relating to the Nature of this subtle and deleterious Poison, or its manner of acting, so as to produce its direful Effects; as so many able Physicians, both ancient *Greeks* and *Arabians*, and many learned Moderns, have so learnedly and judiciously treated on this Subject.[12] From which the Diagnosis of this Disease may be certainly known, though the Prognosis of its Consequences and Effects are not so certainly known as we could wish them to be: since all the greatest Professors of our Art, have lamented, that even in its present improved State, it has scarce once furnished us with a certain *Prophylactic*, or real preventative Cure of those who have been bitten by a real mad Animal; and affords us not one single Instance of a Cure, that can be certainly relied upon, after the Dread of Liquors has appeared and seized those Patients. As the great *Boerhaave* has judiciously observed; and adds, "It is much to be lamented, that after so many Ages past have been thus deplorably sensible of the fruitless Inefficiency in all their former known Methods, they should still neglect the Trial of new ones, different from those of their Predecessors."[13]

To say any thing on those, or any other how much soever extolled Nostrums, is unnecessary; unless we can introduce something that is new, and produce certain undeniable Instances of their Success, so as that they may become useful to Mankind. I shall therefore, after describing the State in which the Bodies of those who died of this Disease, have been found upon Dissection; and then relate the *Prophylactic Method of Cure*, which I have used, and found to be successful, after the persons have been bitten by mad Animals, but before the Hydrophobia came on. And then say something on the *Therapeutic* Method of Cure after those fatal Symptoms are come on; and shall candidly relate such Cases as were very remarkable and have fallen under my own Observation, with Fidelity.

From Dissecting Bodies [of those] who died of this Disease,[14] we are

---

11. In Profess. *Boerhaave's* Aphor. de Cog. et Cur. Morb, and his Lectures published by the learned Baron *Van Sweiten*.

12. *Boerhaave* in locis cit. *Mead* on Poisons. Tulpius Ob. Med. Salius Diversus, Stalpart Van der Weilen, Sauvages, Philos. Transact. Memoir de l'Acad. des Scienc. Curios. Acta Physico-Medic. Curiosr. &c., &c.

13. *Boerhaave's* Lectures on his Aphorisms, by the Baron *Van Sweiten*, de Rab. Canin.

14. Boerhaav. Aphorism. de Cog. &c. Bonet. Sepulemet. Anatom. Tom. I Lib. I &c.

informed, that the Organs of swallowing are usually in an inflamed State; that a viscid Glue-like bilious Matter is found in the Stomach; the Gall bladder filled with black Bile; the Pericardium quite dry; the Lungs incredibly stuffed up with Blood; the Heart filled with Blood, which is often found almost dry; the Arteries filled with Blood; the Veins almost empty; and their Blood very liquid, and will not easily coagulate in the Air, tho' it concreted† but three Days before when taken from a Vein; all the Muscles, Viscera, Brain, Cerebellum, and the spinal Marrow, are found much drier than usual.

From whence I beg leave to observe, that although an Inflammation of the Organs of Swallowing usually, but not always, is found in such dead Bodies; and that Inspection into the Fauces and Throat, informs us, that an Inflammation of those Parts is never found in the Beginning of the Disease, and very seldom, even some time after the Patient has been unable to swallow any Liquids, and in some, not even at the last; so that it is not an Inflammation and Swelling of the Parts that hinders their Swallowing, but the convulsive Spasms of those Parts.

Hence we conclude, that though the first Cause or Bite may be in the remotest Part of the Body, yet the contagious Poison, when it begins to act, and exerts its poisonous Force, it chiefly affects the Nerves of the Gula,† and the Muscles employed in Deglutition, which it so greatly irritates, when they are moved, as to cause violent Spasms and convulsive Contractions in them; from whence proceeds that Impossibility of swallowing any Liquids whatever: And both that glutinous Matter in the Stomach, and the great Dryness in the Blood, Heart, and other Parts above-mentioned, proceed principally from a want of a Supply of Liquids to dilute them, increased by the inward heat, and continual Waste of the Fluids, by Saliva, Urine, Perspiration, and Sweat: and the inflammation of the Gula and the Muscles serving for Deglutition, which is found in some Patients, but not in all, arises from the want of that Supply of Liquids, and Dryness of the Blood, and the frequent convulsive Spasms of those Parts: Hence we must conclude, that this Inflammation of those Parts, is not the Cause of their Inability of Swallowing, but is the Effect of the above-mentioned Causes, and the often repeated convulsive Spasms of those Parts.

As all the Histories of this Disease, give us so many dreadful Accounts of its most fatal Effects, we cannot be too careful and assiduous in using all prudent Methods to prevent them, when any Person has the Misfortune to be infected with its Poison; for I believe that no Man who has seen the dreadful

Issue of this Disease, but would readily prefer a Maiming, if not the Loss of a Limb, to save his Body from so calamitous a Death.

Wherefore, when any Person has the Misfortune to be bitten by a mad Animal, if a Surgeon or an Apothecary be near, it is undoubtedly the safest and most prudent Method, immediately to cut the bitten Part clean out, (if it be in such a Part of the Body, that it can be safely done), then apply a Cupping-glass† over that Wound so soon as possible after, in order to suck out as much of the Poison with the Blood, as you possibly can; after which cauterize the Bottom and all the Sides of the Wound with an actual Cautery,† and dress it with a proper Digestive; then wash the Wound every Day with Salt-water and Vinegar, and keep it open with gentle Escharoticks† for a considerable long time, that it may discharge as much of the Poison as possible. But if the Part bitten be such that it cannot be safely cut out, let it be gently scarified near the Wound, then cupped and cauterized, and dressed, washed, and kept open as above, or cauterized without scarifying.†

Also, great Care should be taken that the Garments of the Person, if torn, or the least daubed with the Slaver of the mad Animal, be burned, and the rest of it be carefully clean washed: Also, that the Straw, Trash, or Bedding, on which the Negroe laid, spit, or slavered, be burned; or the Trash on which the mad Animal laid, slavered, or on which it was killed, be carefully burned, and the Place clean washed; and the Sword or Instrument with which it was killed, be carefully cleaned; for we have Instances of Cattle eating such Straw some Time after, on which the mad Animal had laid, and dying mad soon after, by eating that Straw.

This being done, (or where these Operations have been neglected to be done), if the Patient be of a plethoric Constitution, and has lost little Blood by Cupping; I usually order some Blood to be taken from then, and if their Stomach be foul, a Vomit to be given (if not, it is not necessary), that Evening, and a Musk Bolus of the following Nature after it when going to Bed; with Directions to encourage moderate Sweating that Night, by drinking warm small Whey-wine after it.

℞ *Moschi Orient. gr.* xvi. *Cinnabar. Nativ. levig.* ℥ss. *vel* ℈ii. *Pil. Saponac. gr.* viij. *Camphorii gr* vi. *Bals. Peruv.* q.s. *Misce, fi Bolus.*†

And the next Morning I usually give an antiphlogistic Purge, and in the Evening after, I most commonly order the Patient to bathe in the Sea, (or if that is at too great a Distance, in a cold Bath, or a River), and either plunge himself, or be plunged by the Hands of another Person, quite over Head, and detained under the Water some time; and to repeat that two or three times, then come out and be rubbed dry, and go into Bed, and take the *Musk Bolus* as above, and drink half a Pint of the Infusion of *Rad. Valerian. Sylvest. Cort. Sassafræ,*[†] and as much warm small Wine-whey as he pleases after that, and encourage moderate Sweating all that Night; and to repeat the Bathing in the Sea, and the Musk Bolus after it; as also the Infusion and warm Whey every Night, for three or four Nights more successively, with moderate Sweating each Night. And if the Animal which bit them, was in its last Stage of Madness, or was very rabid or raging when it bit them, I order them to repeat all the same, for six or seven Nights more successively; and also to repeat all the same for three Nights at the next Full, and the next Change of the Moon following. For I have observed frequently, that several Persons (though not all) who were bitten by mad Animals, were more disordered, and were seized with a Heaviness, Dullness, and a Love of Solitude, at the Full and Change of the Moon next following them being bitten, tho' it went off, and they recovered by these Methods and Medicines, and they became perfectly well after.[†]

I have also generally advised these Patients to go into the Sea or cold Bath, the last Morning after this Bathing and Sweating; then to rub themselves dry, and put on their Cloaths without Sweating, and go about their Business or Pleasure, in order to prevent their taking Cold, and bringing on a Fever, which might be of bad consequence at this time.

I am sensible that this prophylactic Method of Cure differs considerably, in several Respects, from that recommended by my much esteemed and learned Master, *Profes. Boerhaave*; and also from that of several other learned Physicians, who have all recommended Bathing in the Sea, but to be performed with such a bustling and terrifying Apparatus, as to excite a Dread and Fear of Suffocation in the Patient; and the repeating those Immersions several times in order to increase that Terror, though he both threatens and supplicates the Performer to the contrary, as the Dutch Sailors have been taught, and usually do. And both *They*[15] and that learned *Professor*,[16] tell us, that it generally was so successful in effecting a Cure, that it *seldom failed*; and I remember that *He* in his Lectures on his Aphorisms,[17] usually gave us several

---

15. Tulpii. Observ. Med. L. 1. Cap. 20, p. 41. Stalpart Van der Wielen Cent. 1 Obs. 100, &c. Dekkers Exercic. Pract. p. 546.

16. Ridley Observat. de Asthm. et Hydrophob. Ob. 25.

17. Vide Baron Van Sweiten, in Aphor. H. Boerhaavi, Vol. IV.

Histories of Cases in which it was successful; but he also gave us some in which it did not succeed, and they died hydrophobous afterwards.

But they seem to ascribe too much to the Terror and Dread, which the Patient is put into by such a frightful Apparatus; nor can I conceive how exciting such a Dread can be of any Service, or any way contribute to the Cure in this Case, where the Dejection of their Spirits, and great Dread which always attends this Disease, are already too great before without the Addition of such a frightful Apparatus; unless it acts by causing them to sweat more copiously after it.

But we can more rationally account for the producing a copious Sweating after cold Bathing, and its being of great Service in this Case: Since we know that cold Immersion braces up, and gives a greater Spring to the Solids, and causes them to act with greater Force on their contained Fluids, and so increasing their Momentum, which will not only attenuate them, but may contribute to comminute† and break the morbid viscid poisonous Matter also, (especially if they dilute plentifully, with such a saponaceous† Liquor as Whey is, at the same time); and all these Causes thus jointly acting, may probably greatly contribute to cast the morbid Matter out of the Body by such copious warm Sweats, as we frequently see are produced after cold Bathing, especially when assisted by the above Methods and Medicines. And I believe that it is from these Causes, thus acting, that cold Immersions have been found to be of so much Service in the prophylactic Cure of this Disease; and I apprehend that if those learned Gentlemen had been with their Patients when they bathed, and made their Observations with greater Accuracy, in respect to their sweating more or less after it, they would have found that those who had the most free continued warm, copious (not profuse) Sweats, received the greatest Benefit from it, and that those who did not so, received the least; because I think that I have found it so, at least in several Cases, which have fallen under my own Observation; some of which I shall now relate.

A Gentlewoman's two Sons, her Housekeeper, and seven Negroes, were all bitten by a mad Dog, in one Morning; a Month after which the Housekeeper died hydrophobous: this alarmed the Family, and they sent for me the next Day; her eldest son, eighteen Years old, was of a sanguine healthful Constitution; the younger one had a weaker Constitution; they were both bitten in their Legs, tho' not very deep; but their Wounds were both healed up and cicatrized two Weeks before I saw them, and they were seemingly well. They did not tell me that the Negroes were also bitten, [nor] did I know it till afterwards.

The eldest Son being more plethoric, was bled, the younger was not, they were both purged the next Morning; then bathed in the Sea, being near it, and took the Musk and Cinnabar Boluses, as above, (the Younger had a little less Quantity of them both, he being but thirteen Years old) and encouraged moderate Sweating, &c. as directed. And five of the seven Negroes that were bitten by the same Dog, had the same Medicines given to them, as I had prescribed for the eldest Son, they being Men, and were treated in the same manner; and both her Sons and all these five Negroes have continued to be very well, without having any Symptom of this Disease ever since, which is now ten Years ago. But the poor hired Negroes, neither had any Medicines or any thing done for them, unless they bathed, and both died rabid, about two Months after the Housekeeper.

Here three of ten Persons, who were all bitten by the same mad Dog, near the same time, and had no Assistance nor Medicines given to them, all died rabid and hydrophobous; and all the seven Persons who took the Medicines and were treated as above, all remain free from any Symptoms of this Disease, and continue to enjoy Health. This is an Experiment which Humanity would forbid any Man to make; and if I had known the State of those two Negroes, I would have procured them Medicines at my own Expense, but was not acquainted with their being bitten. However, it serves to strongly prove, and greatly confirm the Efficacy of this *prophylactic Method of Cure.*[†]

Not long after this, a worthy Lady of great Merit had thirteen of her Negroes bitten by a mad Dog who, by the best Account that I could obtain, was in the last Stage of his Madness when he bit them. They were all treated in the before-mentioned Method, with Variations *pro ratione Ætatis, &c.* of the *Musk* and *Cinnabar, &c.* and have all continued perfectly free from any Symptoms of this Disease, though it was several Years since. And I could mention several more, who had the misfortune to be bitten by mad Dogs[†] since, and by the same Methods and Medicines, have hitherto escaped entirely free from any Appearance of this Disease; neither have I ever yet seen any who pursued this Method regularly, that have ever had any Appearance of this Disease afterwards; which induces me to recommend this Method of *prophylactic Cure* to others.

I must further observe, that in most of the above-mentioned Patients, the Wounds made by the mad Dogs were healed up, and well, some time before any Applications were made; those few whose Wounds were not healed up, had them washed twice a Day with Salt-water and Vinegar, and then dressed with a common Digestive till well. Neither did I make use of any *Mercury*, either internally or externally, but the Cinnabar, which is Ore of Mercury, tho' it has been strongly recommended by several learned Physicians,[18] who have given us several Accounts of its good Success, but generally when it was used with other Medicines at the same time. But the learned Authors also mention several Cases, wherein Mercury was used very liberally both internally and externally; yet it did not succeed, but the Patients died rabid after; so that it does not by any means merit the Name of an infallible Antidote.

Neither durst I wholly depend upon the Assertions of the *Chinese*, tho' they say, that *Musk* and *Cinnabar* is an infallible Remedy in this Case. Their Method of giving them is *Moschi gr* xvj. *Cinnabar. Facitti, Nativi ana* ʒj. *Misce, fi Pulv.*[†] which they give in a little Arrack,[†] and if it does not cause the Patient to sleep and sweat, in three Hours' Time, they repeat the Dose, which always procures Sleep, and a copious Sweat, as Sir *George Cobb*, who first brought an Account of this Remedy from China,[†] informed me, which was about the Time that the great *Boerhaave* died, and it is probable that *he* had not heard of, as *he* has said nothing of it in this Case; but the learned *Baron Van Sweiten* has added an Account of its Effects, to the Lectures on the *Rabies Canina* of that great *Author*, as also on *Mercury*. But the extraordinary Effects, which I have many times seen from giving *Musk* in convulsive Cases, and particularly in violent *Hiccoughs*, which are a convulsive Spasm of the Æsophagus; and this Disease being attended with violent convulsive Spasms of the superior Parts of the Æsophagus and the Muscles serving for Deglutition, were greater Motives for my giving it, than the Recommendations of the *Chinese*, because as much has been said of the Efficacy of several other Antidotes and Nostrums. But I must add, that giving the *Musk* has hitherto answered my Wishes and Expectations; and I cannot but ascribe much more to the Virtues of *Musk* than to *Cinnabar*, though it may probably contribute something; but from what Observations I have made, the Musk seems to do much more by its subtle Parts, both attenuating the circulating Fluids, and the poisonous Matter also, and so carrying it out of the Body, by those copious warm Sweats, which it usually produces, especially when it is assisted by increasing the Vis Vitæ and Momentum of the Fluids, by the previous cold Bathing, just before they take it, and go into Bed, to encourage that Sweating; and by repeating it four

---

18. Desault Differt. sur la Rage. Sauvages Diff. sur la Rage. Philos. Transactions.

or five Nights successively; and as I have found this Method so successful, I cannot but recommend it to others.

Having said thus much on the *prophylactic Method of Cure*, I shall now say something on the *Therapeutic*, or the Method of Cure when the Symptoms of the Disease have already seized the Patient; and the sooner the Cure is attempted, after the first Appearance of its Symptoms, the better, and the more likely it is to prove successful, as the great *Boerhaave* justly observes,[19]

"Curatio verò morbi jam presentis videtur tentanda, maximè in primo gradu; et in initio secund. imprimis quum aliter sunestissimo exitu neglectus plectatur. — Statim post prima signa invadentis mali morbus tractandus, ut summus inflammatorius, mittendo sanguinem ex lato vulnere magni vasis ad animi deliquium usque, &c."†

But inasmuch as the Hydrophobia arises first from the convulsive Spasms of the Gula and Organs of swallowing, and not from an Inflammation of those Parts; neither is it any Inflammation or Swelling in them, that hinders them from drinking Liquids, but the convulsive Spasms of them, which being often and violently repeated, together with a Want of a Supply of diluting Liquors, that produces an Inflammation of those Parts at the last; hence we discover that the Inflammation is the Effect, and not the cause of the Hydrophobia. But as Bleeding may prevent the Inflammation's coming on, and abate those Spasms, it may be necessary in a moderate Degree; and when the Disease is further advanced, it is necessary in a much larger Quantity; and I have found it to be of very great Service. But I think still that the principal Part of the Cure, depends upon the Effect of the Antispasmodics, especially the *Musk*, and their attenuating the morbid Matter, so as to fit it to be carried out of the Body by free copious Sweating, especially in the prophylactic Cure, as also in the beginning of the second Stage of the Disease; which the following Cases seem to confirm.

A young Gentleman near eighteen Years of Age, was bitten by a mad tame Fox, who was bitten by a mad Dog some time before; the Wound was four Inches above his Heel, and bled a little but was healed up in two Week's time. But the next following new Moon, he appeared to be very dull, heavy, and much dejected, but these [symptoms] went off in three or four Day's time; but the next full Moon all these Symptoms returned in a greater Degree,

19. Boerh. Aphoris. de Cog. et Cur. Morb. Aph. 1144.

joined with a strong Desire of Solitude; that Night he did not sleep much, and that much disturbed; his Father desired him to rise, which after some time he did, but put on his Cloaths, and hid himself in a dark Place under the Roof of the House, and said, he could not bear to see any Company, and was not willing to see me when I came there, though well acquainted with him, neither would he see any other Company; I went to him, and told him that he was not well, and desired him to tell me how he was, and if the Fox had not bit him; he said, yes; but there was nothing in that, the Place was well two Weeks since, and he well after that, but now he had an uneasy Sensation and Weight at his Stomach and Breast, was greatly dejected he knew not why, and desired to be alone; I then took him into a private Room, and found that he had all or most of the Symptoms of the first State of this Disease (though he was of a naturally cheerful Disposition) and found that his Disorder solely arose from the Bite of the mad Fox, who had made his escape. I ordered xviij [fluid ounces] of Blood to be taken from him immediately, gave him a Vomit in the Evening, with which he drank Green-tea plentifully, and the following sudorific Bolus at Bed-time, and warm Whey-wine after it, and encouraged a warm breathing Sweat all that night; for the extraordinary Virtues of Musk in this Case, were not known in England at that time, nor till some Years after.

℞ *Mas. Pil. Saponac. gr.* x. *Sal. Succini vol. Camphorii ana gr.* viij. *Tartar. Regenerat. Theriac. Androm. ana* ʒj. *Ol. Sassafræ gut.* ij. *Bals. Peruv. q.s. Misce, fi Bolus.*[†]

The next Morning he took an antiphlogistick Purge, which purged him pretty briskly, and repeated the same Bolus the Night after it; he slept well and sweated freely both these Nights, and was much better the next Day; he went to Scarborough the Day after, where he drank the cooling, nitrous purging Waters of that Spaw every Morning, and bathed in the Sea every Night for five or six Nights, and then every other Night for three Weeks more, and went to Bed after Bathing and took the above Bolus, and drank warm Whey, and encouraged moderate Sweating after it, and returned home perfectly well, and has continued so ever since, which is now above twenty-six Years ago.

A young Man about 20 Years of Age, was bitten by a mad Dog, and neglected to do any thing for it, and was at the full Moon following seized in the same Manner as the Gentleman above; these Symptoms also went off after three Days, but returned the next full Moon following, but considerably aggravated and increased: He then came to me; and finding his Case to be near the same as the other Gentleman's, except that the Load and Oppression at his Stomach was less, and he had more Pain in his Head; I advised the same Method as above, except the Vomit, and repeated the Purge two or three times; as he did not go to Scarborough, he went into a cold Bath, and took a sudorific Bolus, as above, and an Infusion of Valerian and Sassafras after it; and encouraged a free Perspiration, with moderate Sweating after it, by drinking warm Whey after them every Night, for near two Weeks, and was then well: I saw him some Months after perfectly well, and have not seen or heard any thing from him since.

These two Cases were taken at the first Beginning of the Symptoms, in the first Stage of the Disease, before any Appearance of the Hydrophobia came on; and by this attenuating sudorific Method, it and its dreadful Effects were prevented from ever coming on: but I must add, that I should now prefer giving the Musk and Cinnabar as above, from the many extraordinary Effects which I have since seen them have.

Three Years after this, I was called to a Barber's Wife above 20 Miles from me, but being pre-engaged to go ten Miles the contrary Way; and the Apothecary having described her Case and Constitution very well, I gave the following Directions, as I could not see her in time. She had a pretty good Constitution, though not robust and strong; and was bitten by a mad Dog near three Months before: She was seized with the first Symptoms of this Disease, four or five Days before they sent to me, which increased, and the Hydrophobia with the other Symptoms of the Rabies came on, the Day before they sent for me; she could neither drink, nor bear the Sight of any Liquors for some Hours before the Messenger set out on the Journey; and the Rabies was so great, that the Attendants had bound her Hands and Feet to the Posts of the Bed on which she laid; so that the Hydrophobia had been upon her above thirty Hours, before the following Medicines were administered:

I ordered her to be bled *fere ad deliquium Animi,*[†] and added to bleed her as long as they could, not to let her die away; then two Hours after, to plunge her into a large Tub of cold Water, and to immerge[†] her quite over Head two or three times, and to detain her under the Water each time, as long as they could, not to drown her; then to take her out and rub her dry, and put her into Bed, and give her the following soft sudorific Bolus, without offering her any Liquids with it, or for two Hours after it; which she took and swallowed with a little Difficulty; for they can often swallow a soft solid Substance as Food, when they can neither bear to see, or take any Liquids.

℞ *Theriac. Androm.* ℥ss. *Pil. Saponac. Sal. Succini vol. ana* ℈ss. *Camphorii Pulv. gr.* viij. *Ol. Menthæ gut.* i. *Syr. e Mecon. q. s. Misce, fi Bolus molli, ut supra sumend.*[†]

And three Hours after that, or sooner, if the Opiate began to affect her, so that she could bear the Sight of any Liquids, to give her a Draught of an Infusion of *Rad. Valeriani, Cort. Sassafræ,* with *Sal. Nitri, Sal. Diuretic,* sweetened with a little Sugar, and as much warm small Whey-wine after that, as often as she would drink; which she now took and drank with tolerable Ease: And in two Hour's time after the first Draught, *viz.* about four or five Hours after the Bathing, having sweated most of that Time, she fell asleep, and slept four Hours, and sweated freely all that Time, then awakened very sensible and calm; and as she now could drink Liquids with ease, she took a Draught of the above Infusion every three Hours, and drank off the warm Whey very plentifully, and continued the warm breathing Sweat [for] forty-eight Hours, as I had ordered, and repeated the Bolus three times in that time. An antiphlogistic Cathartic was given her the Morning following, which purged her well, and she continued to dilute plentifully with Whey, and repeated the Bolus that Night after the Operation of the Purge; she slept very well that Night and appeared to be very well the next Day, only she was weak and low from such large Evacuations; but that was soon relieved, and her Strength restored by a suitable cooling, diluting, and nutritious Diet, which she took and perfectly recovered: And I saw her about seven Years after that, in perfect Health.

The first Steps towards this Cure were made by the large Bleeding, and giving the Opiate, which greatly contributed to take off the convulsive Spasms, and so enabled the Patient to drink diluting Liquids copiously, whereby the almost dried circulating Fluids, were diluted and attenuated; and this being seconded by cold Immersion, by which the Momentum of the Fluids must be increased and attenuated, which being assisted by the volatile, attenuating, saponaceous Medicine, and diluting plentifully with such a saponaceous Liquor as Whey is known to be, must jointly contribute not only to attenuate the circulating Fluids, but the poisonous morbid Matter also, and so carry it out of the Body by the long continued, free, warm Sweating, as was above advised. At least these were my Reasons for directing this Method of Cure, to which what the great *Boerhaave* has said concerning Bleeding largely, and cold

Bathing in this Case, was not the least Motive to it: This, however, seems to be the most rational way of accounting for their effecting this extraordinary Cure, in so short a time.

The extraordinary Effects of *Musk* when given in large Doses, in this and some other convulsive Spasms, were not then known in England; and as I have always found the above *Prophylactic* Method of Cure so successful, that I have not had an Opportunity of seeing any one Hydrophobus since the above Patient; otherwise I should have given the *Musk* with the *Opium, Sal. Succini & Camphor* instead of the *Theriaca*, because I think it is a much preferable, and in every way a better Medicine in this Case.

And as *Musk* is found by Experience, to be so effectual a Remedy, in the *Prophylactic* Cure of this Disease; have we not just Reasons to hope for its being equally as successful a Remedy in the *Therapeutic* Cure, if taken in proper time? Especially as it is now known to be a more powerful and effectual antispasmodic Medicine, than the above, or any other Medicines that we now know, *Opium* only excepted; and as powerful an Attenuator and Sudorific as them, if not more so; does it not promise to be as successful in the latter, as it is known to be in the former? And if we add *Musk* to the *Opium* as above, after Bleeding largely, and cold Bathing, may we not hope that it may prove to be the *Antidote* against this singular Poison, which the great *Boerhaave* (and all good Men) have wished for, when he says, *Aphoris.* 1146: "*Nec desperandum tamen, ob exempla jam in aliis Venenis constantia, de inveniendo hujus singularis Veneni Antidoto singulari.*"†

Of CHRONICAL DISEASES

HAVING TREATED on such *Acute Diseases* in the preceding Part, as are either peculiar to, or endemial in the West-India Islands, and such Countries as are situated within the Torrid Zone, and are not so frequently seen in most Parts of Europe; I shall here speak of such *Chronical Diseases* as are either indigenous or endemial, in the same warm Countries, and are unknown and never seen but in the hot Climates, except when they are carried by the Sick into the colder Countries.

And I shall begin with the Description of a Disease, which I think I may safely say is new, and has never yet been described by any Author, neither Ancient nor Modern, not even by any of the *Arabian Physicians*; most of whom lived and practiced in the hot Countries of *Persia*, *Syria*, *Arabia*, and *Ægypt*; but of late Years is become endemial and frequent in Barbadoes, and the other West-India Islands.

From the best Accounts that I can obtain, this Malady has been some chance time seen in this Island, near these thirty Years, though but very seldom; and after I came there in 1747, I did but see one Person who had it, in the first four Years of my residing there; and three more in the next three Years: But within the four Years last past, it is become so frequent, that I have seen some Scores of Patients labouring under it, yet it seems not to be in the least infectious or contagious.

The Patient who labours under this Disease, usually first complains of an uneasy Sensation, or slight burning Heat about the Cardia, or upper Mouth of the Stomach; which comes slowly on, and gradually increases, and rises up the *Oesophagus* into the Mouth, without any Fever, or the least feverish Heat, or much Pain attending it; most commonly without any observable Intemperance or Irregularity in living, or without any Surfeit,[†] taking Cold, or any sort of Fever or other Disorder, which it can be attributed to, preceding it, or any manifest or immediate cause, to which it can be ascribed.

Soon after this burning Heat, little small Pustulæ, or Pimples, filled with a clear acrid Lymph, no bigger than a Pin's Head begin to rise; generally first on the End and Sides of the Tongue, which gradually increase in Number, not in Magnitude, and slowly spread under the Tongue, and sometimes to the Palate and Roof of the Mouth, and the Inside of the Lips; and soon after the thin Skin which covers these Pustulæ, slips off, and the Tongue looks red and a little inflamed, though not swelled, yet is almost raw like a Piece of raw Flesh, and is so tender and sore, that the Patient can eat no Food but what is soft and smooth, nor drink any thing that is vinous, spirituous, or the least pungent, without acute Pain; so that some suffer much from the want of proper Food. In some a Ptyalisme[†] comes on, and continues a long time, which is so far from being of any Service, or giving any Relief to the Patient, that on the contrary it drains and exhausts the Fluids of the Body, and greatly wastes and sinks them.

In this State they continue several Days, or Weeks, and sometimes for Months, sometimes a little better, the worse again; and after a considerable time, sometimes longer, and sometimes shorter, the Pustulæ will disappear and the Mouth grow well, without any Medicines or Applications, or any manifest Cause, and continue so for several Days or Weeks; but soon after this, the Patient finds a burning heat in the Oesophagus and Stomach, attended with Ructuses[†] and sometimes Vomitings, by which a clear acrid Lymph, or waterish Phlegm, which is very hot, and most commonly very acid, is brought up; though in some few it is not so acid: This generally continues but a little time before a Diarrhœa comes on, and continues a longer or shorter time in different Patients, and sometimes for a longer or shorter time in the same Person, and in some it continues for many Weeks; and in all it greatly wastes their Flesh and Strength, and sinks their Spirits very much. The Diarrhœa after continuing a longer or shorter Time, sometimes stops without taking any Medicines, or doing any thing to stay it, and the Patient thinks himself better for a short Time, and sometimes for a longer Time; but in general the acrid Humour soon returns to the Mouth again with all the same Symptoms, but somewhat increased or aggravated; and after some stay there, it removes from thence to the Stomach and Bowels again; and thus a Metastasis of the Humour from the Mouth to the Bowels, and *vice versa*, is frequently, and sometimes suddenly made, without any manifest or perceptible Cause. Some chance time, though but seldom, after the Disease has continued a long time, it affects all the *Primæ Viæ* from the Lips to the Anus at the same time, and excoriates the last; and I have observed in one or two Cases, where the Pustulæ appeared about the genital Parts, as we sometimes find the Aphthæ do, as *Hippocrates* observes;[20] and in one or two Cases I observed it to break out like an Impetigo, about the Mouth.

The Patients are all along without any Fever or feverish Heat, and their Pulse is all this Time rather smaller, lower, slower, and more languid than it was when they were in full Health; and their Body and Countenance rather paler and somewhat colder, especially in the extreme Parts, than when they were well: No Thirst, except what the Diarrhœa causes, when it continues long, and that generally moderate. The Patient's Skin is generally dry, all the Time of the Disease, and he perspires very little.

The frequent Metastases, which this acrid Humour makes from the Mouth to the Stomach and Bowels, and from those to the Mouth again, greatly emaciate, weaken and consume the Patient. For when it is in the Mouth, both it and the Tongue are so excoriated, raw, tender and sore, that they can take no Nourishment, but such as is very soft, smooth and mild, and in a liquid Form, without giving them exquisite Pain: and when it is in the Stomach, it

---

20. Hippoc. de Natur. Muliebr. C. 61. Epidem. Lib. 3, &c.

gives a painful burning Sensation, and a frequent gulping up, or vomiting a little clear, acrid, acid Liquor, and their Food also; so that the Stomach can retain and digest nothing but what is very soft, smooth and light, and sometimes not even that. And when the Humour falls upon the Intestines, it produces a Diarrhœa with a Sense of Heat, and sometimes a Griping, (tho' the last not often) and sometimes with hot Stools and a Tenesmus; so that most of the nutritious Juices run off that Way, which greatly wastes and sinks the Patient. These Circumstances continuing, and the Disease frequently changing from place to place, almost continually deprives the Sick of their proper Nourishment, whence a true *Atrophy* is produced, which at the last, either sinks the Patient, or brings on a *Marasmus*,† which soon ends in Death.

This is a true, and I think exact, Description of this Disease,† and its Symptoms, which too often seizes several of the Inhabitants of Barbadoes and, I believe, of the other West-India Islands also, and has been too often fatal to several of them.

The Nature, Symptoms, and Appearance of this Disease, are considerably different from those of the true *Aphthæ*, either of the Ancients or Moderns. The true *Aphthæ* generally are, either attended with a Fever, or immediately follow a putrid Fever, an irregular interknitting Fever, a Dysentery, a Diarrhœa Febrilis, or some other Fever: This comes on gradually, slowly, and almost imperceptibly, and always without any Fever, either preceding or accompanying it. The *Aphthæ* are much larger Pustules, and either suppurate and fill with a concocted Matter and form little Ulcusculæ,† or turn black and gangrenesce: These are much smaller, and fill with a clear acrid Lymph, or Ichor, and then excoriate the Parts; but rarely or never fill with Matter, except here and there a chance Pustula when the Disease has continued long, but never form Ulcusculæ, nor gangrenesce. These usually seize People advanced in Years, rarely Youths, and never Children: The *Aphthæ* most frequently seize Children, rarely Youths, and sometimes People in Years, but most commonly either with, or immediately after they had a Fever:[21] This is never with a fever,

---

21. The great Profess. *Boerhaave* says, that he saw two Women with small Ulcers in their Mouths or Lips like the Aphthæ without a Fever; but he relates this as an uncommon Case. Was it not this Disease?

And [Vincent] *Ketelaer* [Dutch physician, 1627–79] says, that he has seen the Aphthæ in some without a Fever. Were they not scorbutic Ulcusculæ as it was in Zealand?

De Aphthis [*Nostratibus seu Belgarum Sprouw*, 1669], p. 26.

but on the contrary, they generally have a small, low, and languid Pulse, and are usually colder than in Health. The *Aphthæ* are but of a short Duration, and is an acute Disease, and usually either kills the Patient, or they recover in two or three Weeks' time, or less; but this Disease continues with short Intervals of being a little better, then worse again, for several Years, before it puts an end to Life; I am informed that it has continued for eight or nine Years in some Patients before it was fatal; though it has been so to some in less than a Year, when they had lived too freely, or did not seek for proper Assistance.

It also differs considerably, and in many Respects from an *Erysipelas*, or an *Erysipelatoides*;† and also a little in some Respects from an *Impetigo*,† though it is in some Respects most like that, and if it was external would probably produce scaly Scabs on the Skin after a few Pustulæ broke, as I once saw it about the Mouth.

As it is a new Disease, we must give it some Name; shall we call it an *Aphthoides Chronica*, or an *Impetigo Primarum Viarum*? or what? But I will not dispute with any about its Name, as that is only a Dispute about Words; and if any Person will give it a better Name, I will readily agree with him, and thank him also.

As this Disease comes on so slowly, and increases gradually and almost imperceptibly, and continues with little or no Pain, except the Soreness of the Mouth, and sometimes a little Griping in the Bowels, it is too often neglected, or trifled with, till it is far advanced; and even then, it is sometimes difficult to convince the Patients that they are in any Danger from it, or to prevail on them to take such Medicines as are necessary; so that it is too often neglected so long, that it is not in the Power of Medicines, or Art, to save their Lives.

Divers Means, and various methods have been tried to cure this too often fatal Disease, in this unlearned Part of the World; but as they were generally immethodical, and without Success, I shall not mention any of them here.

As I could not meet with any Description, or the least mention of this Disease, in any of the ancient *Greek* or *Arabian Physicians'* Works that are

---

21. (*cont'd.*)

And the learned *Baron Van Swieten* says, that the Aphthæ are rarely or never seen in hot Countries. But he must have been wrongly informed, for I have frequently seen them, especially in Children, and also in several ancient People in Barbadoes, which is in the Torrid Zone, Lat. 13°, tho' they probably may not be so frequent there, as they may be in Zealand; but I never yet saw it, but with a Fever, or immediately after a Fever.

come to our Hands, nor yet in any *modern Author*, I was obliged to get the best Knowledge of it that I could, by carefully observing its Symptoms, and examining what Functions of Life were either impaired, irregularly performed, or obstructed; and from thence endeavour to discover the Nature, Cause, and Diathesis of the Disease; and from thence to deduce the Intentions of Cure, and form the most rational Methods of Practice, to answer those Intentions of Cure, that I could by Observation, inductive Reasoning, and Analogy; and again to improve that by Observation and Experience: which Method I shall now communicate, and leave to others to improve, or find a better if they can.

As this Distemper generally comes imperceptibly on, and often without any apparent manifest Cause, it is difficult to discover what its true *procatartick Cause* is. But as it appears from the Nature, Symptoms, and Diathesis of this Disease, that whatever will diminish the Strength of the *Vis Vitæ*, and lessen the Momentum of the circulating Fluids, and at the same time diminish or obstruct the Quantity of Matter which ought to be carried off by the insensible Perspiration and Sweat, may be the procatartick Cause of this Disease; and these Causes may be various and many; [such] as too great a Delicacy and natural Weakness, or too great a Relaxation of the Solids; taking Cold, using wet Linen, damp Sheets, or too suddenly stopping or obstructing the Perspiration, in such a weak relaxed Constitution; too often and over freely drinking vinous or spirituous Liquors; too great Anxiety, Distress, or Concern of Mind, Grief, *&c.*, and several other Things and Circumstances, which are known to relax the Solids, and diminish the insensible Perspiration at the same time.

It appears then from the small low, weak Pulse, and the languid Motion of the circulating Fluids, and no Fever, but a Coldness and Driness of the Skin, especially of the extreme Parts of the Body, that there is a great Relaxation of the Solids, and consequently a great Diminution of the *Vis Vitæ* and Momentum of the Fluids; the Coldness, Driness, and Roughness of the Patient's Skin, which usually attends this Disease, shews an Obstruction, and great want of Perspiration and Sweat, which in this warm Climate generally are, and should be considerably great in a State of Health. And the Excoriation and Soreness of the Mouth, Tongue, Gula, Stomach, and Intestines, plainly demonstrate, that an acrid Lymph, or sharp Humour is turned upon those Parts, and produces those Effects. From whence it appears that a relaxed State of the Solids, a diminished Momentum of the Fluids, an obstructed Perspiration, and an Acrimony of the Humours arising from thence, and increased by the

Heat of the Climate, are the immediate concurring Causes of this Disease. For it is well known, that the perspirable Matter, or any other excreted Fluid being obstructed and returned upon any other excretory Vessels, soon becomes acrid, and that it must still be rendered more sharp, by Retention and [the] Heat of the Climate.

These being the Causes of this Disease; we must take our Intentions of Cure from them, and they evidently appear to be these:

First: *To cleanse the Primæ Viæ, and open the perspiratory Pores, and restore a free Perspiration and Sweating.*

Secondly: *To correct and carry off the Acrimony of the Humours.*

Thirdly: *To stay the Purging, and strengthen the Tone of the Stomach and Intestines, and assist Nature to expel the Humours from the internal Parts, to the Surface of the Body, that they may be properly carried off their natural way, by Perspiration and Sweat.*

And lastly: *To strengthen the relaxed Solids, and increase the Momentum of the Fluids, and thereby contribute to restore and continue a free Perspiration, and establish Health.*

As the Humours are thus turned upon the *Primæ Viæ*, by the above mentioned Causes, and have had their Afflux that Way for a considerable Time, as is commonly the Case, the Stomach and Bowels, are generally loaded with Phlegm, and are foul; wherefore an *Emetic* is first necessary, both to carry that off and cleanse them, and render the other Medicines more effectual, as also to encourage Perspiration: and here the *Rad. Ipocacuanha pulv.*[†] is undoubtedly the best; and a Dose of torrified Rhubarb with an *Opiate* and *Diaphoretic* after it, is also necessary. And if the Diarrhœa has continued some time; I have always found it necessary to give a small Dose of the *Ipocacuanha pulv. gr. ij vel gr. iij*[†] about five o'Clock in the Evening, and a *Diaphoretic Opiate* after it has operated once or twice, at going to Bed, for six, eight, or ten Evenings, as the Diarrhœa has continued a longer or shorter Time before we begin. But if it be recent, and has not continued so long, a less Number of Doses of the *Ipocacuanha, viz.* five or six may be sufficient, before the *Alteratives,*[†] and *corroborating Diaphoretics* are given to answer the second and third Intentions of Cure: for which I have found the following the most successful, and therefore shall add the Prescription, which the *Physician* may alter as he sees it necessary *pro re nata.*

℞ *Sulph. Antimonii precipitat gr. v. Mercurii calcinat. subtilis. levigat. ℈j. Gum. Guajac. pulv. Extr. Gentianæ ana ℥j. Camphorii ℈ij. Extract. Thebaic. gr.*

x. *Bals. Guajacin. q. s. Misce, fi. Pil.* lx. *de quibus capiat Æger tres omni nocte hora decubit. insuper bib. Infusionis sequentis* ʒij *vel* ʒiij.†

℞ *Rad. Serpent. Virg. Cort. Sassafræ Granator. ana* ʒj. *Cinnamonii* ʒij. *Sal. Absinth* ʒj. *Misce, et infund in vase clauso, in Aq. Bull.* lbijss. *per hor. octo, et cola* lbij. *Colaturæ adde Vini Crocei* ʒj. *Spir. Mindereri* ʒiiij. *Misce, Sumat ut supra, Capiat etiam* ʒij. *omni Mane.*†

Sometimes I have added *Vini Antimon. gut.* xx *vel* xxx.† to each Dose of the Infusion; and during the Time that the Patient takes these Medicines, I order his Body to be well rubbed half an Hour Nights and Mornings, with a Flesh-brush,† or a coarse warm dry Flannel-cloth, in order to encourage a free Perspiration; and use moderate Exercise on Horseback, or in a Chaise† if weak, to increase the Momentum of their Fluids, and invigorate their Solids: Let them also carefully avoid exposing themselves too suddenly to a cool Air, or the damp moist Air of the Night, or to damp Linen.

If the acid Humour affects the Stomach with a burning Heat and Pain, and sour Belchings, as it often does in this Case, giving *Magnesia Alba* ʒj.† in a Draught of Milk and Water sweetened with a little Sugar, in the Morning, corrects the Acidity, and carries it off by a gentle Motion or two; and this may be repeated every third or fourth Morning, as the Acidity returns.

The corroborating diaphoretic Medicines, and this Method, should be continued constantly, till you find that the Momentum of the circulating Fluids is sufficiently invigorated, and the Patient has acquired a constant, regular, equal Warmth, without its being forced by Exercise, &c. And in order to obtain this desired End, it is generally necessary to add a proper Chalybeat, [such] as *Vinum Chalybeat.*† &c. and a little *Cortex Peruv.* to the before-mentioned warming and corroborating Medicines towards the latter End of the Cure, and to continue the Use of them, till they have recovered their Flesh, Colour, and Strength, and are perfectly recovered; otherwise they are subject to relapse, and the Disease return again.

But if the Disease has continued a long time before the Physician is called, as is too frequently the Case here, so that the Patient is much emaciated, and the Diarrhœa has made frequent Returns, and has continued long, and reduced the Sick low, it will be absolutely necessary to repeat the small Doses of the *Ipocacuanha*, and the diaphoretic Opiate, several times, at any time of the Disease, especially when the Diarrhœa returns, and strong corroborating Sudorifics must be constantly given after, till the Diarrhœa is effectually stayed; and if this is not effected, a free Perspiration cannot be restored, and continued, and without both, the Patient cannot perfectly recover. And as solid Medicines are often retained longer in the Stomach and Intestines, than Liquids usually are, we often find that they will answer where the Liquid will not; wherefore when the Disease has proved very obstinate, as the Diarrhœa too often does in this case, after giving ten or twelve small Doses of the *Ipocacuanha*, as before, I have found the following Composition to answer best.

℞ *Electar. e Scordio* ʒj. *Theriac. Androm.* ʒss. *Terræ Japon. Cort. Granator. Pulv. ana* ʒij. *Cinnamomi Pulv.* ʒj. *Sulph. Antimonni præcipit.* ʒij. *Syr. e Mecon. q.s. Misce, fi. Electar. cujus capiat Æger q. Nuc. Mosc. major. omni mane et hora decubitura, sæpiusve urgente Diarrhœa, superbibendo Decoctionis sequent* ʒij.†

℞ *Cort. Granator. Rad. Serpent. Virg. ana* ʒi. *Cort. Cinnam.* ʒij. *Misce, coq. in Aq. Pur.* lbij. *ad* lbiss. *et sub finem Coctionis adde Elect. e Scordio* ʒi. *coq. parum et cola, Colaturæ adde Aq. Cinnamomi, Tinct. Terræ Japon. ana* ʒj. *Syr. e Mecon* ʒss. *Misce, fi. Decoct. ut supra sumend. capiat etiam Cochl. quatuor post singul. Alvi deject. liquidam.*†

The Frictions and Exercise of Riding should be continued at the same time, and the other Precautions observed.

But if notwithstanding the Use of all these Methods and Medicines, the Diarrhœa proves obstinate, and returns, as it sometimes happens; for I know no Disease that is more obstinate, more subject to return, or more difficult to be cured, than this sometimes proves to be: Therefore when this is the Case, and these Methods do not succeed, only for a time when they take the Medicines, and the Diarrhœa continues to return, and the Patient's Skin is still dry, so that he cannot be brought to perspire as freely as he should do; warm Bathing, in some of the natural warm Baths, and corroborating Diaphoreticks at the same time, promise the best Success. But it may be objected that warm Bathing relaxes the Solids, which are already too much relaxed before by the Disease; but seeing that if a free Perspiration cannot be restored, the Distemper cannot be effectually cured, tho' they may seem to be better for some time, yet it will often return again; though I have known many that have recovered perfectly without warm Bathing, yet I have met with some who I apprehended could not, and found it to be so afterwards: For as I met with some Patients whose Situations were such, that they could not go to any of the natural warm Baths; and as we had not any in the Island of Barbadoes, I ordered an artificial warm Bath to be made of common *Sal. Martis* (called green Copperas†) *Sulphur Vivum*,† and warm Water, made as warm as the warm baths at Bath, [England,] are, and added some Aromaticks, in which the Patients bathed, and were well rubbed whilst in the Bath; but I found that it did not answer in several Respects, so well as the natural warm Baths did, therefore if the Patients can conveniently go to them, they are preferable; as they do not relax the Vessels of the Body in general, (though they may relax those on or near to the Surface of it, during the time they are in the Bath,) so much as the artificial Baths do, though they are made but equally as warm; neither are those who bathe in the natural Baths, so subject to take Cold after Bathing, as those who bathe in the artificial Baths are, as I have several times observed;† and it must be granted that the natural warm sulphurous Baths, [such] as those of *Bath*, *Aix la Chapelle*, *Barage*, *Aix in Provence*, and those in *Portugal*; and it is very probable that the warm Baths in *Jamaica*, *Nevis*, and *Carolina*, if they were properly examined by fit Experiments, would be found to be of the same Nature, and probably equally as good as the above-mentioned Baths are; all these natural Baths, greatly exceed all the artificial warm Baths that we can make: For whenever Nature acts the *Chemist*, she far exceeds the greatest Artist, and the ablest *Chemist*. Besides this, those who go to those natural warm Baths, have the Advantage of drinking their Waters daily, during the time of Bathing, whereby the acrid saline Humours may be attenuated, diluted, dissolved, and at least some of them carried off by Sweat and Urine: And what is still of greater Importance, by drinking those Waters, their Solids will be somewhat braced, and the Circulation of their Fluids increased, and consequently a freer Perspiration obtained, and continued. And though warm Bathing may be objected to, as it relaxes the Solids for a time, yet as it contributes to cleanse the obstructed Mouths of the perspiratory Pores and sudorific Ducts, and gently relaxes the Coats of those obstructed Vessels on the Surface of the Body, whilst the Heat of the Bath increases the Momentum of the circulating Fluids, at the same time; they must by thus jointly acting together, more effectually remove the obstructing Cause, and carry it out of the small obstructed Vessels. Since relaxing the Coats of those small Vessels will have the same Effect as increasing their Diameters; and the Momentum of the Blood being increased by the Heat of the Bath, at the same time, must render it the most effectual Method to remove such Obstructions: And Nature may be assisted in this Work, by giving a deobstruent,† diaphoretic Draught, half an Hour before the Patient goes into the Bath. I have found the following to answer this End the best; but it may be altered *pro re nata*.

℞ *Rad. Serpent. Virg.* ℥ss *vel* ℥i. *Theriac. Androm.* ℥ss. *Misce et infund. in Aq. Pur Bull. q.s. ut col.* ℥iss. *Colaturæ adde Sal. Diuretic* ℈i. *Spir. Mindereri* ℥iij. *Vini Crocei* ℥ij. *Syr. Crocei* ℥ij. *Misce, fi. Haust. ut supra sumend.*†

Also rubbing the Patient's Body very well, both when he is in, and after he comes out of the Bath; and then going into a warm Bed, and encouraging a free Perspiration, and moderate Sweating, by drinking warm Bath water, will contribute much to the same Purpose: And the corroborating diaphoretick Medicines before advised, may be continued with the Bath-waters, during the Intervals between the Times of going into the Bath, in order to brace up and strengthen the internal relaxed weak Vessels, and increase the Momentum of the Fluids, and enable Nature to cast out the Humours from the internal Parts, to the Surface of the Body, that they may be carried off by Perspiration in their natural Way. And though warm Bathing may a little relax the Vessels on and near to the Surface of the Body, yet it does not affect the larger internal Vessels, which are not exposed to it, so much as is sometimes apprehended, as I have often observed; but going into the Baths with too great a Plethora, or Fullness of the Vessels, has undoubtedly done much Hurt, and has brought Bathing into some Discredit, and caused it to be much less used than it was formerly.

These Remarks on Bathing and its Effects, especially in this Disease, are not only plausible in Theory, but I have found them to be true in fact; for I advised several Patients who laboured under this Disease, to come to Bath in Somersetshire, and to drink those Waters, but they were not permitted to bathe in the Waters as I advised, though they drank them a considerable and sufficient time, and no doubt took proper Medicines with them, yet they returned full as bad, and some of them worse than when they went; Wherefore I gave the next Patient that came to the Bath, full Directions both to drink the Waters and bathe in them, though he was more reduced and brought lower and weaker, than any of the others were, before he came: He accordingly drank the Waters five or six Weeks, and bathed twelve times in the Bath, and took the before-mentioned corroborating diaphoretick Medicines with them, after taking an Emetick and a Dose of Rhubarb, and returned to the Island perfectly recovered, and grown strong, fat, and jolly: And I could mention some others who have come hither since with the same Disease, and have used the same Methods, and received the same Advantage. As this is a new Disease, which I think has not been described before by any Author, nor probably been seen before in this Country; I mention this, that my Brethren the Physicians of Bath may advise such Patients as labour under this Disease to come thither to bathe, as well as to drink the Waters, if they think fit: *Sed Verbum sat sapienti.*[†]

As to the Use of Gargarisms in this Case, they are of but little Service, except such as are healing, when the Mouth is very sore, as they only serve to repel the Humours from thence to the Stomach and Bowels, and to which they are but too often translated, without any topical Applications; where they produce a Diarrhœa, which is more difficult to be cured; when the strongest Restringents without Diaphoreticks, will, at best, only stop it for a little Time, and it will either upon taking a little Cold, or the least irregular Accident, return again; wherefore I have found it necessary to advise the Patients, especially when they did not come to Bath, [England,] and bathe, to use the restringent diaphoretick Medicines at least once or twice a Day, for some time after the Diarrhœa is totally stayed; in order to strengthen the Tone of the Stomach and Bowels, as well as to invigorate the Momentum of the circulating Fluids, and restore and establish a free Perspiration; for which Purposes I have frequently, towards the latter End of the Cure, added some *Chalybeat*, in order to obtain those desired Effects; for without strengthening the Solids, and restoring a brisker Circulation of the Fluids, and a free Perspiration, I cannot say that I ever yet have known any one perfectly recovered; though by these being restored, I have known many restored to Health.

Of the NYCTALOPIA, *or* NIGHT-BLINDNESS

THE NYCTALOPIA is a Disease which is so frequently seen among the Negroes in this warm Part of the Globe, and as I am informed in Africa also, that it may be justly deemed an indigenous or endemial Disease in the Torrid Zone; though it is but very seldom seen in England, or in the other Parts of Europe.

The great *Hippocrates*, and most of the other *Greek* Physicians, as also the Arabians, have described this Disease very well; though their Commentators and Interpreters[22] seem to have made some Mistake and confounded it with the *Hemeralopes*, which probably arose from their having seldom or never seen it in Europe: But *Galen*,[†] the best Interpreter of some difficult Passages in

---

22. Foesius in Œconom. Hippocrat.

Hippocrates, calls it Νυκταλωπες,[23] Nyctalopes, a Night-blindness; and *Ætius*,[24] who lived at *Amida* in *Mesopotamia*, now a Part of *Persia*, a hotter Country than *Greece*, [and] probably might see it oftener, describes it clearly, and the Ηεμαραλωπες, Hemeralopia or Day-blindness also, i.e. those who cannot see in the Day-time, but see well by Night; likewise both *Paulus Æginet*[25] and *Actuarius*†[26] describe it well. Among the Latins *Pliny*†[27] also mentions it, and the elegant *Celsus*† calls it *Imbecillitas oculorum, ex quo quidem interdiu satis, noctu nihil cerunt*,[28] they see well by Day, but in the Night nothing, or are blind.

This is a Disease which is now frequently seen among the Negroes in the West-India Islands,† and I have seen many; and an ingenious Apothecary there, told me that he had known, six, eight, ten, or twelve Negroes seized with it in some Estates, when the Night came on, so that the other Negroes who could see well were obliged to lead them home, tho' they cold see well in the Day-time to do any Work, so long as the Sun was above the Horizon, but as soon as the Sum was gone down, their Sight began to grow dim; and as the Darkness of the Night approached, that Dimness increased, and they became perfectly dark and blind; and that Blindness continued till the Morning, that the Sun began to rise, with which their Sight returned also, and continued till Night, when they became blind again; and thus they continue to be blind in the Nights, and to see in the Days, for a long Time, if not relieved by proper Remedies: sometimes some of them will recover their Sight for several Nights, and then lose it again, and that for several times.

I could not observe that the Variations of the Weather had any Influence or Effect on this Disease, either in producing, increasing, or abating it; unless a continued clear, dry, hot, Season had some little Effect on them.

This Night-blindness comes on in the Evenings, after the Sun sets, with a misty Dimness, which gradually increases as the Night approaches, till it becomes dark, when their Sight becomes perfectly dark also; and without any Pain, either in the Head or Eyes, or elsewhere; sometimes a Sense of Fullness in the Head, and a small Tinitus Aurium attends it, at other times not, but

---

23. Galenus in Œconom. Hippocrat.
24. Ætius Tetrabill. II Serm. 2. C. 46
25. Paul. Ægineta, Lib. III. Cap. 22.
26. Actuarius, Meth. Med. L. II. C. 7.
27. Pliny, Hist. Nat. VIII. C. 50.
28. Celsus, Lib. VI. Cap. 6.

without any Vertigo or Giddiness; no Oppression or Sickness at the Stomach, or Loss of Appetite, neither any other Complaint but the Loss of Sight; all the Secretions and other Functions of Life seem to be regularly performed; neither do their Eyes appear to be impaired or altered, the Cornea and Pupil appear perfectly clear and well, and the Iris also, which continues to contract a little in the Day-time, and dilate as usual in the Night, yet no Vision is then performed; neither does there appear to be any afflux of Humours to, or any Signs of Inflammation in, the Eyes.

As no external Injury or impediment in the Eye appears, its Cause must be internal; and as no Pain or Inflammation, or any Signs of it, attends it, it [night blindness] does not proceed from any Obstruction of the sanguiferous,† seriferous,† or lymphatic Vessels; therefore it must arise from some male† Affection of the Retina or optic Nerves, or both: And as this is a Disease which is most frequent in the Torrid Zone, where the Reflections of the Rays of Light are strong and vigouous, and the Sun being several Hours every Day almost perpendicular over them, the Angle of Reflection is very acute, and the Rays of Light must be strongly reflected from the Earth and other Bodies into the Eyes, consequently the Sensation of them, and the Vibrations of the Retina and optic Nerves must be great also; and being thus accustomed to such continued strong Vibrations, they become weakened, and their Tone greatly impaired[29] so that they become insensible of the small weak Vibrations of the few inactive Rays of Light which exist in the Night, and move with almost an infinite less Force than those of the Day, there; and when this happens to such Eyes as have a natural Imbecillity† in the Formation of their Nerves, which by the strong continued Vibrations of the Light of the Day there, become in some degree paralytic, and insensible of the small weak Vibrations of the little Quantity of Light of the Night, so that they perceive no Light, and remain blind till the Sun returns in the Morning, and renews the stronger Vibrations of the Light again, and they see.

This seems to be the Cause of this Disease, and this the most rational and satisfactory Way of accounting for it; and as it plainly and clearly accounts

---

29. A Gentleman by riding ten Miles on the Sea-shore near Noon, had his Eyes so weakened by the strong reflected Rays of Light from the white Sand, that he could not see so well to read by Candle-light in the Night for four or five Weeks after, as he did before and after that. And we see something like it in those who are Snow-blind, and cannot see for some time after they come into a House, tho' it be Day-light.

for all its Symptoms and Appearances in a plain, simple Manner, it appears to be true.

The Ημαραλωπες, Hemeralopia, is a Disease which is very seldom seen; they see pretty well in the Night, but very little in the Day, and cannot see any thing when the Sun shines bright. It proceeds from a different and direct contrary Cause [to] the other, *viz.* from too great a Tenderness and Sensibility of the Iris and Retina, for they cannot bear any Degree of Light from the Sun to fall upon their Eyes, but are obliged to shut their Eye-lids close, and so near closed from the Light of the Day when the Sun does shine out, as not to be able to see, as we sometimes see in an Inflammation of the Iris or Retina, tho' no Inflammation is present here, but too great a Sensibility of those Parts, so that they cannot bear the Light of the Day, but can dilate the Pupil of the Eye, and see very well in the Night: I have but had an Opportunity of seeing two Persons who laboured under this Disease.[30]

The Methods of Cure, which have been used in the *Nyctalopia*, are various, and little has been said of the Cure of the *Hemeralopia*, as it is so very seldom seen. That recommended by *Paulus Ægineta*,[31] in the Cure of the first, is judicious and rational, tho' his Method of Diet, and external Applications, may well be omitted, as there is no external Fault in the Eyes, and his external Applications are of too gross a Nature to penetrate much into the Globe of the Eye. Some, from its periodical returning with the Darkness of the Night have supposed it to be of the intermitting kind, and therefore thought it should be treated as such; but its periodical Returns, are solely owing to the periodical Returns of the Darkness of the Night, and not to any thing in the Diathesis of the Disease; and the *Cortex Peruv.* may be of much greater prejudice to the Patient's Constitution in some other Respects, especially as we find that the Methods which increase and are prejudicial in intermitting Fevers, greatly contribute to the Cure of this Disease. For as Paul Ægineta[32] advises, we find by Experience that Bleeding once, to a greater or less

---

30. When I was at the School, I saw a Man who was blind in the Day-time, and laid Wagers with Men who could see, to run Races with them in dark Nights; and got his Wagers, till they found that he could see in the Night, though not in the Day.

It is said that there are a People in Siam, in the East-Indies, and also in Africa, who are subject to this Disease of being blind in the Day-time and seeing well by Night. Modern Univers. History, Vol. VII.

31. *Paulus Ægineta*, Lib. III. Cap. 22.

32. Idem ibid.

Quantity, as the Patient is more or less plethoric, and purging [him] twice or three times with an antiphlogistick attenuating Cathartic, and giving the *Rad. Valerian Sylv. Pulv.*† with its *volatile Tincture* two or three times a Day, in the intermediate Days, and for two or three after the last Purge, generally removes the Disease and restores the Patient his perfect Sight.

I have sometimes ordered their Eyes to be washed with the following, and I think with Advantage:

℞ *Aq. Rosar.* ℥iss. *Vini Antimonial.* ℥ss. *Misce, fi. Collyr. cum quo lavat. Oculis omni nocte hora decubit. et etiam Mane.*†

And it is probable that the subtile Particles of the Antimony may penetrate the Eye, and be of Service in this Case; and not improbably in the *Hemeralopia* also, but I never had an Opportunity of trying it.

Of the ELEPHANTIASIS

T HE ELEPHANTIASIS is also a Disease which is either indigenous or endemial to such Countries as are within the Torrid Zone.†

This Disease was well described by *Abubeter Mohamed Rhazis*,[33] who lived in *Persia* about 850 Years since; and he does not speak of it as a Distemper that was new in his time; therefore we may conclude, that it was well known in *Persia, Arabia, Egypt,* and the other Parts of *Africa* also, as *Lucretius* mentioned it many Ages before that Time, as a Disease of that Quarter of the World. However we are certain that the Negroes first brought it from *Africa*† to the West-Indies, where it is now but too frequent among them, and among the white People also, who are not exempted from it.

But I cannot think with Dr *Town*[34] that this Disease has any Affinity to the *Lepra. Arabum,* tho' several of the *Arabian Physicians,* or rather their Translators, have called the true *Lepra Arabum* by the Name of *Elephantiasis*; but *Rhazis* distinguishes them clearly; and how the other *Arabians* since him, and the *European Physicians* since them again, have confounded their Names, is difficult to determine.

However it is much to be wished, that the *Arabians,* who are the first

33. Rhazis ad Manzor. Division. Lib. Cap. 107. p. 418.
34. Dr *Town* on the *Diseases of the West-Indies,* p. 184.

Physicians that have mentioned this Disease, had more fully described its first Symptoms and Appearance, and the manner of its coming on, and increasing to its full State, more accurately and clearly, than they or any since them have: which Defect, I will endeavour to supply as well as I can, from repeated Observations.

The Patient when apparently in perfect Health, and without any preceding procatartick Cause that he knows of, is first seized with a cold Rigor, like the Fit of an Ague, which continues one, two, or three Hours, with acute Pain in the Head and Back, a Sickness at his Stomach, and sometimes a Vomiting, and great Pain in one of the *inguinal Glands*, sometimes in one, in others in the other inguinal Gland, never in both, and whether it falls on the Right or Left gland the first Time, it generally continues to fall on the same Gland every Fit afterwards: the Rigor is succeeded by a very hot Fever, which usually continues twenty, thirty, or forty-eight Hours, and sometimes longer; the Patient is often delirious, the Pain in the inguinal Gland increases, and it swells and becomes red and hard, rarely or never suppurating: soon after it is thus swelled, a red Stroke runs down the Thigh from the tumefied† Gland, to the Leg, almost an Inch broad, and of a fresh red Colour; the Leg begins to swell, and is much inflamed, and as that Inflammation increases, the Fever abates, and at last goes quite off, most commonly in four or five Days' time; sometimes sooner, at other times later; and in this time the tumefied Gland subsides and comes to its natural State. The morbid Matter being thus cast upon the Leg by this imperfect Crisis, it continues to be much inflamed and swelled for several Days, and then goes gradually quite off; and the Patient seems to be perfectly well again. The Fever makes frequent Returns with all the same Symptoms, and in the same manner, but at no certain periodical times; sometimes twice, thrice, or four times in a Year, especially in the first two or three Years of the Disease; in others once a Month or three Weeks, or oftener; the most frequent Returns that I have ever seen in any Patient, was four times in eleven Days, but then at no certain Periods; it will come sometimes at two or three Weeks' end; and the next time not till three, four, or six Months after, but whenever it returns, the morbid Matter is each time thrown upon the same Leg, on which it chanced to fall the first time.

The Leg most commonly remains longer swelled after each Return of the Fever, than it did in the former Fit; and after several Returns, it continues to remain swelled, after the Inflammation is entirely gone off; and now it begins to appear oedematous, or as if it was anasarcous,† but that the Swelling does not retain the Impression of the Finger so much, or so long, as it will do in a dropsical[†] Case.

By these frequent Returns of the Fever, the Leg is each time more and more tumefied, and the sanguiferous Vessels are distended, the Veins become varicose, and the Swelling increases down from the Knee to the Extremities of the Toes; the Skin of that Leg begins to grow rough and rugged; the Swelling still increases, and the Membrana Cellulosa[†] becomes very thick, hard, callous or semi-cartilaginous in some Places; the Skin grows thicker and scaly, with great Fissures and Chops[†] upon its Surface; these seeming Scales do not dry up and fall off, but adhere fast, and are daily increased and protruded by the increasing Thickness of the Membrana Cellulosa; and the Leg and Foot are thus continually enlarged to an enormous Bulk, when in Size, Shape, and all other external Appearance it exactly resembles the Leg of an Elephant, from whence the Disease takes its Name.

The Patient continues in this Condition many Years, some have lived above twenty Years, with a Leg of this monstrous Magnitude, and their Appetite and Digestion good, except in the Times when the Fever returns; and all their Secretions and Functions of Life have been (at all other times) regularly performed, and they appeared as if in Health, without being sensible of any other Inconveniency of Life, but that of carrying along with them such a troublesome Load of Leg. This Disease and Bulk of Leg is generally confined to one of them, though it is said that there are some very few Instances, where it has affected both at the same time; but I never yet saw one that was so.

I had an Opportunity of seeing one of these Legs, of the largest size, amputated, and afterwards, at my Request, dissected by Mr *Hickes*, an ingenious Surgeon in the Navy. We found the rough, scaly Skin very thick, its small blood Vessels much enlarged; the Membrana Adiposa[†] was exceeding thick, (though the rest of his Body was lean and thin) in the Ankle it cut full two Inches thick, in other Parts of the Leg an Inch and [a] half or more; when cut it looked clear, like the Fat of a Hog, or rather like salted Pork; the Cellulæ[†] of this Membrane were greatly distended, and filled with an oily, fat, gelatinous Substance; about the Ankle and upon the metatarsal Bones it was become semi-cartilaginous, and cut with a grating Noise. The Coats of both the Veins and Arteries were also very considerably enlarged, so that such as were naturally very small Branches of the Artery, were here pretty large Vessels, insomuch, that when he amputated the Leg, he was obliged to take up no fewer than twelve Branches of the Artery with his Needle, though the Leg was taken off above the Knee, and the Swelling (in which the Vessels were much more distended) extended no higher than the Patella, so that the Vessels were distended even in the Thigh, where no Swelling appeared: The Femoral Artery, where it was amputated, was very large, and the Popliteal Nerve was either naturally larger than usual, or its Coats were rendered thicker by the Disease. The Muscles and their Tendons were in their natural State, and the Bones, even those of the Toes, in which there was an Ulcer, were all clean and sound.

From whence it appears, that the morbid Matter of this Disease was solely deposited in the Cellulæ of the Membrana Adiposa, and was not extended or carried into the Cellulæ of [those membranes] which are expanded between the Muscles and their constituent Fibres, but was deposited in the external Cellulæ of that Membrane which contains the Fat, after each Paroxysm of this peculiar Fever; and that the Cause of the monstrous Leg, which gives the Name to this Disease, is the morbid Matter of a Fever which is gradually deposited on the Leg by an imperfect Crisis of each Paroxysm of this peculiar Fever, and is truly the Effect of that Disease; and may most properly be called a Chronical Disease, which arises from an acute one.

I think none of the *Greek Physicians* have given us any Description of this Disease; neither have any of the *Arabians*, except *Mahomed Ebn Zachria Rhazis*,[35] who has described its last or full grown State very well, but not the preceding Fever which produces it: He says, it may be cured in the Beginning of the Disease, but when it is grown inveterate, it is incurable; and the Reason of this, will appear more fully hereafter.

As this Disease is solely produced by the Fever above described, taking that Fever off must consequently prevent the Production of it, if it be taken before the Humours are fixed in the Leg.

An Enquiry into the Nature and Symptoms of this preceding Fever, though it is very uncertain in its Intermissions, and irregular in its Periods, yet it plainly appears to be something of the intermitting Kind; but one which has not been described before by any Author that I could find. It is well known that *Hippocrates* mentions a *Febris Septimana*† as an intermitting Fever whose periodical Returns are regular, but none of any longer Intermission; besides this, the Manner of this fever's going off, by an imperfect Crisis, as above, is

---

35. Rhazis ad Monsor. Division. p. 418.

singular and peculiar to itself. These Considerations first induced me to try the following Method of Cure, as all the other Methods used in these parts were generally found to be unsuccessful; and I found it to answer my Expectations, if the Disease was taken in proper time, before the leg was much enlarged, and the Humours fixed there.

When the Rigor and Fever has seized the Patient, if I find one of the inguinal Glands inflamed, tumefied, hard, and painful, and the red Stroke from it down the Thigh to the Leg, which are the pathognomonic Symptoms of this Disease,[†] and certainly distinguish it from all other Fevers; though we find the Patient very hot, and the Fever pretty high, his Pulse quick, *full, and soft*, though a little delirious: Bleeding ought not to be advised, though I have seen it too often too hastily practiced in this Case; as it hinders Nature from critically discharging the morbid Humours upon the Leg, and sometimes turns it upon the vital Parts, and proves fatal, as I have more than once seen it: But in some particular plethoric Constitutions, where the Fever is very high, the Pulse rapid, strong, *full, and hard,* and the Patient much delirious, ten or twelve Ounces of Blood may be taken away, but not without Caution and Judgment.

But whether you bleed or not, if the Patient has great Sickness at his Stomach, with Vomiting, or much Reaching to vomit, it is necessary to encourage the Vomiting, by drinking Green-tea, Chamomile-flower-tea, or warm Water; and sometimes to assist it by giving *Vini Ipocacuanh.* ʒi. *vel* ʒ ij.[†] in them to assist Nature in her Endeavours; and it is probable that some of the morbid Matter may be discharged that way; however the Action of Vomiting will assist her to cast it off upon the Leg more effectually and sooner; after which an anodyne diaphoretic Bolus may be given with a little Rhubarb, which will give a Motion or two after the two first have had their Effect, and may assist to carry a little more of the Humours off; [such] as:

℞ *Rad. Rhei. Pulv.* ʒi. *Pil. Saponac. gr.* vij. *Camphorii gr.* v. *Sal. Dieuretic.* ϶i. *Syr. e Mecon. q.s. Misce, fi. Bolus ut supra sumendus, superbib. Seri Lactis vinos. tepide copiose, et Sudor. expectat.*[†]

For it is necessary to encourage a free Diaphoresis, and to continue it, by giving some *saline Draughts* after, and diluting plentifully with small Wine-whey, Viburnium-tea,[†] or Sage-tea;[†] both as they abate the Violence of the Fever by Cooling and Sweating, and assist Nature to cast off the morbid Matter both that way, and in her natural way upon the Leg. But if the Patient, either from too great natural Weakness, or by too free Bleeding before we are called in, is too much sunk, and the Pulse be too weak and low, though very quick, we must endeavour to assist nature to cast off the morbid matter, not only by the above-mentioned Methods, but more warming, cardiac, and volatile Medicines must be added; and if the Humours are carried to and affect the Head, bathing their Feet in a warm Decoction of Viburnium (called black Sage[†] here) and Vesicatories must be applied to the Leg into which it used to fall, also, in order to derive[†] the Humour down thither, if possible, or it will prove fatal.

Though the morbid Matter does most commonly fall upon the inguinal Glands, and so into the one Leg or the other; I have sometimes known it fall upon the Arm, each time it came, and in more than one Patient; and I once saw a Patient where this morbid Matter was cast upon the Scalp, the Ears, and the back Part of the Neck; and another wherein the Matter was cast upon the lower Part of the Spina Dorsi,[†] the Os Coxigis,[†] and the lower Part of the Loins, at each time of the return of the Fever, which was attended with all the same Symptoms, as when it falls upon the Leg; and on what Part soever it falls the first time, the morbid Matter is generally cast upon the same Part, in every Return of the Fever afterwards: But these two were very rare, and very uncommon Cases.

As the Leg (or other Part on which the morbid Matter falls) is generally much inflamed and swelled, I usually order it to be fomented with a Fotus of the following kind, two or three Days, and to cover the Part with a warm Flannel after, and keep it sweating, in order to discharge and carry off as much of the morbid matter as we can.

R *Fol. Alceæ, Viburnii, ana* Miij. *Fol. Salvæ, Flor. Sambuci, ana* Mi. *Sapon. Venet.* ʒss. *Sal. Ammoniac. Crud.* ʒ i. *Misce, coq. in Aq. pur.* lbv. *deinde adde Spir. Sacchari, Aceti. Com. ana* ibss. *Misce.*[†]

And after the Fever-fit is entirely gone off, if the Patient's Stomach has not been sufficiently cleansed by the Vomiting, as above, I usually give an Emetic; and as there is a sufficient time before the Return of another Fit, and the following Alteratives also, before I give the Bark; with Variations *pro re nata*.

R *Sulphur. Antimon. præcipit.* ᴣijss. *Mercur. calcinat. levigat.* ᴣss. *Guajac. pulv.* ᴣj. *Bals. Peruv.* q.s. *Misce, fi. Pil.* xl *de quibus capiat Æger quatuor omni nocte hora decubit. insuper bib. Decoct. sequent.* ʒiiij.[†]

R *Rad. Sasaparil.* ʒij. *Sassafr.* ʒj. *Serpent. Virg.* ʒss. *Sal. Dieuretic.* ʒss. m. *coq. in Aq. Pur.* lbiij. *ad* lbij. *et cola, Colaturæ adde Sp. Nitri Dul.* ʒj. *Aq. Juniperi Com.* ʒij. *Misce, Sumat ut supra, capiat etiam* ʒiij. *omni Mane.*[†]

These Medicines being taken, and the Inflammation and Swelling in the Leg (or other Part) gone off, I usually give the *Cortex Peruv.* every three Hours, till the Patient has taken an Ounce and [a] half, or two Ounces, with *Elix. Vitrioli. acid. gut* l *vel* xl.† in Chamomile-flower-tea, after each Dose; and ten Days after taking the last Dose, I give another ounce of the Bark in the same Manner: And as this Disease is very subject to return, I usually order another Ounce of the Bark to be taken in the same manner, a Month after that, and the Patient to go into the cold Bath, or the Sea, two or three times a Week for several Weeks after that again; and this Method, if strictly followed, seldom fails to take the Fever entirely off, and prevent its returning, and consequently the Elephantiasis also.

But as the great Heat of this Climate greatly relaxes the animal Solids, and the People here cannot be prevailed upon to use cold Bathing, as they do in the Eastern hot Countries, and more frequently not to take their Medicines regularly, this Disease is very subject to return, especially when they have suffered it to continue for a considerable long time, before they entered upon this Method of Cure; and then it is usually more difficult to be effectually cured, than it was at the first, before such Return: In this Case, or where the Patient is of a weak, lax, Habit of Body, I always advise them to repeat the Alteratives once, and the Bark, *&c.* also, after it, in the Spring and Autumn following, *viz.* in the Months of April and November, and the cold Bathing after them, as before; which generally answers the desired Effect: But if they neglect this Repetition, the Disease too often returns.

This Method generally succeeds when taken in time, before the Leg be grown too large, and the Disease is strongly fixed there, and has been so a considerable long time: But when this Method has been neglected, or was not known, and the Disease has continued for several Years, so that the Leg is grown very large, and its Membrana Adiposa is become very hard and callous, or almost semi-cartilaginous, it cannot be removed, and we can only say with *Rhazis*, that it is incurable; and nothing but Amputation can relieve them from such a Load of a Leg: But alas! this does not relieve the unhappy Patient from the Disease, unless the Fever be taken off also, as above; for this Operation has been often performed, but always without removing the Disease, for the Fever has certainly returned, and the morbid Matter has constantly fallen upon the other Leg, and produced the same Effects. And whether the above-mentioned Method and Medicines will so effectually succeed after such a long Continuation of the Disease, and the Amputation of the Leg, by eradicating its Cause, and so prevent its coming on the other Leg, or on some other Part of the Body, is what I have not had an Opportunity of experiencing, so as to say it will: But as it is both very reasonable and highly probable that it may, I therefore recommend it to others, that they may try it, and I wish it may succeed.

Some have proposed keeping the End of the Stump, after Amputation, open, in order to discharge the Humours that way, as by an Issue,† and thereby prevent their falling upon the other Leg, &c. It may be tried, but I fear it will not succeed; because so long as the Fever returns, the Humours will be renewed, and must fall somewhere, and the End of the Stump will not be sufficient to receive and discharge them; wherefore the Method above of taking off the Fever, is much more likely to be successful.

Others have tried Fomentations, Frictions,† mercurial Unctions,† and Bandages, in order to reduce those monstrous swelled Legs, but without Success; for when it is become so large, and the Membranes so hard, callous, and semi-cartilaginous, it cannot be reduced nor cured by Art; *quia, extra Artis Limites est.*†

Of the VENA MEDINENSIS, DRACUNCULUS, *or* GUINEA-WORM

THE *VENA MEDINENSIS*, or more properly *Nervus Medinensis*, is another Disease, which is peculiar to some hot Countries, and has been well known for many Ages in *Arabia*, *Persia*, and most probably in *Guinea*, and the southern Parts of *Africa*. *Galen* is the first that mentions it, and calls it *Dracunculus*,[36] but says that he never saw it. But all the *Arabian Physicians* whose Works are come to our Hands, describe it clearly, and their Method of curing it: *Alsaharavius*,† or rather his Translator,† calls it *Vena Exiens*:[37] *Mesuæ*,† or his Translator, calls it *Vena Egrediens*;[38] and *Abulcasim* or *Albucasus*,† *Vena Cruris*;[39] *Haly Abbas*,† *Vena Saniosa*;[40] *Rhazis*,† calls it *Vena Civilis*, and *Vena Medinesis*;[41]

36. Galen. de locis Affect. 6. 3.
37. Alsaharav. Oper. Tract. 28. C. 12. p. 118.
38. Mesuæ Oper. Part 2. S. 2. Cap. 7.
39. Albucas. Lib. 2. Cap. 93.
40. Haly Abbas Theor. Practic.
41. Rhazis. Cont. Tr. 26. T. 2. Cap. I. p. 298.

and *Avicena*† also, or his Translator, calls it *Vena Medinensis*;[42] but all the *Arabian Authors* call it, in their Language *Irk Medini*, i.e. *Nervous Medinensis*, and not *Vena Medinensis*, this being a Mistake in their Translators: The first from its Similitude to a *Nerve*, and *Medini*, of *Medina*, a City in *Arabia*, where it probably was first found, or taken notice of; though it is now no less frequent in some Parts of *Persia*, as Dr *Kempfer* observes, and after *Galen* calls it *Dracunculus*,[43] but in several Parts of *Africa*, and the *West-Indies*, it is commonly called the *Guinea-Worm*, because the Negroes who come from thence, are subject to it, and frequently bring it in their Legs to the West-India Islands.

Though this is called a *Nerve* or *Vein*, because it resembles the first, nevertheless it is a real *Worm*, of a white Colour except its Head, which is blackish; its Shape is round, long, small, and uniform like a Nerve, or a Piece of white round Tape or Bobbin, and not broad or flat as some Authors say. It is found most commonly lodged in the Legs or Thighs, and sometimes in some other Parts of the Body, in, or immediately under the Membrana Cellulosa, or in the Expansions of that Membrane between the Muscles, where it insinuates itself, and is extended to a great Length; and is commonly from one to two Feet and a half long. It does not cause much Pain, till near the Time that it is ready to come out, when the Part where the Head of the Worm, which is always the first protruded, begins to swell, throb, and be inflamed and painful, like a small Boil, generally in some Part of the Leg or Thigh, and sometimes, though very seldom, higher up on the Body. When this Boil breaks, the Head of the Worm, which is of a blackish Colour, is thrust out first, and soon after more of it comes out and hangs down the Leg, till it is extracted in the manner hereafter described.

This Disease proceeds from drinking the Water of stagnating Ponds, in hot Countries, after Droughts and sultry hot Seasons, where the *Ova* or *Animalcula*† of this Worm are contained, as in *Arabia*, *Persia*, the *East* and *West-Indies*; and I am informed that there are some stagnating Ponds in this Island, the washing in or drinking the Waters of which is subject to generate this Worm.

In the Cure of this Disease, both *Rhazis* and *Avicena* advise giving Aloetics† to hasten the Protrusion and Exclusion of the Worms: when the little

---

42. Avicen. Canon Med.
43. Kempfer. Amenitat. Exotic.

Tumours, where the Head of the Worms begin to appear and swell, they hasten their Suppuration with Cataplasms, or other Applications; and when these Tumours break, the End of the Worm being thrust out, they advise it to be tied to a Piece of Lead made in a long Form, and about half a Drachm Weight,[†] that the Worm may not contract and draw itself in again; and roll it round that Piece of Lead a little every Day, till it is all entirely extracted. The Surgeons here use the same Method, only they use a little Piece of Silk, Cotton, or Lint instead of the Lead, about which they roll it daily an Inch or more at a time till it is all extracted, taking great care not to break the Worm, (which Caution the *Arabians* also give) for if they break it, it is exceeding difficult, and sometimes impossible, to recover the End again; in which Case an Abscess, or rather many Abscesses, will be formed, not only at the Place of the Exit of the Worm, but all along the whole winding Meatuses[†] where the dead putrefied Worm remains, which sometimes degenerate into bad Ulcers, and give the Surgeon much Trouble, and the Patient a great deal of Pain.

Giving Aloetics, or other antihelmintic Medicines, as the *Arabians* advise, to dislodge and hasten the Extraction of the Worms, is a judicious Practice; but as these act more immediately on the Primæ Viæ, than on the fleshy Parts and Surface of the Body, the following coarse Composition has been found to be much more efficacious:

℞ *Sulphur. Viv. Rad. Alii ana* ʒj. *Piper. Nigr.* ʒss. *Camphor.* ℨij. *Spir. vinos tenusis* lbij. *Misce, et digere s. a. et cola, Colaturæ capiat Æger Cochl. duo bis vel ter de die.*[†]

The subtile[†] volatile pungent Parts of this inelegant Composition so stimulates and affects these Worms, that they generally endeavour to make their Exit, and draw themselves towards the Surface of the Body, where a small Tumour forms under the Skin, in which they collect and coil themselves up, and die; and the Tumour being opened, they are easily taken out whole; and not only the Worm which first appeared, but all the other Worms of the same sort which are in the Body, do the same; and are thus taken out in the same manner, where they appear. And when the Worms are thus taken out, the Places from whence they were taken, being not much more than Skin deep, soon heal up with any common Digestive, and no further Uneasiness remains in the Parts from whence the Worms were taken, and the Patient enjoys as good a State of Health, as ever he did before.

Of the LEPROSY *of the* ARABIANS

THE LEPRA ARABUM is indisputably a Disease which is peculiar to such Countries as are situated in the Torrid Zone; and was known many Ages since in *Arabia, Persia, and various Parts of Africa*; in which Countries it seems to have been indigenous. Different Names have been given to this Disease by different Authors, which has caused some Mistakes and Confusion among more modern Authors, who probably had never seen it. Most if not all the Greek Physicians, who lived after *Galen*, have mentioned it, [such] as *Aretæus* of *Cappadox*,† *Paulus* of *Ægina*,† and *Ætius* of *Amida*† either call it ἔλεφας, *Elephantia*, or ἐλεφαντίασις, *Elephantiasis*, though it is a very different Distemper from what *Rhazis*, and what we now call an *Elephantiasis*.

Ætius,[44] who lived in *Mesopotamia*, most probably had frequently seen it, and describes it and its Symptoms very well; but it is probable that the other Greek Writers had very seldom or never seen it, as they describe it less accurately than they generally have done other Diseases, with which they were more frequently conversant. *Ebn Zachariah Rhazis*, the oldest of the Arabian Physicians except *Serapion*,† calls it *Lepra*,[45] the *Leprosy*, though *Haly Abbas*, or his Translator, calls it *Elephantia*;[46] *Avicena*[47] gives it both these Names; and the learned Dr *Lommius*,†[48] has given us an elegant and concise Description of this Disease and calls it *Elephantia*; yet several other modern Authors have confounded the Symptoms of this Disease, with those of the *Lepra Grecorum*,† though they are quite different Diseases.

All the above-mentioned Authors, and several others, unanimously agree that this *Leprosy* is a contagious Disease, and that it not only descends from Parents to their Children but that it is communicated from one leprous Person to others with whom he cohabits: and several of these Authors advise, that all leprous Persons be separated from the Commerce† and Converse† of the Sound,† as in the Plague, and to have suitable Places allotted to them to live in, either in an Island, or somewhere near to the Sea-shore, where all Communication with those who are Sound, may be entirely cut off. This

---

44. Ætius Tetra Biblos. Lib. 13.
45. Rhazis Division L. 1. Cap. 120, p. 422.
46. Haly Abbas Theor. L. 8. p. 97. Pract. L. 4. p. 197.
47. Avicen. Can. V. 2. L.4. p. 133 &c.
48. Lommii Observat. Med. pag. 53.

Dreadful Disease was first brought to this and the other Sugar Islands by the Negroes from *Africa*, and is undoubtedly a Native of that Quarter of the World and *Arabia*, and is not originally of the western Part of it; neither was it ever known here, before it was brought hither by the Negroes, among whom it is now too frequent here, and has made its way into several Families of the white People also; and it is much to be feared, that it will spread further in this warm Climate, into many more both white and black Families, if the legislative Powers do not interpose, and endeavour to prevent its spreading, by some suitable, wise, and effectual laws, as we see the French and Spaniards have done.

This terrible Disease generally seizes the Patient insensibly, gradually, and slowly, when he seems to be in perfect Health, without Sickness, Pain, or any Uneasiness, nay, often without the Patient's knowing that he ails any thing, till some other Person observes that numerous Spots begin to appear in various Parts of his Body; first of a yellowish brownish Colour, and soon after begin to turn to a brownish purplish Colour in white People, and to a copper Colour in the Negroes: these Spots usually first appear on the Forehead and Chin, and continue gradually to increase, both in Number and Magnitude, for many Weeks or Months, without the Patient's knowing that he has the Disease. And as these Spots increase, the Skin on or near those Places begins to grow unequally thicker, then hard and rough, with hard Scales, especially on the face, Arms, and Legs, with a Numbness and Difficulty of moving the Fingers and Toes; these Scales are not like those of the *Lepra Grecorum*, nor fall off as those do. The Hairs on all the Parts of the Body gradually fall off, and become thinner. The Respiration gradually grows difficult, and the Voice obscure† and a little hoarse, the Breath fœtid and offensive, the Lobes of the Ears become thick and knotty, the Cheeks large and sometimes tuberous, as also the Forehead and Eyebrows, the Chin is dilated, and all these are of a livid reddish Colour: Their Urine is thick and turbid, like to that of Cattle; their Dispositions of Mind, Sleep, and Dreams are disturbed, like those who are melancholy, and some are suddenly awaked out of their Sleeps as if they were suffocated, which causes them to jump up. All those who labour under this Disease have frequent and strong Dispositions to Venery.† Varicose Veins of a blackish Colour, Warts or knotty Pustules are observed to rise about the Root of the Tongue, under the Eye-lids, and behind the Ears. All these Symptoms gradually and slowly increase, and grow worse as the Disease advances; and the Body becomes lean and deformed, while the Face, Calves of the Legs, and the Feet grow tumid,† and the last most commonly cold and torpid.† Thus the Disease continues to increase and grow worse for many Years; when the Pinnæ of the Nose† being thick and tuberous, and its Cartilage or Septum is corroded and wasted away, or falls down, the Nose becomes thick and flat, so that the Nostrils are in great measure obstructed, and the patient's Voice seems hollow like a *Ventriloqui*.† His Lips grow thick and are reverted; his Eyes are preternaturally round at their inner Angles, their Whites become yellowish, thick and hard, almost like the Nails of one's Fingers, by the Continuance of the Disease. The Hairs fall off the Eye-brows and Eye-lids, which are grown thick, hard and callous, as also from the Chin, and others come up in their Place, but much fewer and smaller; the Ears at last become acute,† and are extenuated and eaten away: the Fingers and Toes are greatly swelled, and crack with dry Fissures, and are sometimes so puffed up, that they are, as it were, buried under the Tumor of themselves and of the Feet. The Muscles are wasted all over the Body; and the Face and Countenance so disfigured with tuberous Knots, as before-mentioned, that it appears deformed and horrid, such as that of a Satyr is imagined to be, or like to that of a Lion; hence the Greeks give this Disease both the Names of *Satyriasm*, and *Leontiasim*. And now when the Disease is arrived at its last Stage, the Voice is exceeding hollow, and violent Ulcers affect the Hands and Feet, and sometimes some other Parts of the Body; and the Skin, and Part of the Flesh of the Feet, is entirely deprived of all Sensation, so that if you pierce them with a Needle, or scald them with boiling Water, or even apply a red-hot Iron to them, they are not sensible of any Pain. And at last the Humours are all become so very acrid, that a small Fever arises, which soon carries off the miserable Patient.

I have here described all the Symptoms which attend this loathsome Disease; not that every Patient who labours under it has every Symptom here described, but some have more, and others have fewer of them; though, in general, they have much the greatest Part of them sooner or later; and in this miserable Condition, often drag on Life for many Years before they die. O the happy Climate of England, which is totally a Stranger to this, and some other miserable Diseases!

From the strictest Enquiry, and most accurate Examination of the Symptoms and Nature of this Disease, as also from anatomical Dissections, it appears that the *Membrana Cellulosa* is the Seat of this Disease, which Membrane it follows almost into every Part of the Body, even into the very

Bones, some Parts of which it tumefies and indurates, and renders useless, whilst it corrodes, consumes, and eats away other Parts, especially the Cartilages, and sometimes the very Bones, when it becomes inveterate.

Hence it appears, that when the Disease has continued a long time, and some Parts are eaten away, and others become useless, and the Humours are become so acrid as to corrode the Bones, and almost destroy the human Frame, no Remedies whatever can possibly cure it, as *Haly Abbas*,[49] and the learned Dr *Lommius*[50] say: *Inveterascentem morbum hunc depelli remediis non posse.*[†]

Yet several ignorant and illiterate Quacks, here, have promised a certain Cure, even at any time of the Disease, but have as constantly failed of Success; for those very Pretensions and Promises, which such Men usually make, are sufficient Proofs that they are both ignorant of the nature of the Disease, and the Power of their Medicines. I grant that the least Hopes of being delivered from so deplorable a Distemper, is some Excuse for the Credulity of the People, and their suffering themselves to be imposed on by such vain, ignorant Boasters. And I mention this, to prevent such Impositions for the future.

But if the Disease be taken in time, *viz*, at the Beginning, and first Appearance of its Symptoms, the Spots above-mentioned, *&c.*, we have sufficient Reasons to believe it may be cured; and I have seen some Instances of its being cured.

Notwithstanding that the Seat of the venereal Disease is allowed to be chiefly in the Expansions of the *Membrana Adiposa vel Cellulosa*, as well as is this Disease; and is principally cured by the Use of Mercury, or the different Preparations of it; yet it is very remarkable that this Disease is so far from being either cured, or relieved by it, that on the contrary it is greatly increased, and all its Symptoms much aggravated by the Use of *Mercurials*. I grant that it seems to abate the Distemper for a little time, but it soon returns with almost double Force and Violence after it: And Antimony, or the best Preparations of it, which are of little Service in the former, are found to be the most efficacious Medicines in the Cure of this Disease, if properly given, and the Disease be taken in time.

When the above-mentioned Spots first appear, either of a yellowish, or brownish purple Colour, in order to distinguish and be certain whether they

---

49. Haly Abbas in loco citat.
50. Lommii Obs. Med. Lib. I. p. 55.

are the true Spots of this Leprosy, or they are Spots of another kind, which are not uncommon in this Climate, and look like them, but proceed from another Cause, and are of no bad Consequence; anoint the Spots gently with a little *Ol. Tartari per deliquium*,[†] and a little after rub it well off, and if the Spots disappear and return not again, they are not leprous Spots, but if they remain, or soon return again after being thus anointed and rubbed, they are the true Leprous Spots, though the Patient finds himself perfectly well in all other Respects, and may continue so for many Months, Wherefore it is necessary to attempt the Cure before the Disease gains further Ground and becomes inveterate.

To which Purpose, if the Patient be of a sanguine plethoric Constitution, it is advisable to bleed, to ten, twelve, or fourteen Ounces; after which an antimonial Vomit should be given; and then let them enter on the following Course of Medicines, and continue it for two or three Months

℞ *Sulph. Antimonii præcipit* ʒiij. *Mercurii. calcinat. levigat* gr. xxx. *Gum. Guajac. pulv.* ʒiii. *Bals. Gujacim. q.s. Ol. Sassafræ gut* xx. *Misce, fi. Pil.* lxxxx. *de quibus capiat Æger tres omni nocte, hora decubitura, superbib. gut* L. *Tinct. Sequentis in* ʒiij. *Decoc. sequentis.*[†]

℞ *Vini Antimonial.* ʒij. *Tinct. Aromatic.* ʒss. *Misce, fi, Tinct. ut supra sumenda.*[†]

℞ *Rad. Sarsaparil.* ʒiij. *Cort. Sassafr.* ʒj. *Sal. Diuretic.* ʒss. *Misce. coq. vase clauso in Aq. Pur.* lbiijss *ad* lbijss. *et cola; Colaturæ adde Tinct. Antimonii* ʒj. *Aq. Juniperi C.* ʒjss. *Sacchar. q.s. Misce, fi. Decoct. ut supra sumend. Bibat etiam hujus Decoct.* ʒiij. *omni Mane cum gut.* L. *Tinct. supra præscript.*[†]

This Method should be continued two Months, or longer if the Spots do not entirely disappear before that time, for it is necessary to continue them for some time after they are gone off. And the Spots should be rubbed well once or twice a Day, with a warm dry Flannel-cloth, first holden a little over the Fumes of burning Sulphur mixed with a little Antimony, and daily continued as long as the Spots remain.

If the Disease does not abate, and the Spots, Torpor,[†] and Numbness decrease, it is sometimes necessary to repeat the antimonial Vomit two or three times during this Course, especially when the Disease is hereditary, or proves very obstinate: And in this Case it is necessary to repeat the whole Course over again two or three Months after, however in the next Spring or Autumn following, or both if the least Symptoms then appear, as we know no Disease that is more obstinate or more difficult to cure. As the infectious Miasmata of this Disease, especially when it is hereditary, are subject to lay as it were quiet and still, without giving the Patient any Uneasiness, or even without shewing any Symptoms or Remains of the Disease, for a Year, or sometimes Years, and then break out and shew its Malignity with Force again; I think it is absolutely necessary to repeat this Course of Medicines every Spring and Autumn, especially when it is obstinate, for two Years, and when it is hereditary, for more Years; for too much Caution cannot be taken against so dreadful and loathsome a Disease. Wherefore I sometimes give something of the following Nature Spring and Autumn after all.

℞ *Antimonii crud. subtilis. levig.* ℥jss. *Tartar. solubil. Sal. Diuretic. Milleped. præparat. pulv. ana* ℥ss. *Zinziber. cond.* ℥ss. *Syr. e Sulph. q. s. Misce, fi. Elect. cujus capiat Æger q. Nuc. Mosc. major mane et hora decubit. insuper bibend. Tinct. supra præscript. Gut. L. in hatustu Decoct. ante præscript.*[†]

As to the dietetic Part of the Cure, it is not only necessary that the Patients live temperately, but there are several things which must be placed among the *Ledentia* in this Disease, from which the Patient must abstain. They must religiously abstain from all Swine's Flesh, and all fat Meats, and every thing that is oily, fat, or greasy, either in Sauces or other ways, and that not only during the Time they are under this Course of Medicines, but for many Years after. They may eat any sort of Flesh-meats at Noon, that are not too fat, too much salted, or too high seasoned, with Roots, Greens, and plain Sauces; but the more plain, simple, and the lighter, and more easily digested they are, the better: They should be also very temperate in the Use of Wine and all spirituous Liquors, and strictly abstain from all kinds of malt Liquors, for they are by no means a proper Drink in the hot Climates, as they are too viscid and glutinous a Liquid, they require more Labour and Action, in order to digest and animalize them, than can be well used here; and as the Heat is great, and we perspire much, and soon, they are carried into the Blood too soon and too crude, before they are half digested and animalized, and often do much hurt, as I have often observed, and mention it here. Small Punch moderately acid, is a much more proper beverage for the hot Climates: Their Diet also Mornings and Nights should be light and easily digested, and gently attenuating and diluting.

These Rules may seem to be too rigid and severe to some, but they are absolutely necessary, if the Patient is obliged to continue in a hot Climate, and yet desires to recover his Health, and live free from this dreadful Disease. It is highly probable, that removing into a colder Climate, may considerably contribute to their Recovery, and re-establishing their Health, especially as a hot Climate is the Parent and Producer of this Disease.

This Method has succeeded, when the Distemper has been taken in time, before it was too far advanced, and too deeply rooted in the Constitution, and the whole Mass of the Fluids too much inquinated; I therefore communicate it to others, that they may either use it, or improve it if they can; and I wish them all Success.

I have here given several *Formulæ* or *Prescriptions*, which are only suited to some Constitutions and Cases, and are only given as a general Plan; and am very sensible that it will be necessary to make some Alterations in them, as well in regard to the different Constitutions, as to the different Ages of the Patients: And so it is in all other Diseases, wherein we must vary from any Rules which can be laid down; but the judicious Physician will from these readily know when, and how far, it is necessary to make such Alterations.

But when this Disease is hereditary, and is arrived to its last Stage, so that the whole cellular Membrane is loaded with the morbid Matter, and the Bones corroded and eaten away, neither this Method, nor any other whatever yet known, can recover such a Patient, nor possibly restore him to Health again; therefore we can only say with *Haly Abbas* and the learned and eloquent Dr *Lommius*, "*Scire tamen licet, inveterascentem Morbem hunc depelli remediis non posse. Nam extra Artis limites est.*"†

Of the LEPROSY of the JOINTS†

THERE IS ANOTHER SPECIES of this Leprosy, which *Haly Abbas* mentions; he says, "*Sunt autem Elephantiæ species duæ.*" The first is that which is described before; "*Altera et secunda, – quam ex humore nigro, quam ex colore generatur rubea adustionem, in hac specie membrorum est comestio et causus; et ab hac nulla sanatur quovis medela.*"†

I cannot find that any of the Greek Physicians, nor yet any of the Arabians, except *Haly Abbas*, mention this kind of Leprosy, unless we suppose that they made no Distinction between this and the preceding Leprosy, and that they speak of them as one Disease; and that they meant this sort of Leprosy, where they mention the falling off of the Limbs, when they are treating on the *Elephantia* or other Leprosy. Dr Town describes this sort of Leprosy, but with the Vulgar calls it the Joint Evil,[51] though it has not the least Appearance or Nature of a Scrophula[†] in it: But I am more surprised to find the same learned Gentleman call it a cutaneous Disease, when it eats the Flesh even to the Bones, and corrodes them also, till the Fingers and Toes drop off Joint by Joint. He also says, that it is a Disease which has not been taken notice of by any Author; but if he had enquired further, he would have found that *Haly Abbas* the *Persian Magus*, had described it almost 800 Years before him: However, the Doctor has described it very well, and justly observes, that it was first brought hither by the Negroes from Guiney in Africa, where it now seizes many of the Negroes, both Natives and those who are imported from Africa; and I may add several white People also, who are Natives; whatever it might do in his tome, which is not much above twenty Years since, I cannot say.

This sort of Leprosy, when it first appears, seizes the Patient in the same Manner, and with the same Symptoms, as the other kind of Leprosy before described; so that it is not possible to tell for a considerable time, whether[†] of them it will prove to be: For when the Patient thinks himself perfectly well, several superficial Spots of a yellowish, brownish, Copper-colour, with a purplish Cast in white People, and of a dark brownish Copper-colour in the Blacks, first appear in several Parts of the Face, especially about the Nose, and soon after on several other Parts of the Body; at first without any Uneasiness or Roughness in the Skin, or any Sense of Pain, and often without the Person's knowing that they have either this, or any other Disease, till told of it by others who see them. These Spots spread by slow Degrees, and increase both in Number and Magnitude, till they cover a considerable Part of the Body, and yet with very little Uneasiness or Pain; and thus they remain gradually and slowly to increase for several Months, and sometimes Years, and then the Fingers and Toes begin to be numb, and gradually but slowly to swell, especially at their Ends, and their Nails are curved inwards, which plainly shew this to be a kind of Leprosy: And thus they continue to grow slowly worse and worse, till their Fingers and Toes begin to ulcerate; and the Ulcers are very small, never digest,[†] nor are much inflamed, but generally look dry, without much Foulness, Matter, or Fœtor, and, being almost insensible, without much Pain: These gradually creep on from one Joint to another, and corrode the Ligaments, Tendons, Nerves, and all the Vessels to the very Bones,

---

51. Dr Town on the West India Diseases.

but without much Pain, all the Parts being benumbed and almost deprived of all Sensation; and that Joint soon drops off easily, and the Ulcers creep on to the next Joints, which soon drop off in the same manner, and so creep on from Joint to Joint, till all the Fingers and Toes are corroded and quite dropt off: It then seizes the Joints of the Carpus and Metatarsus; but before it can erode all those, it also seizes the Trunk of the Body, and breaks out in little small dry Ulcers, with dry Scabs in the Arms, Legs, and most Parts of the Body; and now the Distemper becomes infectious, if it was not so sooner. These small Ulcers never penetrate deep into the muscular Flesh of the Body, but spread and extend themselves on its Surface, in the *Membrana Adiposa*, and discharge a little thin acrid Ichor, which dries up into scaly Scabs, and emaciates the Patient away, sometimes in two or three Years' time, and often is much longer before it puts an end to their miserable Life; for there are some Instances of Patients who have dragged on a miserable loathsome Life for ten or fifteen Years or more, before they died.

The Method of Cure in this, must be the same as in the other kind of Leprosy; for it is no less remarkable in this, than in the other, that all *Mercurials*, however prepared (except the *Mercurius calcinatus*, given in small Doses as an Alterative with Antimonials, as before;) do in this, as well as in the other kind of Leprosy, greatly aggravate all the Symptoms, and increase the Disease: But if it be taken in time, at the first Appearance and Beginning of the Disease, and treated with Antimonials, in the same manner as in the other Leprosy, we have great Reason to hope for Success; though I have not had such Opportunities of trying it in this, as I have had in the other. But when the Disease is hereditary from their Parents, or has been neglected too long, till the Joints are begun to fall off, and all the Fluids so inquinated and infected, we can do no more than say with *Haly Abbas*, That no Remedies yet known, however powerful and efficacious, can prevail against, and cure this Disease.

Of the YAWS†

THAT DISEASE which the Negroes in Africa, and we in the West Indies, from them, call the *Yaws*, is a Native of, and seems to be indigenous in Africa and Arabia; and was first brought from the former by the Negroes into America and its Islands.

This is a Distemper which has been well known for many Ages in Africa, and some of its neighbouring Countries which are situated within the Torrid Zone: But I do not find that any of the *Greek Physicians*, nor yet any of the *Arabians*, do mention it, except *Haly Abbas*, the Persian Magus, who I think has described it in his *Theoria*, cap. 16. lib. 8. and calls it the *Lepra*: He briefly describes it thus: "*Lepra albedo est quæ in exterioribus fit Cutis: Et aliquando in quibusdam sine aliis est membris: Nonnunquam veró in toto fit corpore interdum ut totius fit corporis color albus. – quæ in membro est, si ex mala fit frigida complexione, hæc sunt Signa; quam membrum in quo est, album est colore, itidemque ejus pili; et si cutis phlebotomo vel certe acu pungitur, sanguis ab eo non egreditur humiditas alba.*"[†]

From this short Description of the Disease, and from its being only in some Parts or Members of the Body, and sometimes all over it, on the Skin, and its white Colour, and particularly the Hair's turning white, and upon opening the little Tumours, only a white Humour coming out; I think he meant this Disease which we now call the *Yaws*, an African Name, and not the *Lepra Arabum*, of which he treats in the preceding Chapter, and with the *Greek* and some of the *Arabian Physicians* calls the *Elephantia*, but he calls this *Lepra*; and whether this Disease is not the same with the Leprosy of the Jews, will admit of some Dispute, though it is most probable that it is; but as the Description which Moses their Legislator has given us of their Leprosy,[52] is so very short and undescriptive, it is difficult to determine; though it is more reasonable to suppose that it was this Disease, than the *Lepra Arabum*, and if so, it is a Disease of great Antiquity: Neither can we collect any thing from Moses's Method of curing it;[†] for if the leprous Person did receive any benefit from the Method which Moses prescribes, and has left us, it must have arisen from a miraculous or supernatural Power, and not from his being sprinkled with the Blood of a Sparrow, or any other Bird, nor from any thing else that the Priest did to the Leper; though he was sure of being a considerable Gainer by the Cure.

We are credibly told, that the *Yaws* seldom fail to attack the Negroes in Africa, at one time or other in their Life-time, but most frequently the Children and young People; and that they very rarely or never have it a second time, if they have been perfectly cured the first time, either in their own native Country by their Negro Doctors, or after they arrived here; for the Negroes

---

52. Leviticus, chap. xiii.

have by long Observation and Experience, found out a Method of curing this Disease with the caustic Juices of certain escharotic Plants externally applied, and giving the Juice or Decoctions of others internally, which they keep as a Secret from the white People, but preserve among themselves by Tradition; with which they sometimes perform notable Cures, both in this, and some other Diseases.

This Disease generally makes its first Appearance without any previous Sickness or Pain, and when the Patient thinks himself perfectly well, in very small Pimples no bigger than the Head of a small Pin, and are smooth and level with the Skin; these daily increase and become protuberant Pustules; soon after the Cuticle turns whitish, cracks and rubs off, and a very small Quantity of Serum or clear Ichor exudes out and dries, and becomes white, but neither Pus nor any Quantity of Ichor is found in the Tumour, but a pretty thick, white Slough† appears, and under that a red fungous† Flesh thrusts itself out of the Skin, which gradually increases to different Magnitudes, some not so large as the smallest Wood-strawberry,† some larger; others exceeding the Size of the largest Mulberry,† which last they very much resemble, being red, and composed of little round Knobs as they are: They appear indifferently on all the Parts of the Body, but most frequently, and generally are the largest, about the Groin, private Parts, Anus, under the Arms, and in the Face: And it is remarkable, that in general when the *Yaws* are very large, they are fewer in number; and *è contra*, when they are more numerous, they are generally smaller in Size. And as the *Yaws* are thus increasing and coming to their Height, the black Hairs which grow out of the Places where the *Yaws* are, gradually turn to be perfectly white, like the Hair of an old Man; and the Ichor which ouzes out if the *Yaws*, drying upon the Skin, makes it appear of a whitish Colour, and renders the Patient a disagreeable loathsome Sight: And now the Disease is become very infectious to those who handle or co-habit with them.

All this Time the Patient neither loses his Appetite, Flesh, nor Strength, and otherwise seems to be in good Health; being free from any Pain, or any Uneasiness but what the disagreeable Nastiness of the Sores, and a little Soreness occasions, for they are not painful unless they are roughly touched and rubbed.

The time from their first Appearance in the before-mentioned small Pimples, to their full Height and Growth, is very different in different Constitutions, as they are stronger or weaker, and according to the Negro's being well fed, or the contrary; for when the Negro is strong, lusty, and of a plethoric Habit, and is well fed, the *Yaws* will often arrive at their full Growth, and be as large as a Mulberry in a Month's time from their first Appearance; but when the Negro is weak, low in Flesh, and poorly fed, the *Yaws* will be small, and often no larger than a Strawberry at the End of three Months.

This Disease is known to be infectious, but there is also a peculiar Aptitude in some Constitutions to receive it more readily, than in some others, and probably in the same Person to receive the Infection more readily at one time, than at another time; as is also observed with the Small-pox.

This is a Description of the true natural Appearance of the Disease, when it is left entirely to Nature, and is neither retarded nor hastened by Medicines, nor altered by external Applications; and it will continue in this State a long time, without any material Alteration, if left alone; and what would be the Consequence, if it was left to continue without and Medical Applications, is uncertain, as I have never yet seen one so left without some Attempts to cure it; but it is most probable that the Funguses† in the *Yaws*, would in time become phagedenic† Ulcers, which would corrode and eat away the Flesh even to the Bones, and then produce Nodes, Exostoses, and Caries in them, and at last totally consume and destroy them also, as we see it does when the Disease is wrong treated, and the Cure attempted without Success. For when this is the Case, and the Patient has taken a considerable Quantity of Mercury, or has been salivated,† especially if by Unction, too soon in the Disease, before the morbid Matter was sufficiently cast out to the Surface of the Body, or has been repelled into it by that or other Means; tho' the Skin has been by such Methods sufficiently cleared; yet the Distemper not being thereby effectually eradicated and cured, it will return again, and then becomes exceeding difficult to cure; and if it has made several of those Returns, and has been repelled, and has at last broke out in malignant Ulcers, and corroded the Bones, it is too often incurable. But if the Disease be judiciously treated at the first, it seldom or never proves dangerous, and very rarely difficult to cure.

There is another vile Custom which I must take notice of, which the Surgeons of the Guinea Ships generally practice; that is, upon the first appearance of the *Yaws*, during the Voyage from Guinea, they apply some strong Repellents to them; such as the Juice of roasted Limes mixed with the Rust of Iron, and Sulphur or Gunpowder; by which they repel the morbid Matter into the Blood, where its Acrimony is increased, though they thereby render their Skins clean for a short time, and then rub them with Palm-oil,† which makes soft and look well, when they are imposed upon the Planters for sound, healthful Negroes; but in a few Days or Weeks after they have purchased them, the Virulency of the morbid Matter being increased by the Retention, and the Heat of the Body, the *Yaws* break out again much worse than ever, and are then very difficult to cure, or sometimes incurable.

As this Disease proceeds from a peculiar kind of *infectious Miasmata,* which is first generated in, and is indigenous to the hot Climate of *Africa*; which Nature, when she acts in the most salutiferous† Manner, always casts out on the Surface of the Body, when not hindered by injudicious or male-Practice; it consequently follows that the true Intentions of Cure, are,

First: *To assist Nature to expel all the morbid Matter to the Surface of the Body, that as much of it as possibly can, may be discharged that Way.*

And, Secondly: *To correct the remaining Part, and destroy such Part of it as is not discharged, but remains lodged in those Funguses, and Ulcers, together with them, by the Use of proper Escharotics.*

Wherefore, as soon as the above-mentioned Pimples begin to appear, let the Negro be confined in a House, or separate Room from the rest of the Negroes; or if you are not certain whether it be the *Yaws,* or a sort of *Itch,* which the Negroes call in their Language *Crocrow,* as they much resemble each other at their first Appearance, though they differ greatly soon after; shut the Negro up in a Room for seven Days, and look on him again as the Jews were commanded to do with their *Lepers,* (*Levit.* Ch. xiii) in which time, one may most commonly be certain whether it be the *Yaws* or not; and if it be, it will be necessary to give something of the following Nature, in order to assist Nature to hasten the Expulsion of the morbid Matter, and bring the Yaws to their full Growth.

℞ *Æthiop. Mineral.* ʒjss. *Antimon. Crud. pulv.* ʒj. *Theriac. Androm.* ʒj. *Camphorii pulv* ʒj. *Syr. Zinziber. q.s. Misce. fi. Elect, cujus capiat Æger q. N. Mosc. major. mane et hora decubitura, superbibend. Vini Antimonial. gut. xl. in haustu seri lactis vel Thæ, et contin. donec Tumores* (the Yaws *dict.*) *ad Maturitat.*†

It may certainly be known that the *Yaws* are come to their full Height, by their being at a stand, and neither increasing in their Number or Magnitude: And when you see that they are at a stand, it is a proper time to begin to give Mercurials to raise a Ptyalisme; which is much better done by giving *Calomel* daily than by Unction, in this Disease, lest the latter should carry the morbid Matter from the Skin into the Mass of the Blood again; neither is it prudent to apply any mercurial Unguents to the *Yaws,* for the same Reasons: The best

Method is to give *Calomel gr.* v or vj. twice a Day till a moderate Salivation is raised, and the Patient spits a Pint and a half every twenty-four Hours, and never raise it higher, for few Patients in this hot Climate, can bear a Ptyalisme to be raised so high without danger of sinking under it, or bringing some other bad Symptoms on. By the time that the Salivation is raised to near a Pint and a half, the *Yaws* are generally all covered over with dry scaly Scabs, which then begin to fall off daily in white Scales or Scabs, and usually in ten or twelve Days' time more leave the Skin, smooth, soft, and clean. As soon as the Scabs are fallen off, and the Skin begins to be clean, cease to give any more Mercury, and let the Salivation go off gradually of its own accord; or if it continues too long, give a Dose of Rhubarb, or some other suitable gentle Cathartic.

It frequently happens that after the *Yaws* are in general gone off and healed, and the Skin is become soft and clean, that one, or more large *Yaws* still remain rising high, and are red, knotted, and moist, discharging a little Ichor; this is usually called the Master-yaw, from its being bigger than any of the rest: Some have been so imprudent as to continue, or repeat the Salivation to carry it or them off, to the Prejudice of the Patient; when in reality nothing more is necessary, than totally to destroy that Yaw, or those Yaws, so remaining, and all their contained fungous Flesh, with gentle Escharotics; and then to incarn† and cicatrize the Place with any common Digestive and Desiccative.

Some use the *Lapis Infernalis*,† others a Solution of *Mercur. Sublimat. Corrosiv.* ʒj. *in Spir. Vini Rect.* ʒj.† and gently touch the remaining Yaws with a feather dipp'd in this, twice a Day, till they are all consumed: Others use blue Vitriol,† or a Mixture of *Mercur. Corrosiv. Rubr.* ʒj. *Alum. ust. pulv.* ʒss. *m.*† This last is the gentlest, and safest, and at the same time full as effectual, and therefore is much the best.

During the use of these Escharotics, it is necessary that the Patient take something of the following Nature, in order to expel any remaining morbid Matter, as well as to prevent any of it from being repelled into the Blood by those topical Applications, as also to correct the Acrimony of the Humours, and sweeten† the Blood, and to restore the Patient's perfect Health.

℞ *Ethiop. Mineral.* ʒjss. *Antimon. Crud. pulv.* ʒj. *Theriac. Androm.* ʒss. *Gum. Guaiaci pulv.* ʒiij. *Syr. Commun. q.s. Misce. fi. Electar. Capiat Æger q. Nuc. Mosc. major. Mane Nocteq; insuperbibend. Vini Antimonial. gut.* xl. *vel* l. *in haustu Decoct. Rad. Sarsaparil. et Lign. Sassafræ.*†

These Methods generally succeed, even in the most numerous and worst kind of Yaws, provided they have not been tampered with, and the morbid

Matter frequently repelled, before, or other ways wrong treated. But if after giving the first Medicines, the Yaws are not numerous, nor of a bad kind, and by their coming to Maturity soon, it appears that the morbid Humours are effectually expelled; giving these following Medicines, and using the last escharotic Powder as above, most commonly effectually cures them without a Salivation.†

℞ *Sulph. Antimon. præcipit.* ʒij. *Mercur. Calcinat. levig. gr.* xxiv. *Gum. Guaiac. pulv.* ʒss. *Camphor.* ʒss. *Bals. Guaiacin. q.s. Misce, fi. Pil.* lxx. *de quibus capiat tres omni nocte hora decubit. superbib. Vini Antimonial. gut.* xl. *in haustu Decoct. Rad. Sarsaparil. et Ligni Sassafræ.*†

It sometimes happens, that after the Patient is cured as before, and all the Yaws are entirely gone: and the Skin in every Part of the Body, except the Soles of the Feet, is perfectly soft, smooth, and sound, that Tumours or little hard Swellings will remain on them, which are painful, and so very sore that they can neither stand up nor walk, nor even bear for them to be touched without great Pain. This proceeds from Yaws rising on the Soles of their Feet, and the Skin there being very hard and thick, from their going Bare-foot, so that the Yaws cannot push thro' so thick a callous Skin. This is easily remedied by bathing their Feet in warm Water, and paring off the callous Skin, and then the Yaws will appear, and push themselves out, when they may soon be destroyed by the above escharotic Powder, and the Place cured as in the Master-yaw.

But the worst Circumstances, attending this Disease, proceed from a wrong Method of treating it; either by the Use of strong repelling Applications, or by too hastily giving Mecurials, and bringing on a Salivation, before Nature has sufficiently expelled the morbid Matter to the Surface of the Body, as that is the salutiferous Way she takes, and points out to us to follow, when she is not hindered by wrong Methods and Medicines, which return the morbid Matter into the Blood again, when she has cast it out; when it falls upon some other excretory Passages, by which it never can be carried off, but is cast upon various Parts of the Body, where it produces the most malignant kind of phagedenic Ulcers,† which when they can be come at, are either exceeding difficult to cure, or are sometimes incurable. Or if it falls upon the Bones, and brings on gnawing Pains in the Limbs, with violent nocturnal Pains, like those which attend the venereal Disease, and at last produces Nodes, Exostoses, and Caries in the Bones, which in time eats them away, and the Patient after continuing a long time, sometimes Years, in this miserable Condition, at last dies torpid. This is a most deplorable Case! But if it be taken, when they have only the external Ulcers, and before the Pains in the Bones, with Nodes, Exostoses, and Caries come on and seize them, it may sometimes be cured by the following Method, which has sometimes succeeded when a Salivation has failed. A salivation may be tried in some Cases; but if it does not bring the Ulcers to digest and heal, proceed no farther, but give the following:

℞ *Sulph. Antimon. præcipit.* ʒijss. *Mercurii calcinat. levigat.* ʒss. *Gum. Guaiac. Pulv.* ʒiij. *Bals. Guaiacin. q.s. Camphorii Pulv.* Əij. *Misce, fi. Pil.* lxxx. *de quibus capiat Æger tres omni Nocte, hora decubitura, insuperbibendo Decoctionis sequentis* ʒv.†

℞ *Rad. Sarsaparil.* ʒiiij. *Cort. Sassafræ* ʒj. *Sal. Nitri* ʒss. *Misce, coq. in Aq. Pur.* lbiij. *ad* lbij. *et cola, Colaturæa adde Aq. Juniperi Comp.* ʒiss. *Sacchar. Alb. q.s. Misce, fi. Decoc. ut supra sumenda.*†

℞ *Vini Antimonial.* ʒj. *Tinct. Aromati* ʒ ij. *Misce, Capiat gut.* L. *omni Mane, et hora quarta postmerid. in* ʒv. *Decoct. supra præscript.*†

And the Ulcers may be dressed with this:

℞ *Ung. Basilic. flav.* ʒj. *Mercurii Corrosiv. Rub. levigat.* ʒ i. *Alum. usti pulv.* ʒss. *Misce, fi. Bals. Digest.*†

And when the Ulcers are clean, and begin to incarn, and tend to cicatrize, they may be dressed with this, till they are perfectly healed, and well.

℞ *Empl. Commun. cum Gum. e Minio una* ʒss. *Mercurii Corrosiv. Rubr.* ij. *Alum. ust. Pulv.* ʒss. *Misce, fi. Empl.*†

But when the Bones are affected with Nodes, and are become carious, and are in part eaten away; which most commonly happens to such Bones as are of the most spungy Nature, as are those of the Metacarpus and Fingers, and Metatarsus and the Toes, and the Spine, with the [Epiphyses] of the other Bones, the Case is deplorable† and incurable; nor will Amputation avail even when it is in the Hands, Feet, or in such Parts where that Operation can be performed; because the Humour will soon fall upon some other Parts, and produce the same Effects.

Of the IMPETIGO or RING-WORM†

THE IMPETIGO is a cutaneous Disease, which was well known to the ancient *Greek* and *Arabian Physicians*, and is more or less frequent still in most other Nations; but it is usually so mild and so easily cured in the colder northern Countries, that it may be thought unnecessary to say any thing of it here:

But it is so frequent, and so much worse, and so very troublesome and disagreeable as well as painful a Disease, in the West-India Islands, and in that Part of the Continent of America, which is situated in, or near to the Torrid Zone, that it may not only be said to be indigenous to them, but is often difficult to be cured.

We are told by some of the first Voyagers into this Part of the World, that the original Natives of these Islands were then, and still are, so subject to a cutaneous Disease, which is either this, or one which very much resembles it, which they call in their Language a *Cowrap*; that they have a Tradition among themselves, that one of the seven first People that were created when the World was first made, (for so many they say were at first created) was a *Cowrap*.

From this Tradition we may however conclude that it is a Disease, at least among them, almost as ancient as the Race of Mankind. Though we do not find that they had any of the before described Diseases, which are indigenous to *Africa*, and have been imported with the African Negroes from thence, to these western Parts of the World; though these Parts are as warm as *Africa* is.

The Disease first appears, without any previous Sickness or Pain in any Part of the Body, in some in one Part, in others in another Part, first in many small Pustulæ or Pimples, clustering together, most commonly in or near to a circular Form, the Bigness of a Sixpence or a Shilling, of a reddish Colour, and contain a small Quantity of clear, acrid, saline Lymph; but they soon spread, sometimes to be as large as the Breadth of the Hand, or broader, and itch most intolerably, especially upon the Persons putting off [their] Cloaths at Night, often to such a Degree that human Resolution is not able to restrain their Hands from scratching; and that, or rubbing them briskly, breaks the small Pimples, and the acrid Lymph ouzes out, and causes a Heat and Smarting, and then it dries upon the Skin, and forms whitish Scales or Scabs, which, upon rubbing or scratching, fall off again, and are daily renewed in the same manner, with the same Symptoms of itching, &c. Thus they increase and spread to various Parts of the Body; and sometimes they will leave one Part of the Body and remove to another Part, without any Remedies being applied. And in this State the Disease will continue for many Years, and probably would remain during the Patient's Life, if not removed by proper Remedies.

This is truly a cutaneous Disease, and is thought by many to be contagious, and probably it may be so in its most virulent State; and whether it arises from small Animalculæ, like, or somewhat different from, the Handworm,[†] which is said to cause the Itch, or it arises from the Heat of the Climate which so exalts and semivolatilizes the Salts and oily Particles of the animal Fluids, as to change them from their soft bland semiammoniacal State, to a semivolatile, acrid Nature, which obstruct the sudorofic Ducts and perspiratory Pores of the Skin, where being retained, they are, by the Heat of the Body and the Climate, still rendered more acrid and corroding, and so stimulate the obstructed Ducts and Pores, as to produce those small Pimples and the almost intolerable Itching, and those being broken and torn by scratching, the acrid Lymph ouzes out and forms the Scaly Scabs; and this being daily repeated, increases the Acrimony of the Humours, and the spreading of the Disease to other Parts of the Body. And when the Disease is suffered to continue a long time, as it is sometimes for Years, the Lymph discharged becomes so very acrid that it corrodes the Parts affected deeper, and expands them larger, and at last degenerates sometimes into a *Herpes exedens.*[†] For this is only a more virulent and malignant Degree of the Impetigo.

This being sufficient to produce Disease, without supposing any Animalculæ, it is not necessary to multiply Causes, at least till such are discovered by microscopical Observation; since Nature is observed not to multiply them where one is sufficient, and the Remark made on the Acrimony of the Sweat, &c. before, is sufficient to confirm this. Wherefore the Intentions of Cure are to attenuate, break, and dissolve those viscid, saline, acrid Moleculæ which are detained in, and obstruct those sudorofic Ducts and perspiratory Pores, in the Parts affected, so that they and the obstructed Fluids may be regularly exhaled and carried off.

Now it is well known, that of all the Medicines, whether vegetable, animal, or mineral Substances, that we are yet acquainted with, *Mercury* is a Body[†] which is the most peculiarly adapted and fitted to answer these Intentions of Cure (whether the Disease proceeds from these Causes, or from the supposed Animalculæ) by its great Gravity[†] and early Divisibility into the minutest spherical Particles; and long Experience has also confirmed this.

It may be thought by some Persons, that some Evacuations, [such] as Bleeding and Purging, may be necessary, before we either give Mercury internally, or use it externally; but unless a Plethora indicate them, they are neither of any Service in this, nor in some other cutaneous Diseases; and Purging may divert the Mecurials from the Skin, where they are intended to act, towards the Intestines afterwards, and so do hurt.

If the Disease is recent, and has neither continued long, nor spread much, nor the Humours become very acrid, it is most commonly very easily cured, even with a little *Sulphur* either mixed with a little *Unguent. Simplex*,[†] or with a little *Diapalma*[†] made into a Plaster and applied to the Part affected; or if that be washed with a Lotion made with *Rad. Hellebori Albi*[†] and a little *Vitrioli Albi*[†] infused in Water, and a few Doses of *Lactis Sulphuris*[†] taken inwardly, at the time of using them. But if the Disease has been neglected, and has continued a long time, so that it is become inveterate, and the Lymph or Serum which it discharges is become very acrid and corroding, or where it is degenerated into a *Herpes exedens*, it is difficult to be cured; and applying any Unguents, Lotions, or any repelling Medicines topically, without giving proper internal Medicines at the same time, may be, nay, have been attended with bad Consequences; for some who have injudiciously made use of such repelling Applications, have turned that acrid Humour upon the Bowels, or the Lungs, or on the vital Parts, which have produced very bad Consequences.

Wherefore, tho' the slight easy Things above-mentioned may cure it when it is moderate and recent, in some Constitutions; yet when it has continued a long time, and the Humour is become very acrid, and the Constitution bad, more powerful and active Remedies are required: And I have found something of the following kind to be the most successful.

℞ *Mercurii calcinat. subtilis. levigat.* ℈i. *Sulphur. Antimon. præcipitat.* ℈iv. *vel* v. *Gum. Guaiac. pulv.* ʒj. *Bals. Guaiacim. q. s. Misce, fi. Pil.* xl. *de quibus capiat Æger duas omni nocte hora decubitura.*[†]

℞ *Vini Antimonial.* ℥i. *Tinct. Aromatic.* ℥ss. *m. capiat. gut.* lx. *omni mane in haustu Infusionis Rad. Sarsaparillæ.*[†]

Where the Constitution of the Patient is pretty strong, and the Disease inveterate, he may take the same after the Pills at Night also; and after he has taken them seven or eight Days, he may begin to anoint the Parts affected with a little of the following every other Night, till he has used it four or five times, and continue the Use of the above Pills and Drops at the same time: And if any Appearance of the Spots remain, or return, may just touch them with a very little of the Ointment again, till they are perfectly well. And if these Pills and Drops move the Belly more than once or twice (at most) a Day, I usually give *Extract. Thebaic.* gr. ss.[†] with each Dose of the Pills, or so much as may be found necessary to stop the Purging; in order that they may be carried into the circulating Fluids, and have their proper Effect upon them, and correct and alter the acrid Humours.

It is well known that *Secrets*† and *Nostrums*† have been greatly extolled and quacked upon the Publick, as infallible Remedies for this Disease; [such] as the *Terra Macke-machee*† among the Spaniards; an Infusion of the *Radix Hellebori albi*, with a little *alkaline Salt*† in Water, and a little Milk added to disguise it, by the French; and several more have been strongly recommended by others, but they all in general frequently prove ineffectual, except in a chance case where the Disease is moderate and recent.

However, I must for the good of the Publick, at least in these Parts, recommend the Use of the Flowers of a Shrub, which is frequently found growing in many Parts of this Island,† and has been found by repeated Experience, to be much more effectual in the Cure of this very troublesome tho' seldom dangerous Disorder, than any of the abovementioned Nostrums; and is said, by some Persons, to have succeeded when the Mercurials in various Forms have failed, for which Reason I shall describe this Shrub here below,⁵³

---

53. Sir *Hans Sloane* has described this Shrub in his *Nat. History of Jamaica*, and calls it, *Juglandis folio, fruticosa, siloquosa, foliis pinnatis, costa media membranulis urtique extantibus alata, siliqua quadrangular alata*: And here it is vulgarly called the *French Guava Bush*; tho' it is nothing of the Nature of a Guava, nor any Similitude to it, except in its Leaf, which much more resembles that Leaf, than it does the Walnut.

This Shrub is an annual Shrub, and usually rises to the Height of four, five, or six Feet high; and is of the Class of the *Heptandria Monogynea* of *Linnæus*: It has many small woody Branches, its Leaves stand on short Stems opposite to each other, and are shaped like the Leaves of the Guava-Bush; (*malo punicæ affinis Pomifera* of Sir *Hans Sloane*) the Flowers are many, and stand on the Ends of the Branches, near to each other, which seem to form one oblong large Flower, of an Orange-yellowish Colour, and an uncommon Shape (to which I think the Botanists have not given a Name) which afterwards open and are a little more yellow: The Perianthum consists of one large Orange-coloured Petal, and five more on the Side next the Stem which are smaller, and of a bright yellow Colour, and seem to make a Part of the Corolla: The Corolla consists of five Petals within the Perianthium, of a bright yellow Colour when open, and of an ovato-lanceolate Figure: The Stamina are seven, two larger shaped like the Seeds of the *Fœniculi dulcis*, but a little larger, and a third slenderer and somewhat longer, and four small ones at the Bottom of the Calyx. The Pistil is much longer than the Stamina, and is curvated downwards: The Germen is long and of a square Figure, the Style something shorter, and the Stigma small, consisting of one small Aperture.

The Fruit is the Pistil enlarged into the Form of a long Pod, four, five, or six Inches long, with a Wing running on each Side of the Pod, from one End to the other, which gives it a square Figure, and is first green, but when ripe of a brown blackish Colour, and contains a great Number of flattish cordated Seeds, of a dark brown Colour, with Semi-valves between each.

And as neither the Name which it is vulgarly given it here, nor yet that given it by Sir *Hans Sloane*, are proper or suitable, shall we call it *ntileichen*, as expresses its medicinal Virtues?

that it may be more publickly known, and brought into more frequent Use: They usually rub the Parts affected with the Impetigo, with the whole Flower, or with the Flowers reduced to a fine Pulp in a marble Mortar, very well for two or three Nights, and again afterwards if any Spots or Roughness remain or return, and it seldom or never fails to remove and effectually cure this troublesome and very uneasy Disease; especially if the above Pills and Drops are taken at the same time, tho' the Disease be inveterate and obstinate.

FINIS

Notes

Preface

page 3
Fahrenheit's **Mercurial Thermometer:** Gabriel Daniel Fahrenheit (1686–1736), a German physicist, devised the temperature scale named after him in 1724. He introduced the use of mercury in thermometers in 1714.

Barometer: The mercury barometer was invented by Evangelista Torricelli (1608–47), an Italian physicist, in 1643.

Station: the height (in inches) at which a barometer's mercury column stands.

Torrid Zone: the region of Earth between the Tropics of Cancer (23°28 north) and Capricorn (23°28 south); also called the tropics.

Hygrometer: used to measure relative humidity. Developed by Leonardo da Vinci (1452–1519), the design was refined by Francisco Folli in 1664.

Friend: identifies Andrew Drury's membership, along with Dr Hillary, in the Religious Society of Friends, or Quakers. Dr Hillary had been practising in Bath, England, but had became disenchanted with his situation there. His Quaker friend Dr John Fothergill recommended Barbados to him, on the strength of his father's visits there as a Quaker preacher. On arrival in Barbados in 1747, Dr Hillary presented his "Certificate of removal to Barbados" and was admitted to membership in the Tudor Street Quakers' meeting in Bridgetown.

Andrew Drury: "Andrew Drury, deceased," possibly the father of Dr Hillary's friend, is named in the 1709 will of Thomas Habbin, a Quaker. Joanne Sanders, *Barbados Records, Wills and Administrations*, vol. 3, *1701–1725* (Houston, TX: Sanders Historical Publications, 1981).

Seat: home, estate or plantation, as in "country seat".

Medium: intermediate in position.

page 4
Medium: average or mean. Recording rainfall has been a long-standing enthusiasm in Barbados, particularly among planters, many of whom meticulously measure and

record it daily. It is interesting to speculate that Dr Hillary's reputation may have influenced both the entrenched Barbadian belief that weather and disease are integrally related and the passion for recording levels of rainfall and the small temperature changes that occur daily on the island.

my Practice: In Barbados Dr Hillary's medical practice would have included planters and their families, negro slaves, military personnel stationed on the island and seafaring men whose ships had called at Bridgetown.

different Ages and Constitutions: In noting the potential differences in dosage necessary in patients of different ages and constitutions, Dr Hillary was instinctively recognizing the variation in human drug response based on differences in drug-metabolizing capacity, deterioration in renal function and differences in anthropometry that were not recognized and methodically studied until some fifty years ago, when techniques became available for measuring drug concentrations in blood and the discipline of pharmacokinetics was developed.

buff-like Blood: blood having a "buffy-coat" forms a light buff-coloured layer on the upper part of the clot when centrifuged or, as would have been practised by Dr Hillary, left standing; also called "sizzy".

Bleeding: the letting of blood for an assumed therapeutic purpose, a medical practice observed for centuries that was based on the concept of "letting out the poisons"; also called phlebotomy.

Evacuations: clearing the body of morbid matter, humours and so forth by bleeding, purging, medicines or other artificial means.

determine: to direct or impel towards some destination.

page 5

Form: formula, recipe.

pro re nata: "for the affair born", that is, arisen, according to the circumstances.

Hippocrates: a Greek physician (c. 460–c. 377 BCE) known as the "father of medicine". See G.E.R. Lloyd, ed., *Hippocratic Writings* (Penguin Classics, 1978).

Dr *Huxam*: John Huxham, MD, FRS, FRCP (c. 1692–1768) was an English physician who, like Dr Hillary, was a pupil of Boerhaave. He published *Observationes de aere et morbis epidemicis ab anno MDCCXXVIII ad finem anni MDCCXXXVII (Plymuthi factae)* in London in 1739.

sixth Commandment: "Thou shalt do no murder." There were few effective forms of medical treatment available to Dr Hillary; even digoxin and Aspirin, mainstays of treatment in the early twentieth century, had not yet been isolated, although he did use both opium and quinine. Several of the medications he used were toxic, so his caustic injunction was highly relevant; it resonates today as an eloquent caution to modern physicians and provides a dramatic conclusion to this summary of his beliefs and approaches to medical practice.

Introduction

page 6

situation: geographical position.

epidemical: of diseases of an epidemic character, causing a sudden increase in numbers of persons affected.

endemial: endemic; of diseases generally present in a certain country or district.

size of Barbados: "Its greatest Length from *Goulding's Green*, in *St Lucy's Parish*, to *Ananias Point*, in the *Parish of Christ Church*, is 20¾ Stat. Miles. Its greatest Breadth from *Kirtrige's Point*, in *St Philip's Parish*, to a Point near *Mr Peyne's*, in *St James's Parish* is 13¾ Stat. Miles." G. Hughes, *The Natural History of the Island of Barbados* (London, 1750. Reprint, New York: Arno Press, 1972).

Freestone: a fine-grained coral stone that can be easily cut or sawn

Lime-stone: rock that consists chiefly of carbonate of lime.

Brain-stones: brain coral.

Astroites: star-shaped minerals or fossils.

stalactite: limestone.

Concretions: rocks formed of aggregations of particles around a nucleus.

Mun-jack: also known as Barbados tar or green tar; a tar or pitch found in the Scotland District of Barbados. In his 1657 *True and Exact History of the Island of Barbadoes*, Richard Ligon refers to this material as mountjack. Because of its intense blackness, Barbados tar was exported for use in the manufacture of paint, and it was used as a fuel for trains and sugar factories during the First World War. S. Carrington et al., *A–Z of Barbados Heritage* (Oxford: Macmillan Education, 2003).

six Non-naturals: six things necessary to health but liable, by abuse or accident, to become the cause of disease: air, meat and drink, sleep and waking, motion and rest, excretion and retention, and the affections of the mind.

page 7

vinous: of the nature of wine; made of or prepared with wine.

Efflorescences: morbid redness of the skin, or rashes.

Figure: shape.

cuticle: the epidermis, or outer layer of the skin ("scarf skin").

ouse: ooze.

smart: become acutely painful.

Scurff: a morbid skin condition characterized by the separation of scales.

exanthematous: characterized by eruptive pustules.

vulgarly: commonly.

Midge: a term loosely applied to many small, gnat-like insects.

Vis Vitæ: vital force.

exalts: volatilizes; carries off in vapour form.

alkalizes: renders alkaline.

semi-ammoniacal: of or pertaining to, or of the nature of, ammonia.

acrid: pungent; irritating; corrosive.

page 8

Prickly-heat: Prickly heat, or *Lichen tropicus*, is an inflammatory disorder of the sweat glands prevalent in tropical countries, characterized by eruption of small papules accompanied by a sensation of pricking or burning.

repelled: forced back into the blood or system, as in repressed swellings, eruptions, and the like.

camphorated Spirits: wine impregnated with camphor.

Gruel: a light liquid food made by boiling oatmeal or some other farinaceous substance in milk or water.

Wine-whey: whey made by curdling milk with wine.

Current of cool air . . . wet Places: Draughts, "night-dews" and damp places are all still considered in Barbados to be dangerous causes of chills, pneumonia and even death, possibly the result of publication of Dr Hillary's views.

Salt of Hartshorn: carbonate of ammonia, or smelling salts.

Spirit of Hartshorn: an aqueous solution of ammonia.

depuratory: descriptive of diseases that were supposed to carry off impurities from the system.

yellow putrid Fever: yellow fever. The association between mosquitoes and the spread of yellow fever was not made for another 140 years.

putrid Fevers: typhus or pythogenic fever.

Antiphlogisticks: medicinal preparations possessing anti-inflammatory properties.

page 9

Diaphoresis: perspiration, especially that produced by artificial means.

Languor: mental suffering or distress; affliction of spirit.

want: lack.

putrescent: rotting or becoming putrid.

Diathesis: a permanent (hereditary or acquired) condition of the body that renders it liable to certain diseases or afflictions.

procatarctic Causes: external factors that are the immediate cause of a disease.

page 10

Banjan: *banian*, a loose gown, shirt or jacket commonly worn in India.

Mandareens: mandarins, or Chinese officials, and by extension, other Asian officials.

Indostan: Hindustan, or northern India.

Fop: a man who is foolishly attentive to and vain about his appearance, dress and manners.

Game: wild birds and animals that are pursued and killed by hunting.

page 11

Navigation: sailing or rowing.

dancing: As an ardent Quaker, Dr Hillary would have shunned the "pleasures of society", regarding them as sinful.

different Ages, Strengths, and Constitutions: Here Dr Hillary demonstrates remarkable insight into variations in human drug response, relating dose to age, strength and constitution. These concepts were not rigorously investigated until the middle of the twentieth century, by which time plasma drug concentrations could be measured and dose/concentration effects evaluated.

Indications: suggestions or directions as to the treatment of diseases, derived from the symptoms observed.

Intentions: aims or purposes in a healing process, hence plans or methods of treatment, or *curationis intentio.*

ex ipsa re et ratione: as and when indicated; according to the circumstances.

page 12

Apothecaries: originally those who sold drugs for medicinal purposes; after 1700 they gradually assumed the role of general medical practitioners.

Performance: publication; literary work.

Part I

A.D. 1752

page 13

1752: Prior to 1752 the Julian calendar (introduced in 46 BCE by Julius Cæsar) was in use in England. In 1752 transition to the Gregorian calendar (introduced in 1582 by Pope Gregory) began. This transition necessitated shortening 1752 by ten days, hence Dr Hillary's statement that September 1752 "had but 19 Days in it" (see below). Moreover, the new calendar established 1 January as the beginning of the year; before 1753, the year in England had begun on 25 March.

Ophthalmies: inflammations of the eyes, in particular of the conjunctivæ.

Quincies: inflammations of the throat, tonsillitis or peritonsillar abscess.

Peripneumonies: inflammations of the lungs; pneumonia.

Pleurisies: inflammations of the membranes surrounding the lungs; pleurisy, usually with fluid between the membrane and the lung, which is termed *pleural effusion*.

Starch: a glutinous mass.

Buff-like inflammatory Pellicle: a buff-coloured layer (scum) that forms on the upper part of a clot of coagulated blood.

page 14

antiphlogistic: anti-inflammatory.

Sal. Nitre: saltpetre, or potassium nitrate.

Sal. Ammoniac: ammonium chloride.

diluting: increasing the proportion of water in the blood and other bodily fluids; "thinning" the fluids of the body.

emollient Fomentations, with crude Sal. Ammoniac: application of flannels soaked in hot water containing dissolved ammonium chloride.

The Small Pox: smallpox; variola. "The next Disease worthy our Notice is the Small-Pox; for we are seldom free from it in some Part of the Island or other"; Hughes, *Natural History*, 39. George Washington visited Barbados in November–December 1751, and while on the island he contracted smallpox. Richard B. Goddard, *George Washington's Visit to Barbados, 1751* (Barbados, 1997). Washington's resistance to smallpox while his army was being decimated with it during the Revolutionary War would have played a significant part in the outcome of that war.

page 15

Cholera Morbus: cholera (*morbus* = disease), a deadly diarrhœal disease with associated vomiting and abdominal pain that is caused by a bacterium, *Vibrio choleræ*. It is transmitted via food and water contaminated by fæces from an infected person. Although formerly universal, it is today most prevalent in Africa and Asia, although some 200 sporadic cases have occurred in the United States within the past thirty years.

Apoplexies: sudden neurological impairments due to a cerebrovascular disorder (limited classically to intracranial hæmorrhage); strokes. Dr Hillary's suspicion of a seasonal variation in stroke incidence has continued up to the present day. Many studies suggest a peak of infarctions in the winter months, but all the studies are not consistent. However, it is known that population blood pressure is lower in the summer months.

Palsies: paralysis.

Aphthæ: small ulcers, especially the reddish or whitish spots in the mouth characteristic of aphthous stomatitis, or thrush.

quick: fast; rapid.

high: strong; forceful.

Restringents: medications tending to restrain the action of the bowels.

Notes

not good Practice: This comment shows intuitive sense on Dr Hillary's part. Eighteenth-century medicine relied heavily on bleeding and purging to rid the body of toxins. Dr Hillary appeared to recognize the merit of slowing or "restricting" diarrhoea, but also the value of "letting out the toxins". In this respect his views are consistent with the modern practice of not stopping diarrhoea but maintaining fluid intake.

Mortification: necrosis, or decay.

Rhubarb: the purgative medicinal rootstock of *Rheum* species.

Anodynes: analgesic, or soothing, medications.

Balsamicks: medications possessing soothing and/or healing properties, based on the resinous oily substance extracted from plants of the genus *Impatiens*, family Balsaminaceæ; they include balm of Gilead, of Biblical fame.

Sperm. Cet. Cremor. Lactis: a mixture of spermaceti (the fatty wax found in the head of the sperm whale, *Physeter macrocephalus*) and dairy cream.

Wax Emulsion, with a little Syr. Meconio: an emulsion of beeswax and syrup of opium poppy juice (*Papaver somniferum*).

Primæ Viæ: "first ways", meaning the alimentary canal.

page 16

much Rain: The Caribbean/Atlantic hurricane season extends from June to November, with a peak in September.

Change of Style made this Year: See note on the introduction of the Gregorian calendar in 1752, page 197.

Catarrhous Fever: Most likely influenza, but the emphasis on headache, pains in the limbs and a weak pulse could suggest dengue fever, a viral disease transmitted by the *Aedes ægypti* mosquito, which is endemic in Barbados and the Caribbean. "Catarrhal" refers to a profuse discharge from the nose and eyes, such as attends the common cold.

Phlegm: a viscid fluid secreted by the mucous membranes of the respiratory tract.

languid: faint; weak; lacking in vitality.

extreme Parts: the extremities – the hands and feet.

plethoric: pertaining to plethora, a morbid condition characterized, according to earlier writers, by over-fullness of blood or any other humour, and according to later writers, by an excess of red corpuscles in the blood.

Pectorals: medicines "good for" diseases or afflictions of the chest.

Volatiles: substances characterized by a natural tendency to disperse as vapour; hence substances applied to the skin that evaporate rapidly and contribute to lowering of body temperature.

attenuating: An attenuant was a drug or agent having the property of thinning the humours or secretions.

Vesicatories: sharp, irritating ointments, plasters or other applications used to produce blisters on the skin for a therapeutic purpose.

page 17

ingeminated: repeated.

intermitting: marked by periods of intermission.

quotidian: recurring every day.

remitting: having periods of abatement and exacerbation.

Emetic: a substance capable of eliciting vomiting.

saponaceous: consisting of or containing soap.

Draughts: single doses of liquid medicines.

Sal. Absinth. Succus Limon.: a saline solution of absinthe – a liqueur containing 68 per cent alcohol, wormwood and other herbals – mixed with lemon juice.

Elixir. Vitrioli Acid.: an alcoholic solution of sulphuric acid; tincture of sulphuric acid.

q.s.: *quantum satis* (in a sufficient amount).

Aq. Menthæ: aqueous solution of peppermint.

Cortex Peruv.: an alcoholic liquor impregnated with Peruvian bark (*Cinchona officinalis*) used as a stomachic, or medicine "good for" the stomach. The active ingredient of *Cinchona officinalis* is quinine, which was found to be effective in malarial fever and then widely used in the treatment of fevers of all kinds.

mali Moris: malignant in nature.

Dr *Boerhaave*: Herman Boerhaave (1668–1738) was a professor of medicine at the University of Leyden, Holland, where Dr Hillary studied as a medical student. Boerhaave's teachings influenced medical curricula throughout Europe, but particularly at the University of Edinburgh. It is of interest that Edinburgh's reputation for medical training was so great in Barbados that for more than a hundred years practically every Barbadian doctor was trained there.

latericious: of a brick-red colour, in reference to urinary sediments.

Crisis: a marked or sudden variation in the progress of a disease; also the phenomena accompanying it.

Tertian: a fever characterized by a paroxysm every other (i.e., third) day.

Quartan: a fever characterized by a paroxysm every fourth (in modern reckoning, every third) day.

very rarely or never seen: This is a most accurate observation of Dr Hillary's. Malaria was introduced to Barbados in more than sporadic numbers only in the 1920s and had been successfully eradicated by the 1940s.

page 18

Afflux: a flowing towards a specific site.

Evacuations downwards: bowel movements.

Revulsion: the action of diminishing a morbid condition in one part of the body by acting upon another, for example, by "blistering" or "cupping".

Load: a sensation of fullness.

Loathing: an aversion to or disgust for food.

page 19

Singultus: hiccup.

Tenesmus: a continual inclination to empty the bowels, accompanied by straining, but with little or no discharge.

This Distemper: Sir Christopher Booth considers the above to be a description of tropical sprue; in his biography of Dr Hillary he has credited him with the first description of the condition. Sir Christopher's description led to a mention of Barbados in Avery-Jones's gastroenterology textbook as a country with endemic tropical sprue, although it has not been observed in the island in modern times.

infectious Effluvia: fluid from diarrhoea.

Tunica Villosa Intestinorum: intestinal villi, threadlike projections covering the mucous membrane lining the small intestine, which serve as sites of absorption of fluids and nutrients.

Specifics: remedies that are especially or exclusively efficacious for a particular ailment or part of the body.

page 20

Ipecacuanha: a solution of the roots of *Psychotria ipecacuanha,* which possesses emetic, diaphoretic and purgative properties.

torrified: torrefied; roasted, toasted, scorched or dried by fire.

Stibium Ceratum: "crude antimony mixed with melted wax, or as it is called 'cerated', is an excellent remedy in a diarrhœa or dysentery." Robert James, *Pharmacopoeia Universalis: or, A New Universal English Dispensatory* (London, 1747).

Synochus: a continued or unremitting fever (from the Greek, meaning "joined together").

Rigor: chills.

Languor: listlessness, weakness.

florid: bright red in colour (i.e., arterial blood).

Catarrh: the discharge from the nose and eyes that generally accompanies the common cold, formerly supposed to issue from the brain.

Coryza: nasal discharge such as accompanies the common cold.

Defluction: defluxion, a flow or discharge from the nose.

Rheum: excessive "defluxion" of watery discharge from the nose.

Oxymel Scilliticum: "3 pounds of honey, and 1 quart of vinegar of squills. Boil together to a syrup, observing to scum it during the operation. It is an emetic and expectorant". Vinegar of squills: "1 lb of squills cut small, and 3 quarts of best vinegar. Let them stand to infuse in the sun, then press and strain." James, *English Dispensatory.* Squill is the bulb or root of the sea onion (*Scilla maritima*).

Syr. Scillitic: syrup of squills: "1½ pints of vinegar of squills, 1 ounce of cinnamon, 3½ pounds of sugar. Steep in the vinegar for 3 days, strain and make syrup by adding the sugar." James, *English Dispensatory*.

A.D. 1753

page 22
Angina Inflammatoria: quinsy, or peritonsillar abscess.
Catharticks: medications possessing purgative properties.
Cataplasms: poultices or plasters.
Gargarisms: gargles.
Integuments: coverings.
discussed: dissipated, dispelled or dispersed.
translated: removed from one part of the body to another.

page 23
Attenuant: a medication possessing the property of "thinning" secretions or humours.
Refrigerant: a medication possessing "cooling" properties.
Lentor: clamminess, tenacity or viscidity.
Materia Medica: remedial substances used in the practice of medicine.
Spir. C.C.: Tinctura Chinchonæ Composita (Huxham's tincture of bark): "Take of calisaya bark [bark of *Cinchona calisaya*], in fine powder, 4 ounces; bitter orange peel [*Citrus bigaradia*], 3 ounces; Virginia snakeroot [*Endotheca serpentaria*] in moderately fine powder, 6 drachms; saffron [dried stigmas of *Crocus sativus*], in coarse powder, 2 drachms; cochineal [dried bodies of the insect *Coccus cacti*], in fine powder, 1 drachm; good diluted alcohol [probably brandy], 20 fluid ounces. Form it into a tincture by maceration or percolation, and make 20 ounces of tincture." Anthony Todd Thomson, *The London Dispensatory* (London, 1815).
vel: or (Latin).
Spir. Salis Ammon. Vol.: volatile spirit of sal ammoniac (ammonium chloride dissolved in water).
gr.v. to gr.xv: 5 to 15 grains. One pound (weight) is equivalent to 5,760 grains.
ℨi to ℨji *vel* ℨi: 1 to 2 scruples (20 to 60 grains) or 1 drachm (60 grains).
Decoct. Pectoral: "Decoctum Pectorale: Take of Raisins of the Sun stoned, and Barley, each an ounce; four fat figs; Spring Water, six pints; Boil to four pints, at the end of the decoction adding the root of Florentine Orris [*Iris florentina*] and Liquorice [*Glycyrrhiza glabra*], each half an ounce; of the leaves of the Harts-tongue [*Scolopendrium vulagre*] and Coltsfoot [*Tussilago farfara*, family Compositæ], each an ounce: strain of the Liquor." James, *English Dispensatory*.

Spr. Nitri. Dul.: "Take of Rectified Spirit of Wine, one Quart; of Glauber's Spirit of Nitre [alcoholic solution of potassium nitrate]. Mix them by pouring the Spirit of Wine on the other and distil the mixture with a gentle heat, as long as what comes off will not raise any fermentation with a lixivical salt." James, *English Dispensatory*.

Sprir. Mindereri: an astringent solution of ammonium acetate. "Take any quantity of distilled Vinegar, and add to it by degree, as much of the Spirit of Sal Ammoniac as will put a stop to the effervescence." James, *English Dispensatory*.

Syr. e Meconio: syrup of opium poppy juice (*Papaver somniferum*).

Peripneumonic Fever: fever associated with pneumonia.

Clysters: enemas.

nine or ten Ounces: 255 to 284 cc (cubic centimetres).

sixty or eighty Ounces: 1,704 to 2,272 cc.

page 24

Cardiacs: medications thought to stimulate the heart.

Cordial Waters: beverages thought to invigorate the heart and stimulate the circulation.

Canary and Frontigniac: Canary is a light sweet wine from the Canary Islands. Frontignac is a strong sweet wine made at Frontignan, in the department of Hérault, France, named for the grape from which it is made.

Decoct. Pectoral.: pectoral decoction, a chest mixture. Canary or Frontignac wine, 5 fluid ounces; paregoric elixir (tincture of camphorated opium), ½ fluid ounce; spirit of mindereri (solution of ammonium acetate), 2 fluid ounces; syrup of squill, 1½ fluid ounces. Let the patient take salt of nitre (potassium nitrate, or saltpetre), ½ drachm, and purified crude sal ammoniac (ammonium chloride), 10 grains, mixed in three or four large spoonfuls of the decoction, every three hours.

nervous Fever: febrile illness associated with "nervous" symptoms such as anxiety and restlessness.

Reaching: retching, spitting.

Symptoms: These symptoms are suggestive of dengue fever, but the later severity, with seizures, coma and death, is more indicative of meningitis.

page 25

Torpor: morbid inertia or insensibility; stupor.

Occiput: back of the head.

Coronary Suture: the coronal or transverse suture (commissure) of the skull, separating the frontal and parietal bones; the forehead region.

Watching: wakefulness; insomnia.

Tinnitus Aurium: ringing in the ears.

Deliquium Animi [animæ]: failure of the vital powers; a swoon or fainting fit.

Præcordia: the region of the body about the heart; the front of the thorax.

dosing: dozing.

Excrements: alvine (pertaining to the abdomen or its contents) fæces.

Catchings: glottal catchings – sounds produced by the sudden opening and closing of the glottis – causing stridor, or noisy breathing.

Subsultus Tendinum: a convulsive twitching of muscles and tendons present in certain fevers.

A Vomit: medication to eliciting vomiting, an emetic.

page 26

Tinct. Cantharid: an alcoholic solution of dried "Spanish fly" beetle (*Cantharis vesicatoria*), which possesses diuretic properties.

Sal. C. C. . . . : Tincture of cinchona bark, ½ scruple; lemon juice, 3 fluid drachms; peppermint water, 1½ fluid ounces; spirit of minderi (solution of ammonium acetate), 2 fluid drachms; wine of crocus (*Crocus* spp.), 1 fluid ounce; syrup of crocus, 2 fluid ounces. Mix and make three or four draughts; take every five hours.

gut. **xx:** 10 drops (*guttae*).

page 27

Dr *Sydenham:* Thomas Sydenham (1624–89), an English physician, published *Observations medicæ* in 1676.

Fauces: the cavity at the back of the mouth that leads to the larynx and pharynx.

page 28

Diarrhœa febrilis: diarrhoea accompanied by fever.

dry Belly-ach: Dry belly-ache, which caused "exquisite abdominal pain" (painful gut cramps, with constipation rather than diarrhoea), is the outstanding symptom of chronic lead poisoning. Lead poisoning was endemic in Barbados because of the high lead content of its rum, which was distilled in lead coils. The association became evident from the suffering of those who had drunk "new" rum. The condition was also known as plumber's or painter's colic. J.S. Handler, "Lead Contact and Poisoning in Barbados Slaves: Historical, Chemical, and Biological Evidence", *Social Science History* 10, no. 4 (1986): 399–427.

Cholica Pictonum: "Spasmodic belly-ach is the same as colica poictu: it is seldom seen nowadays in the West Indies. The inhabitants lead more regular lives, eat fresh food, and drink good liquors"; William Wright, MD, in notes to a new edition of James Grainger's 1764 *Essay on the More Common West-India Diseases* (London, 1802).

putrid bilious Fever: yellow fever.

page 29

Miasmata: infectious or noxious vapours from putrescent organic matter; poisonous particles or germs floating in and polluting the atmosphere.

page 30

keeping the Body moderately open: avoiding constipation.

Milleped. viv. . . . : Millipedes (woodlice, *Oniscus asellus*), live, well washed, ½ ounce, bruised in a glass mortar, and sprinkled over an infusion of 8 ounces of liquorice root (*Glycyrrhiza glabra*). Pound thoroughly, then filter. To the filtrate add 2 fluid ounces of fennel seed (*Fœniculum vulgare*) water; nutmeg (*Myristica fragrans*) water and sweet spirit of nitre (ethyl nitrate), ½ fluid ounce of each; tincture of cantharides (Spanish fly, *Cantharis vesicatoria*), 2 fluid ounces; syrup of poppy (*Papaver somniferum*), ½ or 1 fluid ounce. Mix and label: "One spoonful when the cough is troublesome." Increase the dose according to the patient's age.

Stranguary: strangury, or slow, painful urination.

Musk: an odoriferous reddish-brown substance secreted by a gland of the male musk deer (*Moschus moschiferus*) used medicinally as a stimulant and antispasmodic. Musk has been a prized ingredient in perfumes for many years and was previously believed, particularly in traditional Chinese medicine, to be a potent detoxification agent valuable in treating seizures. The active ingredient, muscone, is similar in structure to imipramine, a tricyclic antidepressive drug.

Elix. Paragoric: paregoric elixir, which was camphorated tincture of opium flavoured with aniseed and benzoic acid.

Acetum Camphoratum: camphorated vinegar.

Haustus è Volatilibus Fullerii: an unidentified preparation of Fuller's.

Dr *Huxham*: John Huxham, MD, FRS, FRCP, English physician (c. 1692–1768) who published *An Essay on Fevers* in 1750, as well as *Treatises on Devonshire Colic, Diphtheria and Smallpox.*

Sal. C.C. et Succus Limon: otherwise known as "Huxham's saline draught".

Rad. Ipocacuanh. . . . : ipecacuanha root (*Psychotria ipecacuanha*), 1 or 2 grains, or ipecacuanha wine, 20 or 30 drops.

page 31

Tinct. Thebaic. a gut. v. *ad* x.: tincture (alcoholic solution) of laudanum (opium), 5 to 10 drops.

Rad. Rhei: "compound powder of rhubarb" (Pulvis rhei composita) in the British Pharmacopœia. This remedy was usually called "Gregory's powder", as it was much prescribed by Dr James Gregory, author of *Conspectus Medicinæ Theoreticæ* and a professor of medicine at Edinburgh University, 1790–1821. Pilulæ rhei compostitæ Edin. (compound rhubarb pills): "Take of rhubarb root in powder, *one ounce*;

Socotorine aloes [juice of *Aloe socotrina*], *six drachms*; myrrh [resin extracted from *Commiphora myrrha*], *half an ounce*; volatile oil of peppermint, *half a drachm*. Beat them into a mass with syrup of orange peel. The dose is from grs. x, given twice daily." Thomson, *London Dispensatory*.

Fotus ex. Fol. Menthæ . . . : a poultice of mint leaves and theriac Andromachus (see note, page 205) with a little red wine.

saline Julep: a medicated drink used as a demulcent, "comforting" or gently stimulating mixture, usually sweetened with sugar or honey, although in this instance salted.

page 32

1.33 cubic Inch deep: This was an unusually dry November, as in Barbados it is usually the month with the highest recorded rainfall.

Mediastinum: the membranous middle septum formed by the inner walls of the pleura, separating the right and left lungs.

Pericardium: the membranous sac that encloses the heart and the points at which the great blood vessels connect to the heart.

page 33

Stroke or Contusion: a blow from a hand or a weapon.

Meninges: the three membranes that envelop the brain, called the dura, arachnoid and pia mater.

A.D. 1754

page 34

slow nervous Fever: possibly meningitis or encephalitis.

Startings: sudden involuntary body movements.

page 35

Plymouth: a port city in Devon, in southwest England.

two Quarts: 2.25 litres.

Stypticks: medicinal applications used to arrest hæmorrhage.

volatile Medicines: for example, "smelling salts", which were used as a restorative in cases of faintness or headache.

cordial Nourishment: "strengthening" food.

Vini Crocei: alcoholic extract of crocus (*Crocus sativus*).

Rad. Serpentar. Virg. Confect. Cardiac.: a confection of Virginia snakeroot for heart use, that is, to stimulate the pulse.

page 36
Scrobiculum Cordis: the epigastric fossa, just below the sternum.

page 37
of the Nothus Kind: associated with a south wind (from Notos, the Greek god of the
south wind).
the Town: Bridgetown.

page 38
unconcocted: not digested in the stomach.

page 39
Sal. C.C. vol. Flor. Benzoin: salt of *Cornus cervi* (hartshorn) and benzoin flour.
Theriac. Adrom.: theriac Andromachus, a remedy containing forty or more ingredients
that was supposedly an antidote to all poisons; also known as treacle of Andromachus
or Venice treacle.
emollient Clysters: "soothing" enemas.

page 41
anomalous: irregular; marked by deviation from the natural order.
Piemento leaves: the leaves of *Pimenta officinalis*, or allspice.
Aromaticks: fragrant drugs; substances or plants with a spicy odour; spices.
Fœnigmi: possibly fennel (*Feoeniculum* spp.).
Chalybeats: chalybeates, or medications impregnated with iron.
Febris Ephemera: a slight fever that lasts only a day or two.

page 42
an uncommon wet Year: More rain fell in 1754 than in any year since recording was begun
by the local meteorological institute.
Febricula: slight or temporary attacks of fever of indefinite origin or pathology.

page 43
Imposthumations: purulent swellings or cysts; abscesses.

A.D. 1755

Elephantiasis: elephantiasis filariaiensis, a chronic filarial tropical disease caused by
infection with *Wuchereria bancrofti* that is marked by inflammation and obstruction
of the lymphatics and hypertrophy of the skin and subcutaneous tissues, chiefly

affecting the legs. It was also known as "Barbadoes leg", although it is said that in Barbados it was known as "Guyana leg", being reputedly more common there. Active elephantiasis has not been seen in Barbados for some forty years, but pockets remained in Trinidad and Guyana until more recently.

Red Stroke: lymphangitis, or infection of the lymph channels, manifested by painful subcutaneous red streaks along the course of the vessels.

page 44

scarlet Fever: scarlatina, a streptococcus infection characterized by pharyngitis, tonsillitis and an erythematous rash progressing from the trunk and neck to the limbs.

Erysipelas: acute superficial cellulitis involving the lymphatics of the skin; also known as St Anthony's fire.

Cuticula: the cuticle, or epidermis ("scarf skin").

phthysical: affected by or having a tendency towards phthisis (wasting of the body); consumptive.

page 46

pituitous: characterized by excess mucus.

especially Strangers: putrid bilious (yellow) fever was also known as "strangers' fever" or "Barbados distemper".

page 47

Ipocacuan. viz. gr. iij. in Theriac. Androm. Ði. Vel. ℥ss.: ipecacuanha, 3 grains, in theriac Andromachus, 1 or ½ drachm.

Pedeluvium: footbath.

page 48

concocted: mature; digested.

page 49

catarrhal Fever: This respiratory infection with quinsy, which spread like an epidemic and apparently produced a significant number of deaths, was probably diphtheria. It was a common scourge in Barbados well into the twentieth century, in 1912 severely affecting the grandfather of editor H.S. Fraser. Diphtheria was eliminated with the introduction of the DPT inoculation, which was made compulsory in the 1950s. However, editor J.E. Hutson was involved in the emergency resuscitation of a child with diphtheria in the mid-1960s – described as "probably the last case of diphtheria reported in the island" by the late Sir Albert Graham, senior paediatrician, Queen Elizabeth Hospital, Barbados (personal communication).

Sneiderian Membrane: schneiderian membrane, the mucous membrane lining the nose.

A.D. 1756

page 51
70°F: 21° Celsius, an unusually low temperature rarely observed in Barbados, even in January, using modern maximum/minimum thermometers.

Opisthotonos: muscular spasms involving the neck, back and legs, in which the body is bent backwards. This is a classic and defining feature of severe tetanus, caused by infection with the tetanus bacillus *Clostridium tetani*, usually the result of contamination of an injury or puncture wound by soil or animal manure. It was common in Barbados in the pre-inoculation era. Although tetanus is more common in rainy conditions, Dr Hillary surprisingly attributed it to the dry weather. (The cause was not known until 1884, when Carle and Rattone produced tetanus in a rabbit by injecting it with pus from a human victim).

Tetany: painful muscle spasm.

page 52
Crassamentum: clot, coagulum.

page 53
Manna: sweet pale yellow or whitish juice obtained from incisions in the bark of the Manna ash (*Fraxinus ornus*), used as a laxative.

Tamarinds: pulp of the fruit of *Tamarindus indica*, used as a laxative.

Tinct. vel Extract. Thebaic: tincture or extract of laudanum (opium).

comatous: comatose.

page 55
Antispecticks: antiseptics.

Testacea: medicinal powder made from the shells of shellfish and other shell-bearing animals.

page 56
stercoraceous: consisting of, containing or pertaining to fæces.

Sal. Nitre, Coral. Rubr, vel Pulv. Bolo C. equal Quantities, in the *Julep e Cret.*: salts of nitre, red coral or compound powder of bole (a fine, unctuous clay, usually yellow, red or brown), equal quantities, in chalk julep (chalk, sugar and gum Arabic in water).

Collyrium: a topical remedy for diseases of the eyes; an eye salve or eyewash.

page 59
icterical: pertaining to jaundice (icterus).

Dirt: faeces, stools.

page 60
chilous: containing chyme, the semi-fluid material produced by gastric digestion of food.
Lientery: diarrhœa in which food passes through the bowels partially or wholly undigested.
Choriza: coryza, or common cold.
Sack-whey: wine-whey made from sack, a fortified wine.

A.D. 1757

page 61
my worthy Friend: Andrew Drury (see preface).
Paraphrenitises: Periphrenitis is an inflammation of the diaphragm and the structures around it.

page 62
Alexipharmic Medicines: antidotes or "counter-poisons"; from the Latin/Greek root *alexin* (to ward off).
reduced: weakened, impaired.
hectic Fever: a fever that recurs each day, with profound sweating, chills and facial flushing; formerly associated with consumption (pulmonary tuberculosis).

page 63
something: somewhat.
depuratory Fever: a fever that was supposed to carry off impurities from the body; from the Latin *purare* (to purify).

page 64
Diluents: medications supposed to be capable of thinning body fluids.
Acet. Camphorat, vel Spir. Mindereri: camphorated vinegar or alcoholic solution of ammonium acetate.
erysipelatose: erysipelas-like.
Aræteus Capadox: Aretæus of Cappadocia was a Greek physician (c. 150 CE) and disciple of Hippocrates. In 1554 two of his manuscripts, *On the Causes and Indications of Acute and Chronic Diseases* and *On the Treatment of Acute and Chronic Diseases*, were discovered and translated from the Ionic Greek dialect; these works contain descriptions of pleurisy, diphtheria, tetanus, pneumonia and epilepsy. Aretæus also published the earliest known clear description of diabetes mellitus.

page 65
St Anthony's Fire: erysipelas.

page 66

Sal. Nitri . . . : salts of nitre, 1 drachm, and purified sal ammoniac, 12 or 14 grains, in a
draught of pectoral decoction (containing barley, raisins, figs and liquorice) with sweet
spirit of nitre and solution of ammonium acetate.

page 69

Synochus Fever: continuous or unremitting fever.
Colluvies: foul matter, especially foul discharge as from an ulcer.

page 70

since I came into this Country: Dr Hillary arrived in Barbados in the spring or early
summer of 1747.

page 71

semi-tertian Fever: emytrycke (*emitricia febris*).
continual Fever: "that which sometimes remits, or abates, but never perfectly intermits"
(*Oxford English Dictionary*).
seldom or never seen in this Island: Dr Hillary is again recognizing the rarity of malaria
in Barbados and its occurrence as an imported condition rather than an endemic
disease.

page 72

Flor. Chamæmeli. . . . : chamomile flowers and peppermint leaves, 1 M [minim] of each.
Soak in boiling water, then strain 16 fluid ounces. To the strained liquid add
peppermint water [spirit?], 1½ ounces; salt of wormwood, ½ ounce; syrup of poppy
juice, 1½ ounces; and aromatic sulphuric acid, a sufficient quantity to reduce the alkali
salt to a neutral state. Mix; prescribe a spoonful every three or four hours.
intermitting quotidian Fever: fever occurring every day.
the Bark: decoction of Jesuit's bark, or the bark of *Cinchona officinalis*; in other words,
quinine.

page 73

Elix. Vitrioli. Acid Camphor. aromatic sulphuric acid with camphor.
Rad. Serpent. Virg. . . . : *Virginia serpentaria* root, ½ ounce, and salt of wormwood,
2 drachms. Boil in 20 fluid ounces of distilled water until the volume is 12 fluid ounces.
Strain and add 1 fluid ounce of catechu tincture. Mix; prescribe a 2-ounce dose every
two or three hours, until fits are absent.

A.D. 1758

page 74

concocted Matter: in reference to a boil, maturated, or "brought to a head".

strikes in: of an eruption that disappears from the surface or the extremities with internal effect.

gangrenesce: develop gangrene.

Sphacelus: an area of necrosis or sloughing, from the Greek *sphakelos* (gangrene).

they die: This affliction was possibly meningococcemia and meningitis.

Paraplegia: paralysis of the lower limbs and part or the whole of the trunk.

extended to . . . its Meninges: meningococcal meningitis.

Scepticks: septic or putrefactive substances.

page 75

Cortex. Peruv. . . . : cinchona bark, root of *Serpentaria virginiana*, English saffron, safron in Canary wine, solution of ammonium acetate, tincture of lavender *et cetera*.

The last was an alcoholic solution of flowers of lavender (*Lavandula vera*), cinnamon (bark of *Cinnamonum zeylanicum*), nutmeg (*Myristica fragrans*), cloves (flower buds of *Carophyllus aromaticus*) and red sanders, or sandalwood (*Petrocarpus santalinus*).

Fotus: fomentation, or medicinal wash.

Fol. Piementi . . . : leaves of pimento, viburnum, salvia and rosemary (*Rosmarinus officinalis*), flowers of chamomile and elder *et cetera*.

Digestive: a substance that produces healthy suppuration in a wound or ulcer.

Liniment. Arcæi: ointment of elemi, a resin obtained from various trees, including *Canarium commune*.

***Cataplasm. Maturans*:** a poultice containing figs, yellow basilicon ointment and galbanum, a gum resin obtained from various trees, including *Ferula galbanifula*.

page 76

suffocating Catarrh: This was probably diphtheria.

eccoprotic: producing evacuation of the bowels; mildly purgative.

Part II

Putrid Bilious Fever [Yellow Fever]

page 79

Kingdom of Siam: now Thailand.

the Tropicks: the Tropics of Cancer and Capricorn.

obnoxious to: liable, subject, exposed or open to something harmful or undesirable.

some have objected to this: In *A Treatise concerning the malignant fever in Barbados and the neighbouring islands: with an account of the seasons there, from the year 1734 to 1738,* Henry Warren "concludes it to be a species of the Plague, and that the Infection was unhappily brought to *Martinico* in Bales of Goods from *Marseilles* in the Year 1721". Hughes, *Natural History*, 37.

page 80

late ingenious Author: Dr Henry Warren, cited above.

many years before: "At the time of our arrival [1674], and a month or two after, the sickness raign'd so extreatly, as the living could hardly bury the dead." Richard Ligon, *A True and Exact History of the Island of Barbadoes* (London, 1673), 25. In fact there were major epidemics of yellow fever in the Caribbean by the mid-seventeenth century. Kiple provides a comprehensive history of the introduction of yellow fever from Africa to the Caribbean, including data demonstrating the increased resistance to the disease of African-born slaves as compared to that of Caribbean-born slaves and Europeans. Review of *World Epidemics: A Chronology of Disease from Prehistory to the Era of SARS,* by K.F. Kiple, *Bulletin of the History of Medicine* 49, no. 1 (2005): 173–74. Hence, Dr Hillary is correct in his assertion that yellow fever had previously existed in the Caribbean, although he almost certainly incorrectly diagnosed patients suffering from leptospirosis as having yellow fever.

pestilential: pertaining to pestilence, or infectious and deadly disease, especially of the nature of or pertaining to bubonic plague.

rarely . . . contagious: This observation provides convincing evidence that Dr Hillary was seeing many cases of leptospirosis, a zoonosis (a disease capable of being transmitted between animals and man) transmitted to man chiefly by rats. The rapid spread of yellow fever in an environment supporting a population of *Aedes aegypti* mosquitoes is beyond dispute, however. Since the role of the mosquito in transmitting the disease was not recognized until the late nineteenth/early twentieth century, it is hardly surprising that eighteenth-century physicians considered yellow fever to be a highly contagious disease transmitted from person to person.

Antigua, **and . . . this Island:** Dr Hillary is here indicating his knowledge of previous severe epidemics in Barbados and Antigua while expressing his view that there was something different about the "Putrid Bilious Fever" he was observing at the time.

page 81

Horror: shuddering or shivering.

pathognomic: a term applied to a sign or symptom by which a disease may be known; specifically characteristic or indicative of a disease.

Reachings: spitting blood or phlegm; hawking; retching.

Appearance of Sizeness: sizzy; pertaining to the buffy coat on the surface of coagulated blood in certain conditions.

page 82

Stadium: stage.

dissolved: disintegrated, decomposed (of blood).

Pulse . . . becomes very low: Inability to recognize that repeated vomiting caused severe hypotension (low blood pressure) was a most tragic failure of eighteenth-century medicine, second only to the devastating results of bleeding, the most powerful and deadly weapon of every physician for centuries.

porraceous: green, resembling the colour of leeks.

Deliria: deliriums.

Deliquia: plural form of deliquium, a swoon or fainting fit.

inflamed and red: Conjunctival injection, or redness of the eyes, is a pathognomonic feature of leptospirosis.

duskish: dusky or blackish.

Prognostic: a symptom or indication on which the prognosis is based.

Dr *Town*: Richard Towne, MD, author of *A Treatise of the diseases most frequent in the West Indies, and herein more particularly of those which occur in Barbados* (1726).

suffusion: defluxion or extravasation of a fluid or humour over a portion of the body.

critical: pertaining to the crisis, or turning point, of a disease.

page 83

colliquated: reduced to a thinner consistency (of humours).

vermicular: pertaining to the supposedly undulatory (peristaltic) contractions of arteries.

died immediately: Death in this instance was probably precipitated by cardiac arrhythmia, a common complication of leptospirosis.

ictericious: icteric (pertaining to jaundice).

page 84

Hypoconders: the hypochondria (plural of hypochondrium), either of the superolateral (upper side) regions of the abdomen, overlying the costal (rib) cartilages.

first and second Concoctions: The old physiology recognized three processes – the first concoction, digestion in the stomach and intestines; the second concoction, the process whereby the chyme so formed is converted into blood; and the third concoction, secretion.

Chylification: the production of chyle, a fluid produced by the digestive process.

Sanguification: the formation of or conversion into blood.

inquinated: polluted, corrupted.

Acrimony: irritation; acridity.

page 85

lethiferous: causing or resulting in death (i.e., deadly).

Ichor: a fluid, real or imaginary, likened to the blood of animals.

late ingenious Author: Henry Warren.

upwards and downwards: through both vomit and stools.

page 86

Ounces of Blood: One fluid ounce is equal to 29 cubic centimetres (cc). Bleeding to 20 ounces would result in a blood loss of 580 cc, a considerable amount.

page 87

the only Rules . . . those laid down before: Dr Hillary clearly recognized the dangers of excessive bleeding but found it impossible to abandon that traditional mainstay of contemporary treatment, removal of "putrid humours" from the body by bleeding.

page 88

Draughts of warm Water: a measure that would have been useful for reducing dehydration and hypotension.

Oximel: oxymel, a medicinal drink or syrup compounded from vinegar and honey.

Extract. Thebaic, gr. i vel gr. iss: opium (inspissated juice of *Papaver somniferum* boiled in water and strained), 1 or 1½ grains.

Compass: measure.

Ledentia: medication likely to be harmful.

page 89

Peripneumonia Notha: atypical pneumonia.

colliquative: having the effect of liquefying or dissolving.

page 90

Extract: viscid matter obtained by treating a substance with solvent and then evaporating the solvent.

durst: dared.

Infusion: steeping a substance in water in order to impregnate the liquid with its
properties; also the resulting liquid.

Rad. Serpent. Virg. . . . : Virginia snakeroot, 2 drachms; English saffron, ½ drachm. Mix
and infuse in a closed vessel with sufficient boiling water for an hour so that 6 ounces
can be strained off. Add simple peppermint water (a cordial prepared from leaves of
peppermint, *Mentha piperta*, steeped in water and then distilled), 2 ounces; Madeira
wine, 4 ounces; syrup of saffron (saffron wine and sugar) or syrup of white poppy, 1
ounce; sulphuric acid with cinnamon (bark of *Pimenta acris* [West Indian bay]),
cardamom (seed capsules of *Elettaria cardamomum*), pepper (*Piper nigrum*) and ginger
(rhizome of *Zingiber officinale*). Prescribe two or three spoonfuls every hour or two
hours, or more often if necessary.

page 91

Rad. Serpent.: Virginia snakeroot.

Vinum Croceum: saffron in Canary wine.

Confec. Cardiac.: confectio cardiac (cordial confection), which contained eight spices in
sugar and alcohol.

Elix. Vitrioli: sulphuric acid.

page 92

Cantharides: pharmacopœial name of the dried beetle *Cantharis vesicatoria*, used externally
as a rubefacient and vesicant.

Lentor: clamminess, tenacity or viscidity of the blood.

page 93

sphacelated: gangrenous.

Adjuvantia.: ingredients added to a prescription to aid the operation of the principal
ingredients.

Mannæ Calab. . . . : Calabrian manna, 1½ to 2 ounces; bruised tamarinds, 1 ounce;
vitriolated tartar (potassium sulphate), 10 grains dissolved in whey; Madeira wine,
6 ounces. Strain and add tincture of senna (alcoholic solution of dried leaflets of various
species of *Cassia*), ½ ounce. Mix and divide into two or four parts, of which the patient
takes one every hour until purging occurs.

page 94

Boluses: medicines shaped into balls adapted for swallowing, larger than ordinary pills.

Contraria contrariis medentur: "Contrary are cured by contrary." This phrase arises from
allopathy, an old system of medical practice whose fundamental principle was to cure
disease by inducing actions contrary to or different from those of the disease.

page 95

Cruor: coagulated blood; the portion of the blood that forms a clot.

ferous: wild, savage.

Surgeon to a Guinea Ship: "physician" on a slaving vessel.

page 96

Panada: a dish made by boiling bread in water to a pulp and flavouring it according to taste with sugar, currants, nutmeg and other ingredients.

recovered perfectly well: This patient may have been suffering from acute alcoholic hepatitis, from which he recovered spontaneously.

Celsus: Aulus Cornelius Celsus, a first-century Roman writer. *De Medicina*, the only extant example of his work, was one of the first medical books to be printed, in 1478.

Citò, tutò, et jucundè: safe, fast and agreeable.

page 98

Panis bene [**good bread**] . . .: Light cooking yeast, 4 ounces. Cook in pure water for 1 hour; then, after a time, press through thick lint so that it is liquid. In this manner prepared to 1½ pounds, to which add 1 ounce of lemon, cut into strips; nutmeg rubbed in fine flour, 1 drachm. Method of use: the patient takes 2 or 3 ounces every two hours, sometimes mixed with Madeira wine and sufficient sugar to taste.

Pearl Barley: barley reduced by attrition to small rounded grains, used in making broths and soups.

Rhenish Wine-whey: whey made by curdling milk with Rhine wine.

Hock: a German wine (Hochheimer) produced at Hochheim, on the River Main. The name "hock" was thence extended to other white German wines.

Dry Gripes or Dry Belly-ache [Lead Poisoning]

page 99

Riverius: Lazare Rivière (1589–1665), a French physician, published *The Practice of Physick: Wherein is plainly set forth, The Nature, Cause, Differences, and Several Sorts of Signs: Together with the Cure of all Diseases in the Body of Man* (London, 1658).

first taken notice of: One of the earliest documentations of the link between dry bellyache and its cause, lead poisoning (from rum manufactured in stills containing lead pipes), was made in 1768 by Benjamin Franklin – his contribution to medicine. See, for example, Theodore Diller, "The Writings of Benjamin Franklin Pertaining to Medicine and the Medical Profession", *Aesculapian* 1, nos. 3–4 (June 1909): 156–97.

page 100

Lacteals: lymphatics.

spinal Marrow: spinal cord.

Metastasis: the transfer of a disease from one organ to another.

reverts: reverses.

Misereri mei: literally, "Have mercy on me"; a name for "iliac passion", a form of colic accompanied by stercoraceous vomiting.

page 101

pumped: dry-pumped, that is, having water pumped on a part of the body for curative purposes without immersing the rest of the body.

Liniment Saponac: soap liniment.

Bals. Peruv. gut. xxx: balsam of Peru, 30 drops.

page 102

Bals. Peruv. gut xl *Philon. Londin.*: balsam of Peru, 40 drops, and philonium Londinense (confection of opium), 1 scruple.

Bath-water: curative waters from the spa at Bath, England.

corroborating: strengthening.

Bitter: an alcoholic solution of bitter medicines such as Peruvian bark (quinine), quassia, wormwood, orange peel, etc.

exploded: rejected.

page 103

Bals. Peruv. . . .: balsam of Peru, 20 to 40 drops two or three times daily, in a small amount of sugar.

Method of treating this Disease: "[The] present Method of Cure is universally followed, being both safe and easy, and the Patients run no Danger of either Life or Limbs: For, as soon as Dr *Warren* found, that it was a convulsive Constriction chiefly in the Ilion, he judged that Purges and sharp Clysters must be attended with bad Success, and Emetics, at least, useless, if not hurtful; from whence he concluded, that Anodynes mixed with Antihysterics would be the likeliest Means of Relief: He therefore purified that Method, as necessary to be followed for the Space of Twenty-four Hours: Then he concluded, that the spasmodic Constrictions were over; at which time he ordered some emollient Clyster, and then gave a gentle Purge of some of the bitter Pills, which generally perfected the Cure, only taking some Anodyne for a few Nights successively afterwards." Hughes, *Natural History*, 34.

Opisthotonos: a form of tetanus.

page 104

Extracti Thebaic. . . .: Thebaic extract (extract of opium), 2 or 3 grains. Make a pill.

Philon. Londin. . . . : Confection of opium, 1 scruple; extract of opium, 1 or 2 grains; balsam of Peru, 10 drops. Make a bolus.

Aq. Menthæ Simp. . . . : Simple peppermint water, 1½ fluid ounces; confection of opium, 2 or 3 grains; balsam of Peru, 20 drops; syrup of poppies, ½ fluid ounce. Make a draught to be taken immediately.

lenient Eccoprotic: an emollient laxative.

Compass: measure, dose.

Tart. Vitriolat. . . . : Potassium sulphate, 10 grains; cinnamon oil, 1 drop, or mint oil, 1 drop. Mix as prescribed in a spoonful of mint water and repeat every hour until the vomiting ceases, then prescribe extract of opium as at first.

page 105

Cremor. Tartari. Pulv. . . . : Cream of tartar, 3 drachms; soluble cream of tartar, 1½ drachms; potassium sulphate, 2 scruples; cinnamon oil or mint oil, 3 drops. Mix to make a powder and divide into six parts, which the patient takes every one, two or three hours in a suitable medium of choice.

Posset-drink: hot milk curdled with ale, wine or other liquor, often mixed with sugar, spices and other ingredients.

Rad. Jalapii. . . .: jalap root, 5 or 6 grains.

Paper: dose.

Bals. Peruv. gut. **xv.:** balsam of Peru, 15 drops.

Semicupium: a bath in which only the hips and legs are submerged (a hipbath).

Fol. Althea . . . : Mallow flowers, 3; mint, elder and chamomile flowers, 3 of each; linseed oil, 1 fluid ounce; Venetian soap, 1 ounce. Mix and boil in 8 pounds [pints] water. Then add theriac of Andromachus, 1 ounce; Barbados peas (*Cajanus cajan*), 2 ounces; rum, 1½ pounds [pints]. Mix and make a fomentation with which to warm the belly and abdomen, using a linen rag, every six hours until the pain ceases.

page 106

Decotc. Fotu . . . : Decocted fomentation without additives, 8 fluid ounces; Venetian soap, 1 drachm; Barbados peas, ½ ounce; balsam of Peru, 1 drachm; American castor oil or castor oil, 1½ drachms. Mix and make an enema.

Ung. Dialthea . . . : Marsh mallow ointment and castor oil, 1 fluid ounce each; camphorated opium and balsam of Peru, 1 drachm of each; expressed oil of mace, ½ drachm. Make a liniment and use as above.

Moschi Orient. . . . : Oriental musk, 10 grains, and extract of opium, 2, 3 or 4 grains. Mix and make four pills or make a bolus with sufficient Peruvian balsam.

Nervous: acting upon the nerves or the nervous system.

page 107

Crem. Tart. . . . : Cream of tartar, 1 drachm; potassium tartrate, ½ scruple; and cinnamon oil, 1 drop. Mix and make a powder to be taken first thing in the morning in a draught of whey.

Polenta: porridge.

Malt-liquor: ale, beer or stout.

page 108

Cort. Peruv. . . . : Peruvian bark, coarsely powdered, 1 ounce; Cassumunar ginger (*Curcuma aromatica*) root and best rhubarb, 1½ drachms of each; Peruvian balsam, 2 drachms; and Madeira wine, 2 pints. Leave to soak ("digest") in a warm place, then strain. Of the drained substance let the patient take 3 spoonfuls twice or three times daily on an empty stomach.

chalybeate: spring water impregnated with iron.

Bals. Peruv. Camphor and Extract. Valerian Sylvest.: balsam of Peru, camphor and extract of wild valerian root [*Valeriana* spp.].

to cure it: Although West Indian dry bellyache was recognized by the nineteenth century as associated with consumption of "new" rum, treatment continued to be based on bleeding and the administration of enemas. William Brewer, *The Military and Naval Medical Reference Book* (London, 1841). It is also of significance that the bones of slaves buried at Newton Plantation, Barbados, have been shown to contain very high levels of lead, indicating liberal ingestion of new rum during life. Handler, "Lead Contact and Poisoning"; "Diseases and Medical Disabilities".

DYSENTERY

page 109

Diarrhœa Colliquativa: diarrhoea associated with discharge of stool profuse enough to cause wasting of the body.

Fluxus Hepaticus: diarrhoea associated with discharge of bile.

page 111

sanguiferous Vessels: blood vessels.

Close-stools: chamber pots enclosed in a box; commodes.

page 112

Sanies: thin, foetid pus mixed with serum or blood.

Ichor: watery, acrid discharge.

intermits: stops for a while; "skips" beats.

page 113

corroborate: strengthen; return to normal.

revulse: drag, draw or pull back.

restringes: constipates.

Rad. Rhei. tor. pulv. . . . : Powdered rhubarb root, 1 scruple; electuary of scordium (water germander, *Teucrium scordium*), ½ drachm; thebiac extract (opium in boiling water), 1½ or 2 grains; oil of cinnamon, 1 drop; and syrup of white poppy in sufficient quantity to make a bolus. To be taken one hour after vomiting.

Cort. Restring. Barbad. . . . : Bark of Barbadoes restringent (bastard locust) and mistletoe of the lemon tree, 1 ounce of each, and pomegranate rind, 1½ drachm. Mix. Boil in 2 pounds of spring water to reduce to 1½ pounds and to a fine decoction. Add electuary of scordium, 1 ounce. Boil and strain to 1½ pounds. To the strained liquid add catechu (an astringent containing 40 to 50 per cent tannin) tincture, 1 ounce; sweet spirit of nitre, ½ ounce; purified salts of nitre, ½ ounce; and syrup of white poppy, 1 ounce. Mix and make a decoction of which the patient takes 3 or 4 spoonfuls every three hours or after a single liquid bowel motion.

Bastard Locus: jatoba (*Hymenea coubaril*). "Bastard Locust or Forrest-Tree – This grows to be a large Tree, cloathed with a whitish Bark, red within. The Leaves are of a dark Green, about an inch and an half long, smooth and very blunt pointed. The Bark is used as an Astringent." Hughes, *Natural History*, 149.

Misleto of the Lemon-tree: "*The* MISLETOE, *or* BIRD'S TURD – The origin of this Shrub is a small white Berry, containing a very glutinous milky Juice. These, when ripe are eaten by Birds; and by them voided upon other Trees, where they stick very fast, and soon after germinate. I am apt to believe, that this brownish Juice hath likewise a corrosive Quality, which frets and wears away the outward Bark of the Tree upon which it sticks; by this means opening a Passage for the new tubular Roots of the Berry, to penetrate among those larger Vessels of the Tree, thro' which the nutritious Juices are conveyed. These Roots being thus able to suck Nourishment, the young Sprout soon grows . . . The Leaves of this parasitical Shrub are of a dark Green . . . This grows to about Three Feet high, and bushy, bearing a small white flower, succeeded by a Berry, as described above. The milky Juice, being squeezed out, is made use of to cure Fluxes and Lasks [diarrhœa]. It grows chiefly upon Orange-trees." Ibid., 156. "It may have since disappeared from Barbados although persists elsewhere in the Caribbean." Professor Sean Carrington, University of the West Indies, Cave Hill, Barbados (personal communication).

page 114

here: in England.

Elect. e Scord: electuary of scordium (*Teucrium scordium*).

Bals. Locotel.: Locatelli's balsam. Take of olive oil, 1 pint; Strassburg turpentine and yellow wax, of each ½ pound, red saunders, 6 drachms. Melt the wax with some part of the oil over a gentle fire; then adding the remaining part of the oil and turpentine; afterwards mix in the saunders, previously reduced to a powder, and keep them stirring together until the balsam is cold. This balsam is recommended in erosions of the intestines, the dysentery, haemorrhages, internal bruises and some complaints of the breast. Outwardly it is used for healing and cleansing wounds and ulcers. The dose, when taken internally, is from two scruples to two drachms.

page 116

Electar. e Scord. . . . : Take 1 ounce each of scordium electuary and Locatelli's balsam; spermaceti and powder from a lump of opium, 1½ drachms of each; and a sufficient quantity of syrup of tolu (resinous secretion of *Myroxylon toluifera*). Mix and make an electuary of which the patient takes a quantity the size of a nutmeg every four, five or six hours, emulsified in a drink of 3 tablespoonfuls prepared with wax.

page 117

Secum: cæcum, the first part of the large intestine.

Wax, Sperm, Ceti: spermaceti wax, from the head cavities of the sperm whale (*Physeter macrocephalus*).

Senna: dried leaflets of various species of *Cassia*, used as a cathartic and emetic.

Sal. Polychrestum: potassium sulphate (K_2So_4), "salt of many virtues".

page 118

nourishing Diet: Despite his continuing emphasis on bleeding and purging, Dr Hillary frequently comments on the need for moderation and the use of less vigorous methods, in addition to a nourishing diet.

OPISTHOTONOS AND TETANY [TETANUS]

Bontius: Jacobus Bontius (1592–1631), a Dutch physician, published *De Medicina Indorum* in 1642. It was translated into English as *An Account of the Diseases, Natural History and Medicines of the East Indies* (London, 1796).

Island of *Coos*: Kos, the Greek island that was the birthplace and home of Hippocrates.

page 119

digested: healed.

page 122

Consent: relation of sympathy between one organ or part of the body and another, whereby when one is affected, the other is affected correspondingly.

page 123

Moat: mote; particle of dust.

the same Nerve: the vagus (tenth cranial) nerve, which supplies branches to the stomach and both kidneys.

crural Nerve: nervus interosseus cruris.

page 124

Tolle causam et cessabit effectum: "Accept the cause and stop the effect."

page 125

cut the lacerated Nerve: Dr Hillary's observation that even the smallest contaminated puncture wound may cause tetanus, even after the wound itself has healed, is absolutely correct. His hypothesis that "something" was transmitted throughout the nervous system was intuitively correct and his recommendation of deeper surgical incision of contaminated wounds logical.

Digestive: a digestive ointment; unguentum terebinthinæ compositum.

Moschi Oriental. . . . : Oriental musk, 12 grains; extract of opium, 2 or 3 grains; theriac of Andromachus, 1 scruple; and balsam of Peru, a sufficient quantity to make a bolus. To be taken immediately.

Aq Alex Simp . . . : Simple alexiterial water, 1½ ounces; compound spirit of lavender, 1 drachm; spirit of hartshorn, 30 drops; Oriental musk, 8 grains; extract of opium, 2 grains; balsam of Peru, 10 drops; and syrup of poppy, ½ ounce. Mix and make a draught to be taken immediately.

Extract. Thebaic. . . . : Extract of opium, 2 or 3 grains; Oriental musk, 10 grains; and balsam of Peru, a sufficient quantity to make four pills. To be taken immediately.

Doses of the Opiates: "Opium then is what is chiefly to be relied on, and it is astonishing what quantities of it may be swallowed, without either procuring sleep or affecting the brain." J. Edward Hutson, ed., *On the Treatment and Management of the More Common West-India Diseases, 1750–1802* (Kingston: University of the West Indies Press, 2005), 29.

page 126

Fol. Althæ vel Alcæ. . . . : Flowers of marsh mallow or vervain mallow, 4 measures; sage and elder flowers, 2 measures of each; bruised linseed, 2 pints; Venice soap, 2 pints; and crude sal ammoniac, 1 pint. Mix and boil in a gallon of water. Then add Barbados tar, 3 pints; compound spirit of sugar, ½ pound; and solution of theriac of

Andromachus, 2 pints. Mix and make a fomentation with which to foment the region of the diaphragm, throat and spine, by means of tepid woollen rags, with pharmaceutical skill, every six hours. (Inclusion of Barbados tar in this prescription marks a very early use of tar extract in an oral medication.)

Liniment. Saponac. . . . : Soap liniment, (Volatil. Nervin) and Barbados tar, 1 pint of each; balsam of Peru, 2 fluid drachms; oils of lavender and rosemary, 20 drops of each; and opium, 1 drachm. Mix and make a liniment and use over.

page 127

Aq. Menthæ Simp. . . . : Simple peppermint water and simple alexiterial water, 4 pints of each; Madeira or Canary wine, 4 pints; compound spirit of lavender, ½ pint; tincture of castoreum and volatile aromatic spirit, 2 fluid drachms of each; and syrup of poppies, 1 pint. Mix. Take 2 or 3 spoonfuls in weak spirit.

breathing Sweat: profuse perspiration.

Decoct. Emol. pro Clys. . . . : Emollient decoction for an enema, 8 pints – lentitive electuary and castor oil, 1 pint of each; balsam of Peru, 1 fluid ounce; and Barbados tar, 1 pint. Mix and make an enema.

page 129

Cloaths: clothing.

page 130

pro re nata et pro ratione Ætatis: as often as needed and as indicated by the patient's age.

Seri Lactis . . . : Whey, 2 pints; Venice soap, 1 scruple; Calabrian manna, 2 or 3 ounces; sweet oil of almonds, ½ pint; sweet fennel oil, 2 drops; and balsam of Peru, 5 drops. Mix and make an enema; use as the first injection.

to assist the Operation of the Clyster: Fennel seed water, 3 pints; white magnesia, ½ ounce; prepared crabs' eyes, 1 ounce; syrup of succory with rhubarb, syrup of roses and water, 3 ounces of each. Mix.

Or, fennel seed water, 3 pints; almond soap, ½ ounce; white magnesia, ½ ounce; syrup of succory with rhubarb and best manna, 2 ounces of each; and sweet oil of almonds, 3 ounces. Mix. Prescribe a small spoonful or two according to the age of the patient, every half-hour or hour until the bowels respond.

to abate the convulsive Twitchings: Fennel seed water, 3 pints; white magnesia, ½ ounce; syrup of succory with rhubarb and best manna, 2 ounces of each; Oriental musk, 3 grains; true spirit of hartshorn, 15 drops; and syrup of poppies, ½ pint. Prescribe a small spoonful three or four times a day, or more often if a convulsion or spasm is troublesome.

to prevent the Tetany from coming on: Fennel seed water, 4 drachms; Oriental musk, 1 grain; tincture of opium, 4 drops; and syrup of poppies, 2 drachms. Mix for two doses, one dose to be taken immediately, and repeated if the convulsive spasm returns.

page 131
its Causes: Despite his accurate clinical observations, Dr Hillary, and other contemporary physicians, failed to make the connection with animal manure – the ubiquitous source of the tetanus-causing bacillus, *Clostridium tetani*; this association was not elucidated until the 1880s. With the disappearance of the horse and buggy, widespread wearing of shoes and inoculation against tetanus, the disease has all but disappeared from Barbados.

RABIES

in the West-India Islands: "In or about the Year 1741 a great number of Dogs ran mad; and I observed, that the Temperament of the Air, for many Months before, was very hot. In this season, a great Number of Cattle, being bit by these Dogs, ran mad likewise." Hughes, *Natural History*, 33.

page 132
so many learned Authors: Rabies is one of the oldest infections known to man, well described by the ancients and endemic across the Roman Empire. *Rabies* derives from the Latin *rabere* (to rave), while the name of the causative virus (genus *Lyssavirus*) conveys "madness" in Greek.

Baron Van Swieten: Gerhard van Swieten (1770–72) was a pupil of Boerhaave. In 1745 he became the personal physician of Empress Maria Theresa of Austria and was subsequently granted a baronetcy.

Contagion: In his 1750 *Natural History of the Island of Barbados*, Griffith Hughes used the word "virus" in his description of rabies. However, at the time *virus* was understood to mean "poison" or "venom". Hughes, *Natural History*, 33.

fatally propagated: Rabies, an acute infectious disease of the central nervous system, is usually spread by contamination with virus-laden saliva from the bite of an infected animal. However, rabies can be transmitted by ingestion of infected tissues.

page 133
bye: out of the way.

page 134
hydrophobous: affected with rabies, also known as hydrophobia.

page 135
Priapism: persistent erection of the penis.

page 137
concreted: coagulated.

Gula: external throat.

page 138
Cupping-glass: a cup-shaped vessel applied to the skin in the operation of cupping, a method of drawing blood by scarifying the skin and applying a cupping-glass, the air in which has been rarefied by heat.

Cautery: a heated metallic instrument for burning or searing organic tissue.

Escharoticks: escharotic drugs (powerful caustics).

cauterized without scarifying: Dr Hillary's approach for preventing spread of the poison was sound. Cleansing and cautery of the wound was advocated by the ancients, and it remained the cornerstone of treatment until development of a vaccine. It was the treatment recommended by Sir William Osler in his famous textbook *The Principles and Practice of Medicine*, which was published some years after Louis Pasteur's 1885 demonstration of the first human cure using his vaccine. Osler expressed uncertainty regarding use of this vaccination, even though he mentioned the success of the Pasteur Institute.

Moschi Orient. . . . : Oriental musk, 16 grains; ground local cinnabar, ½ drachm, or soap pill, 13 grains; camphor, 6 grains; and balsam of Peru, a sufficient quantity. Mix and make a bolus.

page 139
Rad. Valerian. Sylvest. Cort. Sasafræ: valerian root (*Valerinia officinalis*) and sassafras bark.

perfectly well after: "Recovery [from rabies] is rare, with death usually associated with progressive respiratory depression and cardiorespiratory failure." *Dorland's Illustrated Medical Dictionary*, 30th ed. (W.B. Saunders, 2003).

page 140
comminute: divide minutely.

saponaceous: soap-like.

page 141
Efficacy of this . . . *Cure*: Dr Hillary draws his conclusions from comparison of three untreated cases (who all died) with seven treated cases (who remained symptom-free), an example of a very early, primitive example of a "controlled trial". Moreover, he recognized that it would have been unethical to wittingly carry out that experiment ("which Humanity would forbid any Man to make").

misfortune to be bitten by mad Dogs: One can only speculate as to whether these patients were truly bitten by a rabid dog. The mortality associated with human rabies was considered to be 100 per cent in the pre-vaccination era.

page 142

Moschi . . . : Musk, 16 grains, and crude mercuric sulphide, locally produced, 1 scruple. Mix and make a powder.

Arrack: a spirituous liquor made from rice and sugar fermented with coconut juice.

Sir *George Cobb*: "An Infallible Cure for the Bite of a mad Dog Brought from Tonquin by Sir George Cobb, Bart: Take 24 grains of Native Cinnabar, 24 grains of Facticious Cinnabar, and 16 grains of Musk. Grind all these together into an exceeding fine Powder, and put it into a small Teacup of Arrack, Rum or Brandy; let it be well mix'd and give it to the Person as soon as possible after the Bite; a Second Dose of the same must be repeated thirty Days after; and a Third may be taken after thirty Days more: But if the Symptoms of Madness appear on the Persons, they must take One of the above Doses immediately, and a Second in an Hour after; and, if wanted, a Third must be given a few hours afterwards." *British Medical Journal*, 15 May 1875, 641.

page 143

Curatio *veró* **morbi** . . . : "But treatment of the disease, when it is already present, seems worth attempting, especially in its first stage and at the beginning of the second [stage] particularly, as otherwise the penalty for neglecting it is a most terrible outcome. Immediately after the first signs of the invading evil the disease should be treated as being highly inflammatory, by letting blood from a broad wound in a large [blood] vessel, even to the point of fainting, etc."

page 144

Mas. Pil. Saponac. . . . : Soap pill, 10 grains; succinic acid; camphor, about 8 grains; regenerated tartar (potassium acid tartrate treated with acetic acid); theriac of Andromachus, about 1 scruple; sassafras oil, 2 drops; and balsam of Peru, a sufficient quantity. Mix and make a bolus.

page 145

fere ad deliquium Animi: almost to the point of fainting.

immerge: immerse, submerge.

page 146

Theriac. Androm. . . . : Theriac of Andromachus, ½ drachm; soap pill; succinic acid, volume about ½ scruple; powdered camphor, 8 grains; peppermint oil, 1 drop; and syrup of poppies, a sufficient quantity. Mix and make a bolus and take as above.

page 17

Nec desperandum tamen . . . : "However, because of precedents already established with regard to other poisons, we should not despair of finding a particular antidote to this particular poison." It is of interest to note that for many years Barbados has been considered rabies-free. However, the neighbouring island of Trinidad is not; Pawan reported transmission of rabies to humans through the bites of vampire bats (*Desmodus rotundus*) in Trinidad in the 1930s.

Chronic Diseases

page 148
Surfeit: gluttonous indulgence in eating or drinking.
Ptyalisme: excessive secretion of saliva.

page 149
Ructuses: eructation, or belching.

page 150
Marasmus: wasting away of the body.
this Disease: See the editors' introduction regarding Sir Christopher Booth's interpretation of this description as being the first published account of tropical sprue. Sir Christopher's analysis of Dr Hillary's observations has led to continuing references to the occurrence of tropical sprue in the West Indies, specifically in Barbados, although today it is not seen there.
Ulcusculæ: ulcers.

page 151
Erysipelatoides: a skin condition resembling erysipelas.
Impetigo: a name given to various pustular diseases of the skin.

page 153
Rad. Ipocacuanha pulv.: powdered ipecacuanha root.
gr. ij *vel gr.* iij: 2 or 3 grains.
Alteratives: medicines that alter the processes of nutrition and reduce them to healthy action.
Sulph. Antimonii precipitat . . . : Precipitated antimony sulphide, 5 grains; finely ground mercuric chloride, 1 scruple; powdered guaiacum gum and extract of gentian, 1 drachm of each; camphor, 2 scruples; extract of opium, 10 grains; and guaiacum balsam, a sufficient quantity. Mix and make fifty pills, of which the patient takes three each night at bedtime, accompanied by 2 or 3 ounces of the following infusion.

Preparations of antimony were used in medicine over several centuries, chiefly for their emetic properties (for example, tartar emetic, a mixture of antimony and potassium tartrate; antimony sulphide). Tartar emetic has a more prolonged emetic action than ipecacuanha but is very toxic; George Wood and Franklin Bache, *Dispensary of the United States of America* (Philadelphia, 1891). The long-hallowed use of antimony preparations beautifully illustrates the maxim of eighteenth-century medical cynics that sometimes the cure can be worse than the disease.

page 154

Rad. Serpent. Virg. . . . : Virginia snakeroot, sassafras bark and pomegranate rind, 1 ounce of each; cinnamon, 2 drachms; and salt of wormwood, 1 drachm. Mix and soak in 2½ pints of boiling water in a closed vessel for eight hours, then strain, reducing the liquid to 2 pints. To the strained liquid add 1 ounce of saffron wine and 2 ounces of ammonium acetate. Mix. The patient takes 2 ounces, with the prescription above, daily.

Vini Antimon. gut. xx *vel* xxx: antimonial wine, 20 or 30 drops.

Flesh-brush: a brush used for rubbing the skin in order to excite the circulation.

Chaise: a light open carriage for one or two persons.

Magnesia Alba ℨj: hydrated magnesium carbonate, 1 drachm. The simple antacid remedy recommended here contrasts markedly with the complex and potentially toxic polypharmacy described above.

Vinum Chalybeat.: wine impregnated with iron.

page 155

Electar. e Scordio . . . : Electuary of scordium, 1 ounce; theriac of Andromachus, ½ ounce; pale catechu and powdered pomegranate peel, 2 drachms of each; powdered cinnamon, 1 drachm; precipitated antimony sulphate, 2 scruples; and syrup of poppies, a sufficient quantity. Mix and make an electuary, of which the patient takes a quantity the size of a nutmeg and, at bedtime, if diarrhoea is troublesome, with the following decoction.

Cort. Granator. . . . : Pomegranate peel and Virginia snakeroot, 1 ounce of each, and cinnamon bark, 2 drachms. Mix and boil in distilled water, reducing from 2 pints to 1½ pints. To the remains add electuary of scordium, 1 ounce; then boil and strain. To the strained liquid add cinnamon water and tincture of catechu, 1 ounce of each, and syrup of poppies, ½ ounce. Mix and make a decoction. The patient is to take four spoonfuls of the above with each liquid bowel movement.

green Copperas: proto-sulphate of iron, or ferrous sulphate ($FeSO_4$).

Sulphur Vivum: wine (sherry) impregnated with sulphur.

page 156

as I have several times observed: "Dr Hillary practiced at Bath [England] from 1743 to 1746 and while there published *An Inquiry into the Contents and Medicinal Virtues of Lincomb Spaw water near Bath.*" J. Edward Hutson, "William Hillary, MD,

Meteorologist and Physician, Barbados, 1752–58", *Journal of the Barbados Museum and Historical Society*, 52 (December 2006): 178.

deobstruent: having the property of removing obstructions by opening the natural passages or pores of the body.

page 157

Rad. Serpent. Virg. . . . : Virginia snakeroot, ½ or 1 drachm, and theriac of Andromachus, ½ drachm. Mix and soak in boiling distilled water, then strain. To the strained liquid add solution of potassium acetate, 1 scruple; tincture of ammonium acetate, 3 ounces; saffron wine, 2 ounces; and syrup of saffron, 2 ounces. Mix and make a draught to be taken as above.

page 158

Sed Verbum sat sapienti: But a word to the wise is enough.

NYCTALOPIA OR NIGHT-BLINDNESS

Galen: Claudius Galenus (c. 130–c. 200 CE), Greek physician and author.

page 159

Actuarius: Joannes Zacharias Actuarius (c. 1275–c. 1328), a Byzantine physician, published *De Methodo Medendi* (On the therapeutic method) and Περί ούρων (On urines).

Pliny: Gaius Plinius Secundus (23–79 CE), known as Pliny the Elder, a Roman military commander, naturalist and author who published *Naturalis Historia*.

Celsus: Aulus Cornelius Celsus (25 BCE–50 CE), a Roman physician and encyclopaedist. He published *De Medicina*, which is famous for its elegant Latin style.

among the Negroes in the West-India Islands: The prevalence of night blindness, which is due to vitamin A deficiency, in the West Indian slave population is not at all surprising given the gross deficiencies of their diets. Vitamin A occurs chiefly in animal products, especially liver, and in green and yellow vegetables.

page 160

sanguiferous: carrying blood.

seriferous: carrying serum.

male: mal-, that is, bad.

Imbecillity: weakness, feebleness.

page 162

Rad. Valerian Sylv. Pulv.: powdered wild valerian root.

Aq. Rosar. . . . : Rose water, 1½ ounces, and antimonial wine, ½ ounce. Mix and make an eye lotion with which to wash the eyes every night at bedtime and also in the morning.

Elephantiasis

within the Torrid Zone: Most cases of elephantiasis are caused by filarial worms (*Filaria bancrofti*), transmitted via mosquito bites. Once endemic in the Caribbean, the disease is now seen rarely in Guyana, although it made a brief reappearance in Trinidad in the 1970s. Joseph Bell, the Scottish surgeon who was the inspiration for Conan Doyle's fictional detective, Sherlock Holmes, once diagnosed the occupation and place of residence of a returning soldier by his elephantiasis, which he knew as "Barbados leg".

brought it from *Africa*: Elephantiasis was one of several African diseases brought to the West Indies during the era of the slave trade.

page 163
tumefied: swollen.

anasarcous: displaying a very puffed appearance; of the subcutaneous cellular tissue of a limb or other large surface of the body.

page 164
dropsical: pertaining to dropsy, which is now thought to have referred to congestive heart failure.

Membrana Cellulosa: connective tissue.

Chops: painful fissures or cracks in the skin.

Membrana Adiposa: the layer of fat underlying the skin.

Cellulæ: Cells, in anatomy, are little sacs or bladders where fluids or other matters are lodged; also called cellulæ. Chambers' *Cyclopaedia* (London, 1751).

page 165
Febris Septimana: a fever that returns after a remission of seven days.

page 166
Symptoms of this Disease: an accurate observation of the lymphangitis attending elephantiasis, even though Dr Hillary had little understanding of the body's lymphatic system.

Vini Ipocacuanh. ℥i. *vel* ℥ij.: ipecacuanha root dissolved in wine (sherry), 1 or 2 drachms.

Rad. Rhei. Pulv. . . . : Powdered rhubarb root, 1 scruple; soap pill, 7 grains; camphor, 5 grains; potassium acetate, 1 scruple; and syrup of poppies, a sufficient quantity. Mix and make a bolus and take as above, with plenty of tepid vinous whey. Will induce perspiration.

Viburnium-tea: a tea brewed from the bark of *Viburnum prunifolium*, thought to contain viburnin, valerianic, oxalic, citric and malic acids, besides other ingredients.

Sage-tea: a tea brewed from *Salvia officinalis*, an aromatic culinary herb formerly much esteemed as a medicinal herb.

page 167

black Sage: *Cordia curassavica*. In some West Indian islands a tea brewed from the leaves is used in the treatment of influenza, fever and insomnia. S. Carrington, *Wild Plants of Barbados* (London: Macmillan Caribbean, 1993), 85.

derive: conduct a stream of water or other fluid from its source into a channel or destination.

Spina Dorsi: spinal column.

Os Coxigis: coccyx.

***Fol. Alceæ* . . . :** Hollyhock leaves and viburnum leaves, 3 minims; elder flowers, 1 minim; Venice soap, ½ ounce; and crude sal ammoniac, 1 ounce. Mix and soak in distilled water, then add rum and ordinary vinegar, 1 pint, and mix well.

***Sulphur. Antimon. præcipit.* . . . :** Precipitated antimony sulphide, 2½ scruples; ground red mercuric oxide, ½ scruple; powdered guaiacum gum, 1 scruple; and Peruvian balsam, a sufficient quantity. Mix and make sixty pills, from which the patient takes four at bedtime with the following decoction.

***Rad. Sasaparil.* . . . :** Sarsaparilla root, 2 ounces; sassafras root, 1 ounce; Virginia snakeroot, ½ ounce; and potassium acetate, ½ ounce. Mix and digest in distilled water, then strain. To the strained liquid add sweet spirit of nitre, 1 ounce, and compound juniper water, 2 ounces. Take with the above every morning.

page 168

***Elix. Vitrioli. acid. gut* l *vel* xl.:** alcoholic solution of vitriolic acid (an acidic solution of iron sulphate), 50 or 60 drops.

page 169

Issue: discharge of blood or other matter from the body.

Frictions: chafing or rubbing the body or limbs.

Unctions: ointments.

***quia, extra Artis Limites est*:** which is beyond the capacity of the medical arts.

Vena Medinensis, Dracunculus or Guinea-Worm

Alsaharavius: Abu al-Qasim (died c. 1013), known in Latin as Abulcasis or Alsaharavius, was "the greatest Muslim surgeon". He published *Al-Tasrif* (Vade-mecum), a medical encyclopaedia in thirty sections, which was translated into Latin, Provençal and Hebrew.

his Translator: Gherardo Cremonese (Gerard of Cremona).

Mesuæ: Yuhanna ibn Masawaih (777–857), an Arab physician and author, was known in Latin as Ioannes Mesuæ.

Abulcasim or *Albucasus:* Abulcasis (see above).

Haly Abbas: Ali ibn Abbas al-Majusi (died 994), an Arab physician and author, published *The Royal Book of All Medicine.*

Rhazis: Abu Bakr Muhammad ibn Zakariya al-Razi (865–925), a Persian physician and author, was known in Latin as Rhazes or Rasis.

page 170

Avicena: Abu Ali al-Husayn ibn Abdallah ibn Sina al-Balakh (980–1037), a Persian author.

Animalcula: animalcule, or microscopic animal.

Aloetics: medicines consisting chiefly of aloes.

page 171

half a Drachm Weight: 30 grains (about 2 grams or 0.07 ounce).

Meatuses: plural form of *meatus*, Latin for way, path or course.

Sulphur. . . . : Sulphur and garlic, 1 ounce; black pepper, ½ ounce; camphor, 2 drachms; and proof spirit, 2 pints. Mix and digest, then strain. The patient takes two spoonfuls of the strained liquid two or three times daily.

subtile: not dense; thin, rarefied; penetrating.

LEPROSY OF THE ARABIANS

page 172

Aretæus of *Cappadox:* Aretæus (Αρεταος) the Cappadocian, a Greek physician and author of the first century CE, who published four pairs of books: *De causis et signis acutorum morborum, De causis et signis duitumorum morborum, De curatione acutorum morobrum* and *De curatione diutumorum morobrum.*

Paulus of *Ægina:* a Byzantine Greek physician (c. 625–c. 690) who published the *Medical Compendium,* in eight books.

Ætius of *Amida:* Aëtius Amidenus (Αέτος), the court physician of Justinian I. He published a medical encyclopaedia, *Tetrabibloi* (Βιβλία Ιατρικά).

Serapion: Yahya ibn Sarafiyun, an Arab medical author known in medieval Europe as Johannes Serapion.

Dr *Lommius:* Jodocus Lommius, or Joost van Lom (c. 1500–c. 1564), a Dutch physician. He published *Medicinalium observationum libri tres.*

Lepra Grecorum: a tubercular disease often mistakenly identified as leprosy.

Commerce: dealing in the affairs of life.

Converse: manner of life; "conversation".

Sound: healthy.

page 173

obscure: indistinct; difficult to understand.

Venery: indulgence in sexual desire.

page 174

tumid: swollen.

torpid: devoid of the power of motion or feeling.

Pinnæ of the Nose: the allæ, or lateral cartilages of the nose.

Ventriloqui: plural form of *ventriloquus*, a ventriloquist.

acute: sharply pointed.

page 175

Inveterascentem morbum hunc depelli remediis non posse: "If this disease becomes chronic it cannot be driven out by any remedies."

page 176

Ol. Tartari per deliquium: potassium carbonate, for use after fainting.

Sulph. Antimonii præcipit . . . : Precipitated antimony sulphide, 3 drachms; ground red mercuric oxide, 30 grains; powdered guaiacum gum, 3 drachms; and guaiacum balsam, a sufficient quantity. Mix and make ninety pills, of which the patient takes three every night at bedtime, with 50 drops of the following decoction.

Vini Antimonial. . . . : Antimonial wine, 2 ounces, and aromatic tincture, ½ ounce. Mix, make a tincture and take as above.

Rad. Sarsaparil. . . . : Sarsaparilla root, 3 ounces; sassafras root, 1 ounce; and potassium acetate, ½ ounce. Boil in a covered vessel with distilled water; strain. To the strained liquid add antimonial tincture, 1 ounce; compound juniper water, 1½ ounces; and a sufficient quantity of sugar. Mix and make a decoction, then take as above. Also take a decoction of this with 50 drops of the tincture prescribed above.

Torpor: insensibility, lack of feeling.

page 177

Antimonii crud. . . . : Crude antimony, finely powdered, 1½ ounces; potassium tartrate and powdered woodlice, of each ½ ounce; and ginger root, ½ ounce. Mix and make an electuary of which the patient takes a quantity the size of a nutmeg with 50 drops of the previously prescribed tincture.

page 178

Scire tamen licet . . . : "But you should know that if this disease becomes chronic it cannot be driven out by any remedies; it is beyond the limit of [medical] skill."

LEPROSY OF THE JOINTS

LEPROSY of the JOINTS: the so-called Joint-Evil (*Elephantiasis græcorum*), a tubercular disease often mistakenly identified with leprosy.

Altera et secunda . . . : In this instance Dr Hillary has misquoted Haly Abbas. The quotation should read: "*Sunt autem Elephantiæ species duæ . . . . Altera et secunda est quæ ex humore fit nigro qui ex coleræ generatur rubeæ adjustione; in hac specie membrorum est comestio et casus, et ab hac nulla sanatur quis medela.*" [There are two kinds of elephantiasis . . . . The other, the second kind, is one which results from a black humor which is produced by the burning off of red bile; in this kind the limbs are eaten away and fall off, and there is no remedy by which anyone is cured of it.] Haly Abbas, *Liber totius medicinæ* (c. 960).

page 179

Scrophula: scrofula (also known as struma or the king's evil), a constitutional disease characterized by chronic enlargement and degeneration of the lymphatic glands.

whether: which of the two.

digest: suppurate.

YAWS

page 180

YAWS: a non-venereal, systemic infectious disease caused by the spirochete *Treponema pertenue*.

page 181

Lepra albedo est . . . : "Leprosy is a whiteness that occurs on the outside of the skin; sometimes it occurs in some limbs but not in others; sometimes in the whole body so that the colour of the whole body is white. – With regard to that which is in a limb, if it comes about from an evil cold complexion, these are the signs: when the limb in which it is present is white in colour, and likewise its hairs, and when, if the skin pierced by a lancet, or indeed a needle, it is not blood that comes out but a white fluid."

Moses's Method: see Leviticus 14:1–7.

page 182
fungous: resembling a fungus in texture; spongy.
Wood-strawberry: the common wild strawberry (*Fragaria vesca*).
Mulberry: the fruit of the black mulberry (*Morus nigra*).

page 183
Funguses: morbid spongy growths, such as exuberant granulation in a wound.
phagedenic: progressive, rapidly spreading, sloughing.
salivated: stimulated (usually by use of mercury) to produce an excessive quantity of saliva.
Palm-oil: oil derived from the fruit pulp of the oil palm of West Africa (*Elæsis guineensis*).

page 184
salutiferous: promoting or conducive to health.
Æthiop. Mineral. . . . : Ethiop's mineral (black mercuric sulphide), 1½ ounces; crude
   antimony, powdered, 1 ounce; treacle of Andromachus (Venice treacle), 1 ounce;
   powdered camphor, 1 drachm; and syrup of ginger, a sufficient quantity. Mix and
   make an electuary, of which the patient takes a quantity the size of a nutmeg in the
   morning and at bedtime, with 40 drops of antimonial wine in a draught of whey, and
   continues until the swellings (yaws) are ripe.

page 185
incarn: induce healing.
Lapis Infernalis: the "infernal stone", or silver caustic.
Mercur. Sublimat. Corrosiv. . . . : Mercuric chloride, 1 drachm, dissolved in 1 ounce of
   rectified wine.
blue Vitriol: copper sulphate.
Mercur. Corrosiv. . . . : Mercuric chloride, 1 drachm, and powdered burnt alum,
   ½ drachm.
sweeten: free from taint, purify; bring into a wholesome condition.
Ethiop. Mineral. . . . : Ethiop's mineral (black mercuric sulphide), 1½ ounces; crude
   antimony, powdered, 1 ounce; treacle of Andromachus, ½ ounce; powdered guaiacum
   gum, 3 drachms; and ordinary syrup, a sufficient quantity. Mix and make an electuary.
   Take a quantity the size of a walnut, morning and night, with 40 or 50 drops of a
   draught of decoction of sarsaparilla and sassafras wood.

page 186
cures them without a Salivation: The natural progression of yaws is such that the primary
   and secondary lesions disappear spontaneously (hence the implication of a cure), while
   tertiary lesions appear, when they do, five or even ten years later.

Sulph. Antimon. præcipit. . . . : Precipitated antimony sulphide, 2 drachms; ground red mercuric oxide, 24 grains; powdered guaiacum gum, ½ ounce; camphor, ½ ounce; and guaiacum balsam, a sufficient quantity. Mix and make seventy pills, of which the patient takes three every night at bedtime with antimonial wine, 40 drops, in a draught or decoction of sarsaparilla and sassafras wood.

phagedenic Ulcers: chronic painful ulcers, usually seen on the lower limbs of malnourished children in the tropics; also called tropical ulcers.

page 187

Sulph. Antimon. præcipit. . . . : Precipitated antimony sulphide, 2½ drachms; ground red mercuric oxide, ½ drachm; powdered guaiacum gum, 3 drachms; guaiacum balsam, a sufficient quantity; and powdered camphor, 2 scruples. Mix and make eighty pills, of which the patient takes three every night at bedtime, accompanied by 5 ounces of the following decoction.

Rad. Sarsaparil. . . . : Sarsaparilla root, 3 ounces; sassafras wood, 1 ounce; and sodium nitrate, ½ ounce. Mix and boil in distilled water, reducing from 3 to 2 pints, and strain. To the strained liquid add compound juniper water, 1½ ounces, and sugar, a sufficient quantity. Mix and make a decoction for the patient to take.

Vini Antimonial. . . . : Antimonial wine, 1 ounce, and aromatic tincture, 2 drachms. Mix; take 50 drops every morning and at four o'clock in the afternoon, in 5 ounces of the above prescribed decoction.

Ung. Basilic. flav. . . . : Yellow basilicon ointment, 1 ounce; fine red mercuric chloride, 1 drachm; and powdered burnt alum, ½ drachm. Mix and make a digesting balsam.

Empl. Commun. . . . : Ordinary plaster with gum of red lead, 1½ ounces; red mercuric chloride, 2 scruples; and powdered burnt alum ½ drachm. Mix and make a plaster.

deplorable: given up as hopeless.

IMPETIGO OR RING-WORM

IMPETIGO *or* RING-WORM: Dr Hillary seems to have failed to distinguish impetigo, which he describes accurately with its characteristic pustules and readily infective nature, from ringworm. The latter is not pustular unless scratched and infected, is caused by a fungus, and is much more likely to become chronic if not adequately treated.

page 189

Handworm: the itch insect, or scabies, (*Sarcoptes scabiei*), which burrows into the hands.

Herpes exedens: serpigo, a general term for creeping or spreading skin diseases, especially ringworm.

Body: a distinct form or kind of matter; one of the seven "bodies terrestrial" (the seven ancient metals) answering to the seven heavenly bodies (the sun, the moon and five old planets).

Gravity: weight.

page 190

Unguent. Simplex: simple ointment.

Diapalma: palm oil, litharge (protoxide of lead) and zinc sulphate.

Rad. Hellebori Albi: root of white hellebore (*Veratrum album*).

Vitrioli Albi: white vitriol, or zinc sulphate.

Lactis Sulphuris: precipitated sulphur.

Mercurii calcinat. . . . : Red mercuric oxide, finely ground; precipitated antimony sulphide or guaiacum gum, powdered; and guaiacum balsam. Mix and make forty pills, of which the patient takes two every night at bedtime.

Vini Antimonial. . . . : Antimonial wine, 1 pint, and aromatic tincture, ½ pint. Mix and take 60 drops every morning in a draught of sarsaparilla root.

Extract. Thebaic. **gr. ss.:** extract of opium, ½ grain.

page 191

Secrets: "infallible" prescriptions.

Nostrums: quack remedies; patent medicines.

Terra Macke-machee: possibly a preparation made from papier-mâché.

alkaline Salt: natron (*natrum*), or sesquicarbonate of soda.

Flowers of a Shrub: "*The* FRENCH GUAVA, [*Senna occidentalis*]. This is a shrubby Plant, whose main Stalk hath a strong ligneous Texture. Its Side-branches are cloathed with several Pair of large oval winged Leaves, the upper Stalks ending in upright Spikes, which are covered for three Inches in Length with pendulous yellow Flowers, not ill-resembling those of the Aloe Plant. These are succeeded by several blackish long Pods, whose several partitional Cells inclose a great many round blackish Seeds. A Decoction of this Plant, or an Ointment made of a Mixture of its Juices, is looked upon to be of great Use to cure and dry up any cutaneous Eruptions. This flourishes about *Christmas*, and loves a rich Soil, as well as a shady Place to grow in." Hughes, *Natural History*, 202.

Selected Bibliography

Adams, A.R.D., and B.G. Maegraith. *Clinical Tropical Diseases*. 2nd ed. Oxford: Blackwell Scientific Publishers, 1960.

Booth, Christopher C. "A Pupil of Boerhaave". In *Doctors in Science and Society: Essays of a Clinical Scientist*. London: British Medical Journal, 1987.

Carrington, S., A. Forde, H. Fraser and J. Gilmore. *A–Z of Barbados Heritage*. Oxford: Macmillan Education, 2003.

Dunn, R. *Sugar and Slaves*. New York: W.W. Norton, 1973.

Hughes, G. *The Natural History of the Island of Barbados*. London, 1750. Reprint, New York: Arno Press, 1972.

Ligon, R. *A True and Exact History of the Island of Barbadoes*. London: Peter Parker, 1657. Reprint, London: Frank Cass, 1976.

Sanders, Joanne. *Barbados Records, Wills and Administrations*. Vol. 3, *1701–1725*. Houston: Sanders Historical Publications, 1981.

Sheridan, R. *Doctors and Slaves: A Medical and Demographic History of Slavery in the British West Indies, 1680–1834*. Cambridge: Cambridge University Press, 1985.

Index

*Entries appearing in **bold** are those originally indexed by Dr Hillary.*

www.ingramcontent.com/pod-product-compliance
Lightning Source LLC
Chambersburg PA
CBHW020210290326

41948CB00022B/267/J